CHEMISTRY OF SYNTHETIC DRUGS

Dr. Snigdha Singh

ALLIED HEALTH PRESS

Chemistry of Synthetic Drugs

Author: **Dr. Snigdha Singh**

Allied Health Press
4164 Lakeshore Road
Burlington ON L7L 1A4
Canada
www.alliedhealthpress.com
Email: orders@arclereducation.com

ISBN: 978-1-77956-275-3

ABOUT THE AUTHOR

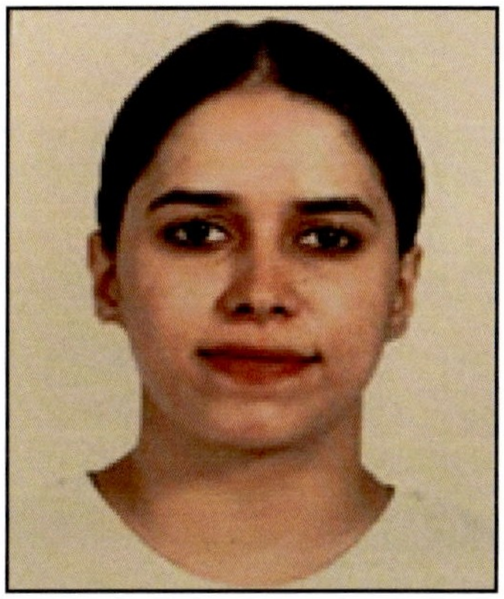

Dr. Snigdha Singh was born and raised in Delhi, India. She received her B.Sc. degree from Hindu College in 2013 and M.Tech. degree (Chemical Synthesis and Process Technologies) in 2016 from University of Delhi, India. She completed her doctoral studies on medicinal chemistry from University of Delhi in the year 2021 under the supervision of Prof. Ramesh Chandra. During PhD research, Snigdha majorly worked on the synthesis of biologically active small heterocyclic molecules. In 2018, She received Indo-Italy PhD Exchange Scholarship awarded by the MHRD, Govt. of India to carry out research at the University of Siena, Italy for a period of nine months.

Later in 2020, She was one of the few students who were awarded Indo-UK Newton Bhabha Scholarship by the British Council (U.K.) to carry out research at the University of Oxford, U.K. She worked on natural product synthesis to treat Leishmaniasis. She received various young scientist travel awards to attend International Conferences.

In 2021, after her doctoral studies Snigdha worked as a guest scientist at the Humboldt University of Berlin to work on the Synthesis of potential analogs for ACER3 activity. In 2023, She also went to Rensselaer Polytechnic Institute as Postdoctoral Research Associate to work on Design and Synthesis of Neuropathic Inhibitors.

In June 2023, Snigdha joined the Department of Chemistry, University of Delhi as an Assistant Professor. Her research interest lies in the areas of development of novel small heterocyclic molecules as potent anticancer, antimalarial and antibacterial agents, their binding interaction with blood proteins and synthesis of metallic nanoparticles for organic applications and drug delivery in cancer cell lines. To illustrate, she has to her credit one international patent, 3 Books; 2 book chapters and more than 32 original Scientific Research Papers in International journals of repute.

Word Roots, Prefixes, and Suffixes by Chapter

Chapter 1 Introduction to Synthetic Drugs

anti-: against or opposing

psycho-: the mind or mental processes

-amine: a compound derived from ammonia

-cycline: a class of antibiotics

phenyl-: benzene ring attached to another group or molecule

entheo-: altered state of consciousness.

Chapter 2 Chemistry of Synthetic Drugs

-caine: local anesthetic

cef -, ceph-: cephalosporin antibiotic

-cillin: penicillin antibiotic

-cycline: tetracycline antibiotic

-fenac: NSAID

-mycin: antibiotic; antibacterial

-olone: corticosteroid

pred-: corticosteroid

-profen: NSAID

Chapter 3 Designer Drugs: History and Evolution

bi-: Bifurcation

brady-: Bradycardia

cardio-: Cardioversion

-centesis: Thoracocentesis

cephal-: Cephalic

contra-: Contraindicated

-cyst: Cystoscopy

-cyt(e,o)-: Cytoplasm

dys-: Dysuria

Chapter 4 Stimulants: Amphetamines and Cathinones

-azine: Phenothiazines

-azole: Azole antifungals

-cillin: Penicillin antibiotics

-fungin: Echinocandins

Chapter 5 Hallucinogens: Psychedelic and Dissociative Drugs

-ectomy: : Hysterectomy

endo-: Endometrium

erythr(o)-: Erythrocyte

extra-: Extracellular

gastr(o)-: Gastro

gen(esis)-: Pathogen

Chapter 6 Synthetic Cannabinoids

Cannabin: pertaining to cannabis

-oid: resembling, derived from

Syn-: together, with

-thetic: pertaining to production or creation

-in: a compound

-s: plural

Chapter 7 Opioids: Synthetic Analgesics and Analogs

-asone: dexamethasone

-bital: phenobarbital; secobarbital

-cillin: methicillin

-fenac: diclofenac

-mycin: erythromycin

parin; -parin: heparin

-phylline: aminophylline

-profen: ibuprofen

vir; -vir: ritonavir

-zepam: lorazepam

Chapter 8 Designer Steroids and Performance-Enhancing Drugs

andro-: man or male

abol-: abolition or destruction

glyc/o-: sugar

hemat/o: blood

anti-: against

-itis: inflammation

-oid: resembling

-rrhage: excessive bleeding

-um: structure

Chapter 9 Synthetic Club Drugs

-bital: barbiturate (sedative)

-caine: local anesthetic

cort: corticosteroid

-dipine: calcium channel blocker

-phylline: xanthine derivative (bronchodilator)

-lamide: carbonic anhydrase inhibitor

-mycin: antibiotic; antibacterial

Chapter 10 Emerging Trends in Synthetic Drug Design

Apo-: apoptosis

-aemia: bacteraemia

Brachy-: brachycephalic

Brady: bradycardia

Brev-: Brevundimonas diminuta

-bacillus, bacilli: Bacillus

Table of Contents

LIST OF FIGURES

opposed to the latter (IC_{50} >10,000 nM). However, in a synaptosomal release assay, mephedrone (**26**) and 4-MEC (**54**) were similar in potency to evoke release from SERT (EC_{50} *ca.* 100 nM), whereas 4-MePPP (**55**) was inactive. In contrast, mephedrone was an effective releaser at DAT (EC_{50} = 39 nM), whereas 4-MEC (**54**) and 4-MePPP (**55**) were inactive (Reith et al., 2015). The overall conclusion was that changing the nature of the N-alkyl substituent of cathinone analogs has a profound influence on their actions; 4-MEC (**54**) is a SERT-releasing agent/DAT blocker, whereas 4-MePPP (**55**) is a selective DAT blocker.

LIST OF TABLES

PREFACE

Synthetic drugs are engineered to mimic the effects of illicit substances, but they possess distinctly different chemical structures. The manufacturers of these drugs frequently modify their chemical formulas in an attempt to circumvent legal regulations, allowing some to be marketed as "legal" alternatives that are seemingly safe and acceptable compared to their illicit counterparts. However, the reality of synthetic drugs is far from benign.

The challenges associated with the illicit manufacture, trafficking, and non-medical use of synthetic drugs are longstanding global issues. Innovations in the pharmaceutical and chemical industries have significantly contributed to the proliferation of new synthetic drugs. Since the early twentieth century, the introduction of synthetic pharmaceuticals such as tranquilizers, stimulants, and anesthetics has not only advanced medical science but also opened up new avenues for unauthorized drug supply and consumption. This has led to the emergence of new mind-altering substances that have often bypassed legal controls.

The enactment of the Convention on Psychotropic Substances in 1971, in which member states concurred on imposing stricter regulations over certain synthetic drugs, many of which were developed within the pharmaceutical industry, underscored the considerable harm associated with the non-medical use of synthetic drugs during the twentieth century. Despite these controls, the last decade has seen a significant increase in the proliferation of synthetic drugs within global markets.

Among the synthetic substances, amphetamine-type stimulants (ATS), particularly methamphetamine and MDMA (ecstasy), have established strong global markets. Methamphetamine, in particular, is probably the most widely manufactured and consumed synthetic drug worldwide, with its use continuing to rise across regions such as Southeast Asia, North America, South-West Asia, Africa, and Europe. Additionally, synthetic cannabinoids (SCBs) represent a broad and ever-evolving class of compounds, which persist in appearing across global drug markets, further complicating the efforts to regulate and control these substances.

The book "Chemistry of Synthetic Drugs" comprehensively explores the chemical foundations, methodologies, and implications of synthetic drug production, emphasizing the science behind their design, synthesis, and action mechanisms. This text aims to bridge the gap between theoretical chemistry principles and their practical applications in the field of medicinal and pharmaceutical chemistry, particularly concerning synthetic substances.

The primary purpose of this book is to educate and inform readers about the complex chemical processes involved in the creation of synthetic drugs. It deals with the molecular structures, chemical properties, and synthesis techniques that define these compounds. By detailing the pathways from compound discovery to drug development and market introduction, the book provides a thorough understanding of the lifecycle of synthetic drugs. It also addresses the legal and ethical dimensions of synthetic drug production, offering insights into the regulatory landscape and the challenges posed by new psychoactive substances.

"Chemistry of Synthetic Drugs" is designed to serve as a foundational text for students in pharmaceutical sciences, chemistry, and related fields, equipping them with the necessary knowledge to engage in or critique synthetic drug development. Beyond its academic utility, the book is an invaluable resource for professionals in the pharmaceutical industry, including chemists, pharmacologists, and regulatory affairs specialists. It offers advanced knowledge of the latest trends and technologies in drug synthesis, providing professionals with insights that can drive innovation and adherence to best practices in drug development. This book is a textbook, guide for ongoing professional development, and a reference source for established professionals navigating the dynamic field of synthetic drug chemistry.

Chapter

INTRODUCTION TO SYNTHETIC DRUGS

1

Contents

Introduction

Drugs that have been artificially modified from naturally occurring substances and have the ability to have both therapeutic and psychoactive effects are referred to as synthetic drugs.

The chemical structures of synthetic drugs differ from those of the illegal substances they are intended to replace. To try and stay ahead of the law, synthetic drugs producers alter their chemical structures on a regular basis.producers of Certain synthetic drugs may be promoted as "safe," "legal," and acceptable substitutes for illegal drugs. This does not imply that they are safe or lawful, though.

Synthetic medications have psychotropic properties that can treat insomnia in a medical context. The majority of synthetic drugs have poorly understood pharmacology and side effects due to a lack of human studies and clinical trials. Consult a professional before using synthetic drugs as misuse can be lethal.

Orientation and Directional Terms

Term	Definition	Illustration
Insomnia	Insomnia is a common sleep disorder that can make it hard to fall asleep or stay asleep. It also can cause you to wake up too early and not be able to get back to sleep. You may still feel tired when you wake up.	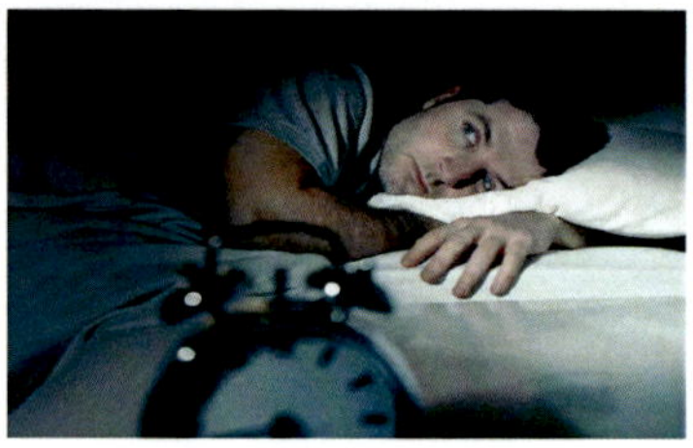
Synthetic cannabinoid receptor agonists (SCRAs)	SCRAs are heterogeneous compounds originally intended as probes of the endogenous cannabinoid system or as potential therapeutic agents.	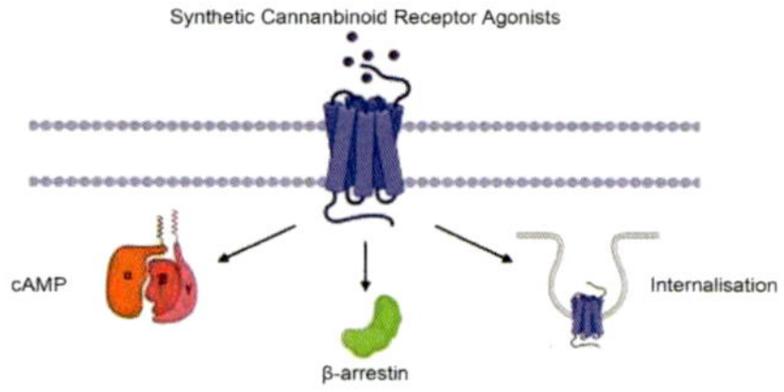
Pharmacokinetics (PK)	Pharmacokinetics (PK) is the study of how the body interacts with administered substances for the entire duration of exposure (medications for the sake of this article). This is closely related to but distinctly different from pharmacodynamics, which examines the drug's effect on the body more closely	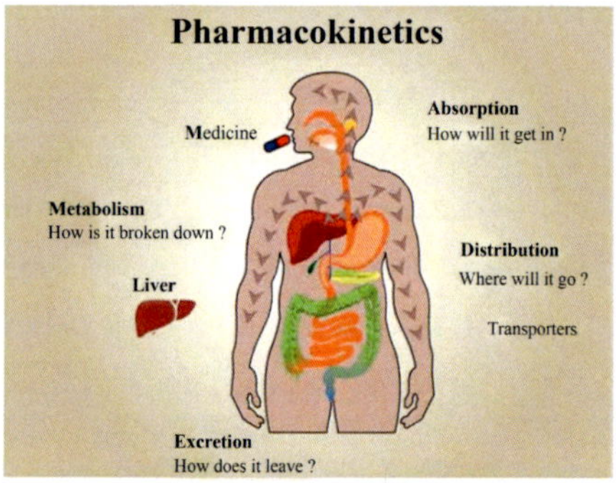
Phenethylamine	Phenethylamine is an organic compound, natural monoamine alkaloid, and trace amine, which acts as a central nervous system stimulant in humans.	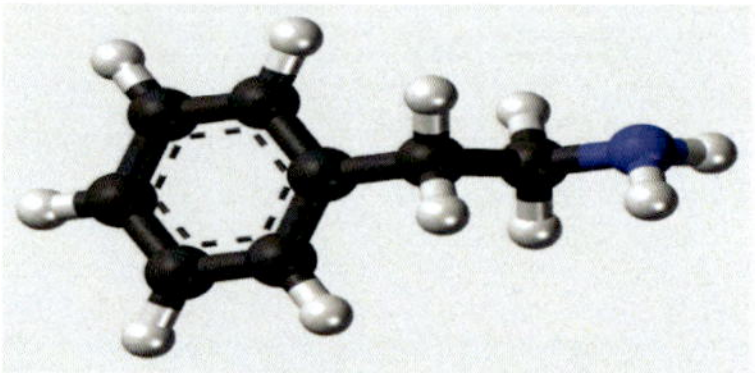
Structure-activity relationship (SAR)	Structure-Activity Relationship (SAR) is an approach designed to find relationships between chemical structure (or structural-related properties) and biological activity (or target property) of studied compounds.	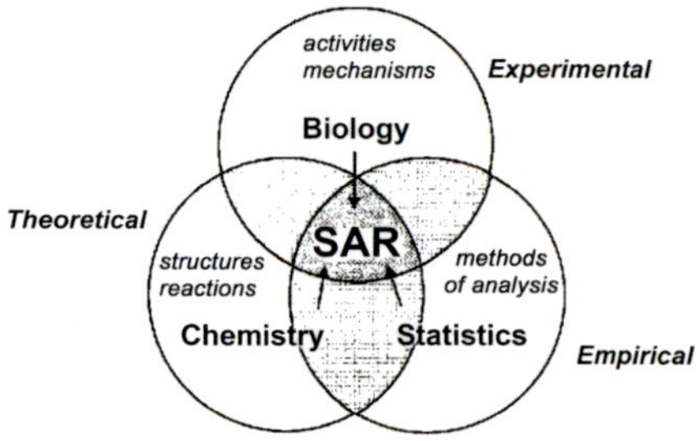

1.1 Types of Drugs

There are mainly two types of drugs.

- Drugs obtained from natural products
- Synthetic drugs

1.1.1 Drugs Obtained from Natural Products

The world has been using a variety of natural products for medicinal purposes since the beginning of time. These goods, which came from plant, animal, and mineral sources, occasionally had remarkable efficacy. The Assyrian herbal of the seventh century BC contains a list of medicinal plants, indicating that the use of medicinal plants dates back to that time. In a similar vein, the Chinese emperor Shen Nung (2800 BC) wrote about the use of Egyptian papyrus from Ebers and the arrangement of medicinal plants in 1550 BC.

For centuries, the Greeks studied medicinal plants. Around 75 BC, Dioscorides penned the De Materia Medica manuscript, which included a list of about 600 medicinal plants. The discovery of several valuable medicinal plants in the "New World" contributed significantly to the eradication of superstitions from early medicine during the Age of Herbals, which lasted from 1488 to 1682.

Nowadays, more than 25% of common medications contain at least one plant-derived ingredient. For instance, over 5,000 plant families have been identified as having alkaloids, such as morphine and codeine (Opium); quinine from Peruvian bark; atropine, scopolamine, podophyllin, mandragorin, and hyoscyamine from belladonna; emetine from Ipecac; nicotine from tobacco; caffeine from coffee and tea; and glycosides, which are substances that have one or more sugar molecules attached to one or more non-sugar molecules, such as digitoxin from Digitalis or Foxglove, ginsenosides, or panaxosides from Ginseng.

Even today, plants are a significant source of novel drugs and lead compounds (Walsh et al., 2020). However, random screening is not always successful due to the wide variety of possible natural sources present in the world. Ethnopharmacology, which screens traditional local remedies, provides the foundation of a more methodical approach.

After a material with an active compound is found through screening, the challenge is to extract it, purify it, and determine its pharmacological activity. However, there may be ecological issues if a drug's usable amounts are removed from their marine or terrestrial sources. The Pacific Yew Tree's bark provided the initial source of the anticancer drug Taxol. However, the massive destruction of the tree that would accompany the production of large amounts of Taxol from this source would upset the ecological balance.

1.1.2 Synthetic Drugs

The development of medications began with this diverse array of plant-based pharmaceutically active compounds. Many pharmaceuticals have biological origins, and alkaloids, in particular, are where they may be found. Chemists have used the clarity of their structures as a springboard to create related compounds. In this regard, cocaine, atropine, and morphine are especially good examples since compounds derived from them have demonstrated clinically demonstrated local anesthetic, antispasmodic, and marked analgesic properties, respectively. The new compounds' physiological characteristics appear to be comparable to the compound to which they are structurally related in each of these instances.

Pharmacologists now test prospective sources biologically to ascertain the type and potency of their pharmacological activity before making many discoveries. These screening initiatives could be aimed or haphazard. Regardless of their structural makeup, all substances and compounds are tested in random screening. The antibiotics streptomycin and tetracycline were found as a result of the random screening of soil sample collections (walsh et al., 2020).

Following the identification of compounds with pharmacological activity of interest by a screening program, the active compound is isolated and utilized as a lead compound to produce related analogs. These substances go through additional screening procedures. The most promising of these compounds are analogs, which are then created and put through the screening process. Several iterations of this process of selective screening and analog synthesis may be required before a potentially helpful medication is discovered.

The synthetic compounds created from lead are referred to as its analogues, while the compounds that served as the foundation for the development are now known as lead compounds. A medicinal chemist's job primarily entails finding novel lead compounds with particular medicinal qualities and creating safer and more potent analogs from both new and known compounds. Therefore, many scientific disciplines are linked by medicinal chemistry.

The goal of creating novel synthetic drug compounds has led to the integration of medicinal chemistry with numerous other fields, including molecular biology and biochemistry. Collaborating in groups with scientists from diverse fields beyond chemistry is a requirement in the field of medicinal chemistry. Biochemistry, computer-aided design, X-ray crystallography, metabolism and pharmacokinetics, clinical, and franchise management, pharmaceutics, legal and regulatory affairs, and process research chemistry are some of these fields. A team of scientists from various disciplines, such as biologists, toxicologists, pharmacologists, theoretical chemists, microbiologists, and biopharmacists, is typically assembled by chemists. Together, this team develops the most economical and ecologically friendly production methods while synthesizing and testing novel pharmaceutical products using advanced analytical techniques.

A combination of systematic research and luck goes into the development of a new medication. Drugs and lead compounds derived from natural sources, including plants, animals, trees, and microorganisms, were the initial ingredients. Although they weren't used until the middle of the 20th century, marine sources are now valuable sources as well. Although most lead compounds are now produced in laboratories, natural sources remain significant. The biochemistry of the pathogenic condition is taken into consideration when determining the nature of these synthetic compounds.

Paul Ehrlich was the first to rationally develop synthetic drugs, he realized at the start of the 20th century that a drug's evaluation should take into account both its beneficial and toxic properties. More potent medications exhibited a higher selectivity for the target microorganisms relative to their host. As a result, the selectivity and efficacy of drugs were expressed.

Before a suitable compound is produced, hundreds of compounds must be synthesized and tested; in fact, one compound out of every 1000 synthesized is suitable for medical use.

1.2 Synthetic Drug: An Overview

Synthetic drug discovery and proliferation have been facilitated by advancements in the chemical and pharmaceutical industries. Drugs classified as "synthetic" are those that are produced chemically as opposed to coming from natural sources. Their purpose is to imitate the effects of popular drugs like stimulants, opioids, and cannabinoids.

1.2.1 Common Synthetic Drugs

Synthetic cannabinoids

Naphthoylindoles, naphthylmethylindoles, naphthoypyrroles, naphthylmethylindenes, phenylacetylindoles, cyclohexylphenols, and classical cannabinoids are the seven main structural groups. The structures of synthetic and classical cannabinoids are different (Janssen et al., 1999). There are several popular SCBs on the market, including JWH-250, a phenylacetylindole, and JWH-018, the most well-known naphthoylindole (Brents et al., 2011). For the past ten years, they have been offered for sale as recreational drugs under the brand name "Spice" (Atwood, 2010).

Phenethylamines

There are two types of phenolethylamines: ring-substituted and non-ring-substituted. "D-series" and "2C-series" are examples of ring-substituted phenethylamines, whereas "benzodifurans" and paramethoxymethamphetamine (PMMA) are examples of common non-ring-substituted phenethylamines (Khan et al., 2012).

Novel benzodiazepines (Xanax)

Xanax is a brand name for Alprazolam, a generic drug made from benzodiazepines.

1.2.2 Adverse Effects

Because there are few human studies and synthetic drugs typically contain other chemicals in variable concentrations, it is difficult to determine the adverse effects of these medications.

In addition to psychological issues, tachyarrhythmia, seizures, and possible cancer, SCBs can lead to cardiovascular issues. Prolonged usage of SCBs has been associated with addiction and withdrawal symptoms, such as cognitive impairments (like difficulty thinking), excessive perspiration, central nervous system disturbances, and gastrointestinal disturbances (like nausea and vomiting).

Depending on the medication, phenethylamines can have different side effects. Compared to other phenylethylamines, "D series" have longer-lasting effects, such as tachycardia. The "2C series" has entactogenic and hallucinogenic effects at high doses. Suicidal thoughts and disruptions in the central nervous system can be brought on by alprazolam.

1.2.3 Pharmacology: Pharmacodynamics/Mechanism of Action (MOA)

By attaching to the cannabinoid receptors CB_1 and CB_2, SCBs function as Synthetic Cannabinoid Receptor Antagonists (SCRA). When it binds to the CB_1 receptor, it phosphorylates the receptor, which attracts β-arrestins 1 and 2, which causes the cell to lose its responsiveness and internalize (endocytose) the molecules. Acute inhibition of synaptic neurotransmitter release is caused by the dissociation of the βγ subunits of pertussis toxin-sensitive G proteins (Gi /Go) from the α subunit (Giα) upon stimulation of the CB_1 receptor. β-arrestin has the ability to activate mitogen-activated protein kinase, which can result in extracellular effects. Inotropic transient receptor potential channels are activated by SCBs when they bind to receptors other than CB_1 and CB_2, which results in cell membrane depolarization and Ca^{2+} influx.

Stimulants and hallucinogens alike, phenethylamines are indirectly acting as sympathomimetic amines. Monoamine neurotransmitters like dopamine, serotonin, and noradrenaline, which cause vasoconstriction and blood pressure elevation, can have their levels and actions modulated by stimulants. For instance, the vasoconstriction effect can be reached by amphetamine at 10-100 μM. Psychedelics, or hallucinogens, have the ability to mediate particular serotonin-receptor activities and induce hallucinations. They might also possess residual stimulant properties. In contrast to human pharmacology, phenethylamines have been shown in certain animal studies to exhibit negative inotropism in isolated rat heart tissues because they stimulate TAAR1.

Alprazolam binds to members of the pentameric ligand-gated ion channel (PLGIC) superfamily, which are GABA type-A benzodiazepine receptor sites. It acts extrasynaptically to mediate tonic inhibition as well as phasic inhibition. After attachment, the receptors undergo conformational changes that stabilize them and cause the production of inhibitory signals.

1.2.4 Pharmacokinetics

Smoking is the method of delivering SCBs. In a human study, one male and one female had serum concentrations of 8.1 and 10.2 μg/L, respectively, after five minutes of receiving 50 μg/kg smoked JWH-018; these concentrations decreased to 4.6 and 6.1 μg/L after fifteen minutes, indicating that JWH-018's biological half-life is brief. There are thirteen phase 1 metabolites found. Most common metabolites of SCBs are monohydroxylated and dihydrodiol. The conjugation of JWH-018 and JWH-073 metabolites was mainly carried out by UDP-glucuronosyltransferases, UGT1A1, UGT1A3, UGT1A9, UGT1A10, and UGT2B7 isoenzymes, which also exhibited a strong affinity for hydroxylated metabolites (Km=12–18 mmol/L). CYP2C9 was the main mediator of the generation of JWH-018-N-4- and 5-hydroxypentyl (JWH-018 metabolites), with CYP1A2 and CYP2C19 following. JWH-018-N-4-hydroxypentyl synthesis was catalyzed by CYP3A4, albeit with less activity than CYP1A2 and CP2C19. Urine is the primary excretion of the drugs (Brents et al., 2011).

Phenethylamines are absorbed through ingestion and have first-order kinetics with a half-life of five to ten minutes. Due to their short biological half-lives, the medications have a low concentration in the brain. Because phenethylamine is not very stable, measuring the plasma concentration can be challenging. Two different metabolic pathways are possible. The first potential route involves the metabolism of free primary and secondary amines by MAO-B, an intracellular enzyme that is primarily found in the brain and is tightly bound to the outer membrane of mitochondria. Because of MAO-B's selectivity for non-polar aromatic amines, phenylacetic acid is formed during this process. The sympathetic neurotransmitter noradrenaline and secondary amines are then produced when the metabolites are N-methylated by either phenylethanolamine-N-methyltransferase (PNMT), which is located in the adrenal medulla or non-specific N-methyltransferase (NMT). The second potential mechanism involves the medication being deamined by semi-carbazide-sensitive amine oxidases, which are present in vascular tissue and have a metabolism akin to that of MAO. The medication is resistant to deamination in the stomach due to an alpha-methyl side chain. Urine and feces are the primary excretions of the drugs.

Alprazolam has a high oral bioavailability (84–91 %), taking one to two hours to reach its maximum plasma concentration (Cmax). The Cmax increases by 25% when taken with food.

Asian patients have a 25% longer half-life than Caucasian patients in terms of race. In healthy adult patients, the half-life of the extended-release formulation is 10.7–15.7 hours. After oral administration, alprazolam has a volume distribution of 0.8–1.3 L/kg. It can cross the blood-brain barrier and has an

80% protein binding (mostly albumin-bound) in plasma. It is metabolized by a number of CYP450 enzymes, such as CYP2C9, CYP3A4, CYP3A5, and CYP3A7, to less potent forms. The majority of alprazolam metabolism is carried out by CYP3A-mediated hydroxylation. The binding affinity of the parent drug is 20% for 4-hydroxyalprazolam, 66% for alpha-hydroxyalprazolam, and less than 1% for the benzophenone metabolite. The majority of the medication is eliminated in urine as unaltered Alprazolam. Less than 10% of the dosage is excreted as 4- and alpha-hydroxyalprazolam.

1.2.5 Chemistry

Detection in body fluids

Drugs must have specific reference data from the target drug in order to be detected in bodily fluids. The inability of spectrometers to detect structurally modified illegal substances due to a lack of reference data is a common trap in the detection of New Psychoactive Substances (NPS) (Evans and Sedefov, 2018). Immunoassay is another method of drug detection that uses active antibodies to selectively identify the drug of interest. The original antibodies will react differently to a structurally modified drug, leading to false positive or negative results.

Structure-activity relationship

Synthetic cannabinoids

Members of the aminoalkylindole class of SCBs were first identified in 2008. Because of a chemist by the name of John W., it was given the name "JWH.". In the 1960s, Huffman synthesized them. The majority of SCBs are agonists to the CB1 (Type I) and CB2 (Type II) cannabinoid receptors because they structurally resemble 9-tetrahydrocannabinol (THC) (Chin et al., 1999). The central nervous system expresses CB1, which is primarily in charge of the psychoactive effect. These three parts make up a typical agonist: head, linker core, and tail. The drug's affinity for cannabinoid receptors will change if the structures of any of the constituents are changed. For example, the affinity for CB1 increases when a nitrile or fluoride group is added to the carbon chains. Additionally, the aromatic rings of the aminoalkylindole class contribute to the enhancement of affinity by stabilizing the CB1 receptors through the formation of a hydrophobic cavity (Hutter et al., 2012). Aims are made to modify the structure as laws tighten under the supervision of the Early Warning System (EWS), leading to the creation of new analogs like adamantylindoles (APINACA) and cyclopropylindoles (UR-144).

Novel benzodiazepines

Novel benzodiazepine analogs have the potential to be antibacterial. The isoxazolyl analogs with the p-chlorophenyl group (p-ClC6H4) attached have proven to be the most effective agent against the majority of the strains when tested against different bacterial strains. Moreover, the inhibitory effect against bacteria will be strengthened by the attachment of heterocyclic rings like furan and thiophene, as well as electron-withdrawing groups. Novel benzodiazepines have the ability to bind to the human dopamine transporter D_3 and modulate the central nervous system. The binding affinity of imidazole diazepines towards human dopamine D_3 receptors is increased in their enantiomers that have either a methyl (CH_3) or a propyl group attached.

Phenylethylamine

Phenylethylamine is generally made up of an aromatic ring that is joined to an amine group that is two carbons away. The substitutions made at the alpha and beta carbon positions distinguish each type of phenylethylamine from the others. Amphetamines are compounds that can modulate the 5HT-2A serotonin receptors when a methyl group is attached at the alpha position. The triggered receptors eventually result in hallucinations. The agonists need to have a primary amine, a methoxy group, and hydrophobic functional groups in order to guarantee adequate binding.

1.3 Structure-Activity Relationship (Sar)

SAR is a method for relating a drug's or toxic chemical's effects on an animal, plant, or the environment to its molecular structure.

A SAR connects a drug's characteristics or chemical structure to a characteristic, outcome, or biological activity connected to that material. It is a branch of medicinal chemistry in which the chemical structure of bioactive chemical compounds is altered to modify their potency effect, or activity.

Medicinal chemists test the biological effects of introducing new chemical groups into biological compounds using synthesis-based chemical techniques. Every theory based on molecules starts with the fundamental premise that molecules with similar properties will behave similarly. A compound's reactivities, physical characteristics, and chemical makeup are entirely determined by its structure. By connecting the chemical structure to biological activity, the compound's interaction with a biological system establishes its biological and toxicological characteristics. These changes can be implemented by chemists through qualitative and quantitative modeling techniques (Valento and Lebin, 2017).

Creating a SAR involves an effort to comprehend and make visible how the chemical structure encodes and determines characteristics that are pertinent to an activity. The biological characteristics of novel compounds are frequently deduced from those of analogous, already-existing materials, the actions and risks of which are well-established. Although they are frequently too expensive and time-consuming to be used for the entire spectrum of chemicals, animal and in vitro testing is still crucial for the real investigations of risk assessment and regulatory action. Chemical structure and qualitative biological activity are related through computer-based modeling techniques known as SAR and Quantitative Structure Activity Relationship (QSAR), which have been used in a wide range of problem contexts.

1.3.1 Importance of Structure Activity Relationship

SARs have long been used in the chemical and pharmaceutical industries to create compounds and medications with qualities that are desirable to consumers. This has been especially true in the field of drug design, where substances with desired therapeutic and pharmacologic properties are sought after. SAR is being applied in a variety of ways to forecast ecological and human health impacts in the field of environmental health protection. In addition to predicting and characterizing chemical toxicity for commercial use as a component of their desirable properties, it is even being used to assist the industry in designing safer chemicals. One way to identify the structural components of a lead compound that contribute to both its positive and negative effects is to look at the surface area ratios (SARs) of the compound and its analogs. With the use of this knowledge, a new medication with fewer side effects, enhanced activity, or a different activity from the one currently on the market could be created.

In relating structure to activity, the main aim of SAR is:

i) To develop an understanding of a class of molecules that are active

ii) To find out what determines relative activity

iii) To know what distinguishes these from inactive classes.

SAR encompasses a wide range of tasks, such as formal mathematical associations of properties and activity measures, expert judgment, and considerations of chemical similarity and diversity. In the end, the ability to connect SAR to mechanism allows for the creation of a scientific justification to explain why different compounds have different activities. This is the most reliable scientific foundation for predicting novel, unproven chemical compounds' activities.

1.3.2 Quantitative Structure-Activity Relationship

Quantitative SARs, or QSAR, are based on the fundamental premise that chemicals that are similar share enough mechanistic elements.

The creation of a relationship between structural characteristics and the desired property is known as quantitative SARs, or QSAR, and it enables the prediction of property values for novel candidate structures (Wiley et al., 2011).

These properties include

- Measures of potency
- Strength of binding of the drug to an active site
- Inhibition of enzyme
- Prediction of ADMET properties (Absorption, distribution, metabolism, excretion and toxicity).

3D-Quantitative Structure Activity Relationship (QSAR)

3D-QSAR methods are a class of structure-activity methods that take into account the 3D structure of modeled compounds in spatial relation to one another. These techniques look for spatially localized characteristics among a range of molecules that are correlated with activity and serve as prerequisites for complementarity and ligand binding to a putative receptor binding site.

These procedures extend the QSAR approach in three dimensions by selecting one specific geometry for each modelled compound, either manually or automatically, and superimposing the results using the molecular scaffold, the pharmacophore, or the molecular field method.

1.4 Understanding Clandestine Synthetic Drugs

Drug abuse trends often exhibit cyclical behavior, with specific drugs or patterns of use resurfacing at various times and/or locations. Comprehending these patterns and their fundamental dynamics can thus aid in enhancing policy measures and prompt responses to the recurrence of issues that have already been identified. Unlike the extensive history of abuse of plant-based drugs like heroin and cocaine, the rise of synthetic drug use among predominantly young consumers in the past decade has become a worldwide concern. The popularity of certain psychoactive drugs within specific subcultures has led to a rapid global distribution of clandestine synthetic drugs. However, the scale of the issue varies significantly in different regions and among different consumer groups.

1.4.1 Clandestine Synthetic Drugs: Evolution of a Problem

From 'plant-based' to 'synthetic' drugs

The use of unprocessed plant materials with

comparatively low psychoactive potency for ceremonial, spiritual, or therapeutic purposes led to the gradual evolution of the current drug problem. Natural science and pharmaceutical technology have advanced, making it feasible to refine the (psycho)active components of crude plant products (opium and coca leaf, respectively), such as cocaine and morphine. More dependable and focused medical applications were made possible by the availability of the pure active principle; however, the therapeutic use of those compounds was still reliant on the availability of the plant's raw material. Only when pharmaceutical research and industry grew to a respectable scale and degree of sophistication in the late 19th and early 20th centuries did the synthetic production of therapeutic drugs start to challenge the extraction of active principles from natural raw materials in terms of cost-effectiveness. Consequently, many of those medications became accessible to large segments of society at low cost. This was made possible by the ability to manufacture the pure active principles of several traditionally used plant-based products in laboratories worldwide, mostly using readily available and inexpensive chemical starting materials.

The next phase of the evolutionary process was the hunt for medications with comparable or identical therapeutic effects but greater potency or improved specificity, that is, with fewer unwanted side effects. Drug design, also referred to as drug modeling, is the process of changing the chemical structure of a parent molecule that has been thoroughly studied. It is a fundamental idea in contemporary pharmaceutical research and industrial production. Fentanyl, a class of synthetic opioids used in anesthesia and as analgesics (painkillers), are an example of modern synthetic drugs based on the structural properties of morphine.

A general enthusiasm for almost all new products characterized the early days of synthetic pharmaceutical drugs. This resulted in somewhat careless use of these drugs, along with the accessibility of certain medications, sloppy prescribing procedures, and/or over prescription prescription-n. Over time, people started to become more conscious of and concerned about the possible risks connected to the widespread use of some psychoactive medications.

Regulations were implemented, medical use was progressively discouraged, and then it began to decline. The primary source of supply for non-medical use then shifted from the legal to the illegal market due to diversion.

The creation of covert laboratories resulted from the tightening and enlarging of control measures. Here, illicit manufacturers created counterfeit versions of the desired products using the same chemicals used in the pharmaceutical industry to satisfy illicit demand.

The "design" of new drugs based on the chemical structure of a parent substance that produced the desired effects marked the final stage in the evolution of the contemporary drug problem.

This idea is a lot like the one used in pharmaceutical research. However, the goal of covert manufacturers is to produce drugs with pharmacological profiles that the user population is interested in, whereas the pharmaceutical industry aims to develop safer drugs or to increase specificity for a specific type of desired therapeutic effect.

The urge to produce drugs that evade national and/or international control regimes to break the law and escape punishment is another motivator for clandestine manufacturers. Since these illegally produced, so-called "designer drugs" are not just illegally produced copies of already-existing substances but are wholly original works created in the clandestine sector, they are also sometimes referred to as "synthetic drugs of the second generation."

There are five major classes of designer drugs:

- synthetic opioids,
- Phencyclidine (PCP) derivatives,
- Tryptamines,
- Methaqualone derivatives, and
- Phenylalkylamines (PAAs).

The majority of synthetic opioids share chemical similarities with either pethidine (meperidine) or fentanyl. As the supply of heroin decreased in the late 1970s and early 1980s, fentanyls started to be available on the streets. As a result, they were sold as "synthetic heroin," despite having hundreds of times the potency of actual heroin. Due to their extreme potency, fentanyls caused numerous overdose deaths and quickly lost favor. Pethidines are the second class of synthetic opioid derivatives that are being modified covertly. The most significant designer drug disaster to date has been linked to pethidine abuse. In the early 1980s, young intravenous drug abusers developed irreversible Parkinsonism as a result of a neurotoxic reaction to a pethidine by-product. Drug control organizations first became aware of PCP derivatives in the latter half of the 1960s. PCP derivatives are based on the molecule of the general anesthetic PCP. Their use never really took off because of their potent hallucinogenic and frequently bizarre effects. Another class of hallucinogenic substances that is amenable to structural alteration is tryptamines. Their chemical structure is similar to that of lysergic acid diethylamide (LSD), and they were also quite popular in the 1960s "psychedelic" era. Even though they are relatively simple to synthesize, covert modifications of the central nervous system depressant methaqualone are not very common in the streets. In contrast, since the mid-1960s, phenylalkylamines—a class of substances related to amphetamine through their chemical structure—have been observed in multiple waves on the streets. The most recent wave began when different amphetamine-type stimulants (ATS) entered the dance drug scene in the middle of the 1980s and early 1990s. The ATS phenomenon, in all its manifestations, is representative of the peculiarities associated with the supply and demand of illicit synthetic drugs for a variety of reasons (Janssen et al., 1999).

Amphetamine-type stimulants: a case scenario

Social and geographical spread of amphetamine-type stimulants abuse

Considered the parent drugs of the ATS group, amphetamine and methamphetamine, were first used in medicine in the 1930s. However, soon after, they were being used for non-medical purposes. The Second World War saw soldiers use instruments, and this, along with lax prescribing, contributed to the subsequent public abuse epidemic. The abuse began with certain occupational groups, then spread to athletes, students, and finally, recreational users. Certain countries, particularly those in northern Europe and Japan, saw a rise in the prevalence of chronic abuse within a core group of heavy abusers. Epidemics of non-instrumental ATS use typically began in the avant-garde and progressed through the middle classes before settling into the margins.

Geographically speaking, ATS abuse progressively extended from a small number of nations, such as Sweden, Japan, and the United States, to nearby nations in those regions, and eventually to additional regions. Abuse of ATS has been seen as a global phenomenon since the mid-1990s, following the beginning of the "ecstasy" epidemic in Europe, albeit with different substances being more common in different regions of the world. The use of ATS for recreational purposes is currently most common in a number of developed nations, especially in Europe. However, it is also rapidly spreading to other regions, especially South-East Asia, where it was previously more common for instrumental purposes, such as long-distance truck drivers.

Sources of supply

Overprescribing and careless prescribing practices contributed to the non-medical use of ATS during the early days when amphetamines were thought to be a cure-all for a variety of illnesses. Following the introduction of regulatory restrictions and the growing concern over the possible risks associated with the widespread use of ATS, large-scale diversion from the licit trade quickly emerged as the main source of supply to meet non-medical demand. The implementation of stricter regulations on various conventional ATS starting in the early 1970s resulted in the phenomenon commonly referred to as the "balloon" effect, which is the transfer of supply from one source to another. The "balloon effect" in this context refers to the movement of resources from the legal to the illegal domain, which has resulted in the covert production of substances such as methamphetamine and amphetamine and eventually structurally altered designer ATS.

An additional aspect of the "balloon" effect emerged with the expansion of control measures to include the production of starting materials. This involved the transition from one well-established precursor to another and the subsequent relocation of covert manufacturing to a neighboring nation with laxer control measures. Such "ballooning" is exemplified by the 1980s transition in the United States from 1-phenyl-2-propanone (P2P; also known as benzyl methyl ketone, or BMK) to ephedrine as the primary precursor for methamphetamine synthesis and the subsequent relocation of covert methamphetamine manufacturing to Mexico. An additional instance of "ballooning," associated with the implementation of more stringent regulations, is the historical transfer of methamphetamine production from Japan to Korea, the Philippines, and eventually China starting in the 1950s.

These days, clandestine synthesis serves as the primary source of ATS supply for the black market in the majority of regions with high consumption rates. Advanced phases of "innovative" covert drug design are presently being carried out in Europe and, to a lesser degree, in Australia and North America. The production of synthetic drugs in secret has progressed to the initial phase in a number of Asian nations. These drugs include methamphetamine and, more recently, ecstasy. On the other hand, oversupply persists in many developing nations, especially those in Africa and Latin America, where access to pharmaceuticals through unregulated channels and loose prescribing guidelines are commonplace. There's a chance that those areas will witness a replay of what happened in Europe, the US, and Japan in the 1960s and 1970s: an abundance of the substance may be followed by covert synthesis, which starts with pharmaceutical drug imitation and ends with the production of structurally related "designer ATS."

1.4.2 Clandestine Synthetic Drugs vis-à-vis Plant-Based Drugs

We examine the intricate interplay between incentives and disincentives on the supply and demand sides for various drug kinds against the backdrop of the ATS case scenario previously mentioned. It also examines some of the fundamental features that influence the supply and demand for drugs, emphasizing the key distinctions between synthetic and plant-based drugs (as demonstrated by the examples of heroin and cocaine).

Access to and availability of the necessary starting materials are critical supply-side factors for a clandestine operator. While the manufacturing of synthetic drugs usually requires starting materials that are readily available worldwide, the production of traditional plant-based drugs, such as heroin and cocaine, depends on natural raw materials produced in specific geographical locations. The desired end product can be created in a few straightforward reaction steps, and the chemicals involved are typically inexpensive. Risks related to the preservation of cultivation areas do not exist, nor are labor-intensive and drawn-out harvesting, extraction, and isolation processes necessary.

The availability of information and the necessary scientific and technical know-how is another crucial component. Synthetic drug manufacturing recipes can be easily obtained online or through specialized underground literature (Walsh et al., 2020). The spread of covert drug synthesis is actually greatly aided by contemporary information technology, which answers common queries like which chemical precursors to use, where to obtain them, how to avoid detection, and how to set up a basic "kitchen" laboratory. The fact that a typical synthesis involves relatively little technology and a small number of reaction steps makes all of this worse. Yields from synthesis are typically high.

The past 10 years have seen a global spread of some synthetic drugs, which can also be linked to financial incentives that influence their production, trafficking, and eventual abuse. From a supply perspective, synthetic drugs are often more profitable in consumer markets than either heroin or cocaine. The production of synthetic drugs is not limited to any particular region; it can happen in close proximity to the final site of consumption. This means that practically all of a synthetic drug's retail price stays in the area where it is used. Additionally, because it permits smaller-scale trafficking, the proximity of locations for covert production and consumption lowers the chance of discovery, for instance, at border crossings. Compared to the production of heroin or cocaine illegally, the fact that synthetic drug laboratories are less noticeable lowers the overall risks for covert operators.

On the demand side, several factors affect a user's final decision to select a specific drug. The drugs own pharmacological properties, i.e., insofar as they are known to the user, the drug's desired effects balanced against its risks and unfavorable side effects most likely play a big part. Comparably, drugs that are appropriate for delivery methods other than intravenous injection and—more and more—methods other than smoking also appear to be contributing factors. The perception and social portrayal of specific drugs, as well as the accessibility and availability of substitute substances, are additional factors. Cultural, social, and economic factors are also taken into account. As a result, the demand side of the equation is more complicated than the supply side, and customer preferences are subject to change.

1.4.3 Approaches to the Control of Clandestine Synthetic Drugs

The need to maintain the availability of drugs used for legal, medical purposes while preventing their diversion into illicit markets serves as the foundation for the global drug control system. The need to preserve the legal trade in those substances for medical purposes has been considered in the formulation of procedures to expand control measures to new substances. They comprise estimates for the quantities required for medical and research purposes, as well as a monitoring system of legal transactions involving specific substances connected to production, inventories, trade, and use. Any discrepancy or alteration in such a system would be obvious and eventually lead to caution and corrective action, preventing the leakage of a controlled substance into unapproved channels.

Clandestine synthetic drugs challenge the current drug control system in several ways:

- First of all, because they are produced covertly, there is no legal market for them, and the conventional drug control system is unable to keep an eye on their distribution.
- Second, because of the so-called "substance-by-substance scheduling approach," the introduction of new substances that are not covered by the conventions' schedules cannot be promptly addressed with the necessary actions because their production, trafficking, and abuse are not currently considered "illicit," meaning they are not crimes. This makes it possible to conduct covert "research" or experimentation on specific drugs within a class of drugs that have comparable pharmacological profiles.
- Thirdly, typically insufficient data are available for the necessary scheduling assessments due to the covert nature of the substances in question. Because the process of incorporating them into the control system is so drawn out, illicit manufacturers are able to sell their goods for a while without worrying about being immediately prosecuted.

The international community has worked to reinforce the current drug control system, which primarily targets finished goods, by enacting legislation that addresses diversion as well as the illegal use of raw materials and other chemicals needed for covert drug production. This was accomplished through the 1988 Convention. The majority of drug control strategies now include precursor control as a fundamental component. It is especially crucial in the case of synthetic drugs because of their versatility in the production process and the abundance of starting materials that can be used in their place.

Furthermore, there had been no global system for the control of precursors for synthetic drugs—not even for the most basic materials—prior to the 1988 Convention's implementation. This is not the case for plant-based drugs, where the 1988 Convention only regulates the chemicals needed for the extraction and purification processes. Instead, the same international control regime covers immediate starting materials (coca leaf, opium), intermediates (coca paste, morphine), and end products (cocaine, heroin).

Precursors are difficult to regulate to a particularly tight degree due to their many acceptable uses and the often high volumes of licit trade. Furthermore, a great number of businesses worldwide produce and trade a large number of precursors, in contrast to the majority of end products. As a result, there are numerous legal supply sources, that help covert operators (i) quickly adjust to the imposition of stricter regulations in important supplier and transit nations and (ii) place orders with multiple suppliers worldwide at once. Routes for trafficking and diversion are therefore, very adaptable. The multiplicity of shipping routes via several middlemen in various nations, which are used to conceal the shipments' ultimate destination, further complicates the efficient tracking of precursor movements.

An additional trend that has emerged in recent years is the growing use of legally obtained, non-controlled substances in the illicit drug trade as replacements for precursors that are already regulated. From the standpoint of drug control, this development raises two issues. Strict regulation of the licit trade of these substances is impractical due to the abundance of viable substitutes, and many of those substitutes have even more acceptable applications than the "traditional" precursor substances. When it comes to synthetic drugs, the situation is more concerning than it is for plant-based ones because even some of the most necessary precursors can be replaced by uncontrolled precursors or synthesized "down the chain" from an uncontrolled pre-precursor. While a sufficient supply of opium or coca leaf, respectively, is always necessary for their manufacture, only the chemicals for the isolation, conversion, and purification of heroin and cocaine, respectively, can be substituted with non-controlled alternatives.

1.4.4 The Development of a Trend - Demand Pull or Supply Push?

Choices for certain substances (or classes of substances) are the outcome of intricate interactions between social, cultural, economic, and other elements. As a result, they change over time and within and between nations. A new drug trend typically appears when manufacturers investigate the market through covert means and is then embraced by consumers. For a new drug to become popular, it must first satisfy consumer preferences in a particular time and sociocultural context. Consequently, in an expanding market, demand may eventually overtake supply as the primary driver. Globally, the majority of new trends in synthetic drug use started in Western nations—most notably the United States—and then made their way to less developed nations.

Changes in societal perceptions of a particular substance are somewhat associated with shifts in drug preferences. This can be partially attributed to the availability of more thorough, precise, and up-to-date information about the risks and adverse effects of using a given substance. Every new generation of drug users appears to rediscover the pleasurable effects of a particular drug in the absence of a sub-cultural memory of the risks associated with its usage. This, along with the later rediscovery and information-sharing regarding detrimental health and psychological effects, is a component of the cyclical pattern that most illicit drug epidemics share.

When it comes to traditional plant-based medications, any new developments are mainly restricted to altering the drug's delivery method (e.g., cocaine and crack cocaine or heroin hydrochloride and heroin base). As a result, customers can only choose from a small selection of products. Contrarily, synthetic drugs make it possible to covertly alter a "successful" drug molecule, usually without altering the desired pharmacological effects for the consumer, which opens up access to a whole class of related substances. Because of their adaptability, synthetic drugs can be a godsend for law enforcement and forensic chemists but also a great fit for situations where trends and fashions change quickly.

From a supply and demand perspective, globalization and the internationalization of societies seem to have played a role in fostering an atmosphere that has enabled the illicit trade of synthetic drugs.

On the demand side, there are at least three phenomena that can be observed over the last decade:

(i). Changes in social structures in many societies around the world, which lead, among other things, to an emphasis on individual success and performance;

(ii). A growing global trend towards fashionable lifestyles, short-lived amusement, and a 'consumption culture' which trusts in 'pills' as universal remedies; and

(iii). The spread of modern communication technology

The last phenomenon adds to the speed at which synthetic drugs spread and the convergence of consumption patterns across borders, even though the first two phenomena—instrumental/occupational use for the purpose of achieving goals and recreational/social use—may translate into distinct consumption patterns. The media landscape and contemporary communication technologies, particularly the Internet, facilitate the globalization of fashion trends and increase public access to detailed information about a range of drugs, including side effects, availability, and cost comparisons.

From the demand perspective

The social backdrop of the 1990s youth's "mass culture" provides insight into the current state of affairs surrounding the recreational use of psychoactive drugs. Since the early 1990s, the use of synthetic drugs has not been linked to specific social classes of drug users, nor does it seem to have any political connotations. Rather, the core of that drug culture in many countries appears to be pleasure-seeking, amusement, and fun in a controlled way without any perceived impact on work performance. As a result, the use of some psychoactive drugs has spread widely, with schoolchildren, college students, and high school students growing up in a culture where drug availability is normalized and drug use is nearly constant. In many countries, the use of certain synthetic drugs as symbols of a stylish lifestyle has made them an essential part of mainstream youth culture. Synthetic drugs appear to be prized for promoting socializing, communication, and a sense of integration and belonging among large segments of the population, including younger and younger segments of all social strata. This is especially the case for the stimulant-heavy drugs that were first connected to the dance community. But for many users, the drug itself—or its particular pharmacological effect—may be less significant than how it fits into their overall lifestyle.

Drug type

Only a few drug classes can meet the current requirements of the synthetic drug market in terms of pharmacological effects. Thesedrugs improve function, change or improve sensory perception, aid in interpersonal communication, and promote socialization. Synthetic drugs with calming effects that tend to isolate the user do not seem to be in line with today's youth values. The general pharmacology of medications used for the (sub)cultural phenomena closely associated with the dance drug scene remains the same, i.e., a combination of stimulation and enhancement of sensory perception. Aside from their pharmacological effects, the inherent qualities of the substances themselves—such as how quickly they take effect and how long they last—also play a role in whether or not they are suitable for a particular consumer demographic. The duration of action of the "ideal" future synthetic drug should not be too long, ideally a few hours; it should not cause a "hangover" the next day; and it should meet the criteria of oral bioavailability, i.e., it must be effective when taken by mouth, perhaps by smoking, though smoking is becoming less socially acceptable in many societies. These criteria are based on the current trend of dance or lifestyle drugs.

While many ATS do not fit those criteria, many synthetic drugs do. Given the reputation and social acceptance some established drugs have gained in the dance drug market, it is reasonable to assume that they will remain accessible and continue to spread outside of the dance scene. The term "ecstasy" has come to be associated with a recreational drug in tablet form, and its reputation, in particular, has led to the marketing of several other substances under the same name. While certain substances, such as amphetamine and LSD, that are marketed under the name "ecstasy" are also available as distinct substances under their names, many other substances, particularly those that are related to one another chemically and pharmacologically, lack a distinct market and consumer identity. Gammahydroxybutyrate, or GHB, is another substance that could be abused more quickly and extensively in the future. Despite having no structural connection to ATS, GHB entered the market by effectively utilizing the "ecstasy analogy" marketing concept. Users refer to it as "liquid ecstasy" or "the ultimate drug" when they are at a dance. It is said to increase sexual pleasure, induce euphoria and hallucinations, and have no "come-down" effect.

Polydrug use is common in environments where drug availability is constantly changing, and there are many different drugs and drug combinations available at the same time. This type of drug use entails the purposeful mixing of drugs to change, intensify, or prolong specific effects or to lessen the side effects of the primary drug taken. Combining illegal drugs with some legal medications is another factor. This is especially true for medications that slow down the illegal drug's metabolism in the body, extending and/or intensifying its effects. Such consumption patterns carry significant additional risks, some of which are potentially fatal due to unpredictable interactions with other therapeutic agents and even normal biological processes within the body.

The variety of drugs that produce the effects that are popular among today's "youth cultures" and that are often used concurrently include stimulants, hallucinogens, ecstasy, and related substances. Hallucinogens will remain, top contenders, when it comes to substance classes that users in the recreational drug scene may be interested in exploring. History demonstrates that users who find ecstasy's effects unappealing may go on to use hallucinogens after first using ecstasy. After that, they either start using hallucinogens directly or start using mixtures that contain them. It is important to consider the resurgence of LSD in this context, which occurred in the mid-1990s. Younger consumers are drawn to LSD because it is usually inexpensive, easy to obtain, and gives a long-lasting high. Since LSD is typically available at a much lower strength per dosage unit than it was in the 1960s, it may also encourage young users to experiment with other mild hallucinogens. Tryptamines are one class of hallucinogens that could grow in popularity. Tryptamines are a class of drug that, when smoked or injected, produces short-lived, powerful "trips." While most countries have prohibited the use of tryptamines since the early 1970s, there are rumors that some partygoers are trying tryptamines instead of LSD. Tryptamines do have some disadvantages, though, including the way they are administered. For some of them to have pharmacological effects, they must be smoked, snorted, or injected. Furthermore, a lot of them are far more hallucinogenic than ecstasy at typical dosage levels. Because of this, they might not be as popular among young people as other party drugs, unless their pharmacological disadvantage is offset by a low cost.

In light of the general consumer preferences underlying the current wave of synthetic drug abuse, it appears unlikely that substances belonging to other chemical or pharmacological classes will be consumed as widely in the near future.

Geographical trends

Geographically speaking, as living standards rise and purchasing power grows in free-market economies, it is reasonable to anticipate an increase in the demand for dance and performance-enhancing drugs. In some communities, the rise of the middle class and the growing popularity of foreign fashions may increase the risk of synthetic drug use. It is expected that the use of synthetic drugs will spread both vertically and horizontally within individual regions or countries, i.e., from wealthier to poorer social classes, as well as from big cities to smaller towns and rural areas. Declining prices resulting from market expansion could also play a role in this development.

South and South-East Asian nations have already seen a rise in the use of "ecstasy" and related ATS. For instance, the demand for synthetic drugs in nightclubs, dance halls, and karaoke bars is growing in China, particularly in Hong Kong, Shanghai, Canton, and the "special economic zones.". For comparable causes, i. e. As synthetic drugs are perceived as more contemporary and typically cost less than traditional drugs, it is also reasonable to anticipate that their use will continue in Eastern Europe. The demand for synthetic drugs may rise even more in several South American nations where young people have recently taken a fancy to "ecstasy."

From the supply perspective

From a supply perspective, synthetic drugs allow underground chemists to monitor changes in a consumer market that is influenced by fashion trends and where the drug itself is less important than the customs and myths surrounding its use. A covert chemist, however, would typically prefer not to substitute a less effective medicine for a more effective one that is well-liked by the general public unless absolutely necessary, as in the case of the unavailability of precursor chemicals. A covert chemist will typically create the medications that yield the largest profits and the fewest chances of being discovered among a group of related substances as long as they stay within the parameters of consumer acceptance and preferences. As a result, the emphasis will be on compounds with the highest potencies that can be produced, to the greatest extent feasible, from unreliable starting materials.

Drug type

Due to their low risk and high financial rewards, a number of the substances and substance classes that appeal to recreational drug users also appeal to covert manufacturers. This is especially true for certain artificial stimulants and hallucinogens, as they present chances for pharmacological design and structural alteration. However, there is some risk involved in developing a completely "new" substance class because consumer acceptance is a factor outside the direct control of covert manufacturers.

As a consequence, future trends are likely to evolve from what is already discernable today:

- increased availability of traditional ATS, such as amphetamine and methamphetamine, to be used for their performance-enhancing effects;
- re-emergence of other ATS already banned in most countries as a consequence of previous periods of abuse; and/or
- increase in consumption of new designer ATS or of substances that have so far only appeared sporadically in illicit markets. The so-called phenethylamines (PEAs), which are close chemical relatives of ATS not controlled in most countries, and which can be expected to produce similar effects, can be included in this category

Tryptamines, that cause hallucinations, are the only other pharmacological drug class amenable to structural modification, similar to ATS, and that might also be appealing to consumers in the near future are.

Geographical trends

For the majority of the past ten years, Western Europe has been the primary illicit manufacturing region for amphetamine and other substances similar to ecstasy in the world. Large-scale production is generally expected to continue in Europe as long as ATS consumption persists there. 'Marketing activities' appear to be expanding from regional to international consumer markets, such as North America, Australia/New Zealand, South Africa, Asia, and South America, at the same time.

The expansion of drug manufacturing into Eastern Europe, the Baltic States, and the CIS Member States is also expected to persist due to the unstable economic conditions in many of those nations, the easy access to labor and precursors, expertise, and technical capabilities for drug synthesis, and low cost of labor.

In South-East Asia, the illicit production of synthetic drugs is also on the rise, as traditional heroin-producing groups are increasingly venturing into the production of ATS, particularly methamphetamine. Even though a large portion of these goods are intended for regional consumption, a growing amount of South East Asian methamphetamine seizures—mostly from Thailand—have occurred in Europe and, more recently, the US. This suggests a reversal of a long-standing trend in which "ecstasy" was being exported from Europe to South-East Asia. Additionally, there are now hints that underground producers in Southeast Asia might soon be able to create premium "ecstasy" on par with that which is imported from Europe. Consequently, prices should decline, making the medication more accessible to a wider range of people. This could be a problem, especially in China, where seizure data show that the nation is increasingly significant as a hub for the distribution of different synthetic drugs.

In some Latin American nations where the demand for "ecstasy" is already developing, a similar trend to that observed in South-East Asia may eventually also emerge. In contrast, Africa—apart from South Africa, that is—does not seem to be in danger of becoming a major hub for the production of illicit synthetic drugs anytime soon since pharmaceuticals are still accessible there through unregulated channels or parallel markets.

As previously mentioned, the drugs themselves, their representation, and inherent qualities—like general pharmacology, suitability for a particular mode of administration, duration of action, etc.— primarily drive trends on the demand side. In addition to the drugs themselves, other supply-side variables also affect the patterns of illicit production and trafficking. Regarding the manufacturing side, these could be things like the emphasis and intensity of regulatory and law enforcement efforts, the expertise of covert chemists, and the sophistication of their labs. Among the issues pertaining to trafficking is the crucial one of "marketing," or the capacity of covert operators to "market" their wares.

1.4.5 Clandestine Synthetic Drugs and Links with Organized Crime

A concerning trend in the recent history of illicit synthetic drug use is the growing organization and integration of the drug's production and distribution into global organized crime networks. A covert synthetic drug "industry" with extensive production and global distribution networks is emerging, propelled by enormous profits.

Similar to the phenomenon of polydrug abuse, "market opportunities" are also likely to cause a spike in polydrug trafficking and distribution. Information gathered by intelligence services in several western European nations also indicates that offenders who have committed violent crimes and brought in traditional drugs are becoming more and more involved in the manufacture and sale of synthetic drugs. A small number of criminal "investors" from Western Europe take advantage of the job and economic conditions in Eastern Europe. They take orders for markets overseas, invest the required funds, deliver the precursor chemicals for making ATS, and use front companies to launder profits. Given their access to substantial amounts of readily available funds, there is also a chance that criminal organizations will buy fully equipped, formerly state-owned properties to engage in extensive, covert production of synthetic drugs. Additionally, there are signs that criminal groups are beginning to take over the establishments that host big dance parties and serve synthetic drug sales to control the drug's retail distribution.

From a historical standpoint, it seems that the trafficking of precursor chemicals was often the first step in the expansion of criminal groups involved in the production and distribution of plant-based drugs into synthetic drugs. This type of trafficking has always been multistage and international in nature, in contrast to the distribution of synthetic end products. For a long time, it has been hypothesized that the two markets are actually connected and that the same groups may be involved in both activities due to similarities in the trafficking patterns of plant-based drugs. The next phase is the distribution of synthetic end products, which is currently taking place in a number of locations across the globe. It is now widely accepted that the illegal markets for synthetic and plant-based drugs are already entwined in some areas. For instance, criminal organizations in North America that were previously mostly engaged in the trafficking of cocaine and cannabis from Mexico appear to be using their current networks of distribution to provide methamphetamine to the US market, facilitating the drug's faster national spread (Zhang et al., 2002). Some reports state that drug trafficking organizations in Mexico are becoming more and more involved in the illegal trade of "ecstasy," exchanging cocaine from Latin America for "ecstasy" that is produced in Europe. The emergence of connections between illegal activities in heroin and ATS, both at the manufacturing and trafficking levels, is another similar development that can be observed in heroin networks in East and South-East Asia. Heroin and ATS are increasingly produced in the same labs and disseminated through the same channels.

1.5 Pharmacological and Toxicological Effects of Synthetic Cannabinoids and their Metabolites

In the USA, young adults have taken SCBs as recreational drugs with great popularity. The use of these drugs began in Europe, where they were sold under the brand name Spice. They swiftly expanded to the USA, where they were sold under the brand name K2. SCBs are most frequently added to herbal mixtures (like incense or potpourri) to be smoked, though they are occasionally offered for commercial distribution as capsules, tablets, and powders. Commercial SCB products are widely accessible online and can still be purchased at "brick and mortar" stores like convenience stores and head shops, even in spite of regulatory efforts to restrict their availability. Clever marketing strategies, typically involving bright packaging and deceptive labeling intended to present a safe herbal blend that is "not intended for human consumption," are responsible for their widespread distribution. These dishonest marketing strategies were used to avoid facing consequences for selling drugs of abuse, but it is unlikely that disputes over product labels would obstruct criminal proceedings resulting from the sale of illegal substances. Crucially, it seems that the marketing of these goods is intended expressly to mislead consumers into believing that they are safe, "natural," and acceptable substitutes for cannabis.

Scientists and legislators have expressed a great deal of interest in examining the pharmacological similarities between SCBs and Δ^9-tetrahydrocannabinol (Δ^9-THC), the primary psychoactive ingredient in marijuana (Huestis, 2005). According to reports, SCBs have different intrinsic activity in comparison to Δ^9-THC and have higher binding affinity at both CB1 and CB2 cannabinoid receptor (CBR) subtypes. These findings have been observed in both animal studies and cellular assays. When it comes to a variety of in vitro and in vivo tests, SCBs are fully effective at both CBRs, in contrast to Δ^9-THC, which continuously shows partial agonist efficacy in vitro (Chin et al., 1999). Furthermore, SCB metabolites frequently have a higher affinity for CBR than Δ^9-THC and can have different pharmacological and toxicological effects from Δ^9-THC. These active metabolites may account for the higher rates of morbidity and death linked to exposure to SCBs than are generally observed with marijuana. The pharmacological and toxicological effects associated with SCB metabolism will be covered in the remaining sections of this chapter, with a focus on the active metabolites in particular. It will be demonstrated that these compounds are not safe, have a more potent toxicological profile than marijuana, and shouldn't be used as a legitimate substitute for cannabis.

1.5.1 Synthetic Cannabinoid Metabolism

Metabolism of xenobiotics occurs through several biotransformation pathways which are conserved across species and quite old from an evolutionary perspective. The goal of drug metabolism is to detoxify potentially harmful compounds, removing them from the circulation and ultimately excreting them from the body altogether. The liver plays a major role in this detoxification process. Sometimes, metabolism can create metabolic intermediates that can cause toxicity on their own, or it can activate inert compounds—the idea of a "pro-drug". Generally speaking, the hepatic cytochrome P450 (CYP) enzyme system is the first step in the oxidative metabolism of xenobiotics (Watanabe, 2007). From there, a class of enzymes known as UGTs, conjugates the metabolites with glucuronic acid, a sugar moiety. After that, the metabolites are sufficiently soluble to be expelled from the body.

The reference standard for comprehending the pharmacokinetics of cannabinoids has been the metabolism of Δ^9-THC. The first step in the metabolism of Δ^9-THC by human hepatic microsomes is oxidation by CYP subtypes 2C9 and 3A4. To put it briefly, the only psychoactive metabolite of Δ^9-THC is 11-hydroxy-Δ^9-THC, which is produced by CPY2C9 hydroxylation of Δ^9-THC. The remaining hydroxyl groups in Δ^9-THC can be further oxidized to produce carboxylic acids at various positions along the alkyl side chain. These metabolites have no biological effect. The primary metabolite excreted in human urine, O-ester glucuronide, is formed when the active metabolite 11-hydroxy-Δ^9-THC is further oxidized, eliminating any pharmacological activity and producing 11-nor-9-carboxy-Δ^9-THC.

In the early 2000s, initial reports of SCB metabolism emerged with a focus on in vitro metabolism of CBR ligands (11R)-2-methyl-11-[(morpholin-4-yl)methyl]-3-(naphthalene-1-carbonyl)-9-oxa-1-azatricyclo[6.3.1.0^{4,12}] dodeca-2,4(12),5,7-tetraene (WIN-55,212-2), 1-[2-(morpholin-4-yl)ethyl]-2-methyl-3-(4-methoxybenzoyl)-6-iodoindole (AM-630), and

(2-methyl-1-propyl-1H-indol-3-yl)-1-naphthalenyl-methanone (JWH-015). The emphasis has since shifted to the in vivo metabolism of the frequently abused CBR ligand naphthalen-1-yl-(1-pentylindol-3-yl)methanone (JWH-018) and its analogs as a result of the recreational use of SCBs. Urine samples taken from three persons who had smoked a commercial product containing JWH-018 were the first to contain JWH-018 metabolites (Rajasekaran et al., 2013). The oxidation of the indole ring or the N-alkyl chain produces mono-hydroxylated compounds, which are the primary phase I metabolites. Phase II glucuronide conjugates are the predominant form of urine excretion of phase I JWH-018 metabolites, as confirmed by gas and liquid chromatography mass spectrometry (GC-MS and LC-MS/MS). The metabolism of JWH-018 to its 4-hydroxyindole metabolite and related glucuronide conjugate is shown in Figure 1.1.

Further studies revealed that human hepatic microsomes incubated with JWH-018, urine specimens from individuals using Spice/K2 products, and rats administered JWH-018, naphthalen-1-yl-(1-butylindol-3-yl)methanone (JWH-073), or 2-(2-methoxyphenyl)-1-(1-pentylindol-3-yl)ethanone (JWH-250) formed phase I mono-hydroxylated metabolites and phase II glucuronides. All of these investigations supported the idea that the main excretion of these SCBs' urinary metabolites is a single hydroxylation followed by glucuronidation (Zhang et al., 2004).

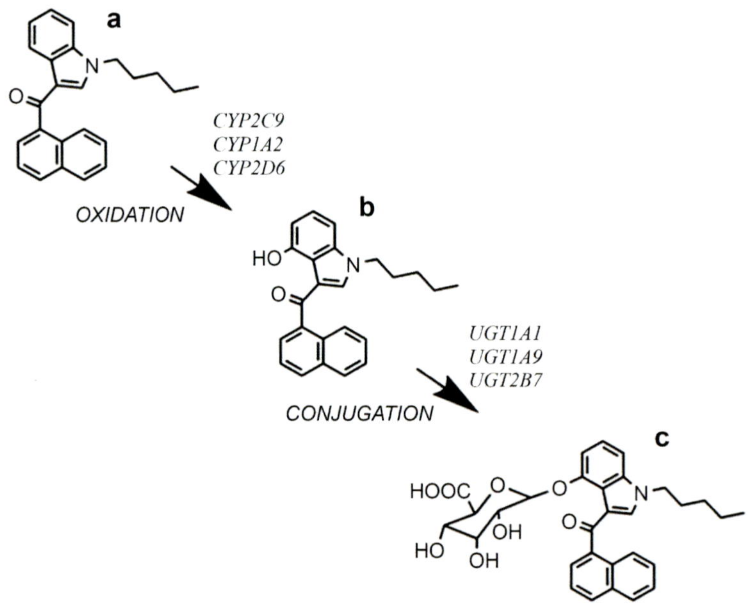

Figure 1.1. Metabolism of the synthetic cannabinoid (SCB) JWH-018.

Source: https://www.ncbi.nlm.nih.gov/pmc/articles/PMC5392241/

Reference standards for identifying particular JWH-018 and JWH-073 metabolites were not developed until 2011, which made it possible to perform quantitative LC-MS measurements both in vitro and in vivo. Human urine samples were taken from subjects who had consumed JWH-018 or a combination of JWH-018 and JWH-073. The analysis showed that the metabolites detected in the urine were mostly excreted as glucuronic acid conjugates and present in high concentrations. Numerous other laboratories have confirmed these results.

It is widely acknowledged that the production of hydroxylated metabolites in humans indicates the involvement of CYPs in the biotransformation of SCBs. According to in vitro metabolism studies, hepatic CYP subtypes 2C9 and 1A2 oxidize SCBs JWH-018 and its fluorinated analogue 1-[(5-fluoropentyl)-1H-indol-3-yl]-(naphthalen-1-yl)methanone (AM-2201). CYPs are widely expressed in the body in a tissue-specific way outside of the liver. Since the intestines also exhibit high expression of CYP2C9, intestinal CYP2C9 is probably involved in the metabolism of SCBs when they are consumed orally. Because of its high lung expression, CYP1A2 is probably in charge of how smoked SCBs are metabolized (Chimalakonda, 2011). Evidence suggests that CYP2D6 is involved in the metabolism of JWH-018 and AM-2201 in the brain, particularly in the cortex, hippocampus, and cerebellum—regions known for their high levels of CB1R expression. More so than in the liver, CYP2D6 is probably involved in controlling the concentrations of these SCBs and their active metabolites in the brain.

The excretion of SCBs in urine is thought to be primarily facilitated by glucuronic acid conjugation, as evidenced by the high concentrations of glucuronide metabolites found in urine specimens from those who consumed the drug and the absence of any traces in serum. Major UGT isoforms UGT1A1, UGT1A9, and UGT2B7 in the liver form JWH-018 and JWH-073 metabolites. Moreover, extrahepatic UGT isoforms implicated in metabolism include UGT1A10, UGT1A3 and UGT2B7 expressed in the brain and liver, and UGT1A7 expressed in the lung. Significantly, the primary isoforms of human UGT1A3 and UGT2B7 are in charge of producing the principal metabolites of JWH-018 and JWH-073 that are discovered in urine. Similar to CYP2D6, UGT1A3 and UGT2B7 may be involved in controlling the amounts of SCBs and their active metabolites in the brain at the CB1 receptor. This is because these UGT isoforms are also expressed in the brain.

1.5.2 Synthetic Cannabinoid Cellular Signaling

The metabolites generated by SCBs JWH-018 and JWH-073 have been characterized as a result of the pharmacological profiling of Δ^9-THC. JWH-018 and JWH-073, like the phytocannabinoid Δ^9-THC, have a strong affinity for the CB1 and CB2Rs. Figure 1.2 displays the chemical structures for JWH-073, which includes many of the related SBCs covered in this chapter.

Emerging SCBs found in commercial preparations also have high affinity for the CB1 and CB2Rs, including 2-[(1S,3R)-3-hydroxycyclo-hexyl]-5-(2-methyloctan-2-yl) phenol (CP-47,497), (1-pentylindol-3-yl) naphtha-len-1-ylmethane (JWH-175), 1-([(1E)-3-pentylinden-1-ylidine]methyl)naphthalene (JWH-176), (1-pentylindol-3-yl)-(2,2,3,3-tetramethylcyclopropyl)metha-none (UR-144), naphthalen-1-yl-(1-pentylpyrrol-3-yl) methanone (JWH-030), 2-(2-methoxyphenyl)-1-(1-pentylindol-3-yl)ethanone (JWH-250), N-(1-adamantyl)-1-pentylindazole-3-carboxamide (APINACA, or AKB48), and 1-[(N-methylpiperidin-2-yl)methyl]-3-(adamant-1-oyl)indole (AM-1248) . Furthermore, most commercial SCB products display high potency and efficacy as CB1R agonists both in vitro and in vivo, including JWH-018, JWH-073, AM-1248, CP-55,940, WIN-55,512-2, and (6aR,10aR)-9-(hydroxymethyl)-6,6-dimethyl-3-(2-methyloctan-2-yl)-6H,6aH,7H,10H,10aH-benzo[c]isochro-men-1-ol (HU-210) (Moran et al., 2011).

The existence of highly affinity and completely effective CB1 agonists in these commercial products may be the cause of the abuse potential of SCB products. For example, Δ^9-THC has a partial in vitro efficacy in comparison to JWH-018 and JWH-073, which have a full efficacy. Crucially, not all in vitro or ex vivo tests are able to distinguish between THC and SCBs' varying levels of efficacy. A fascinating study by Hoffman and colleagues showed that THC and SCBs were equally effective in an electrophysiological test that measured the inhibition of transmitter release.

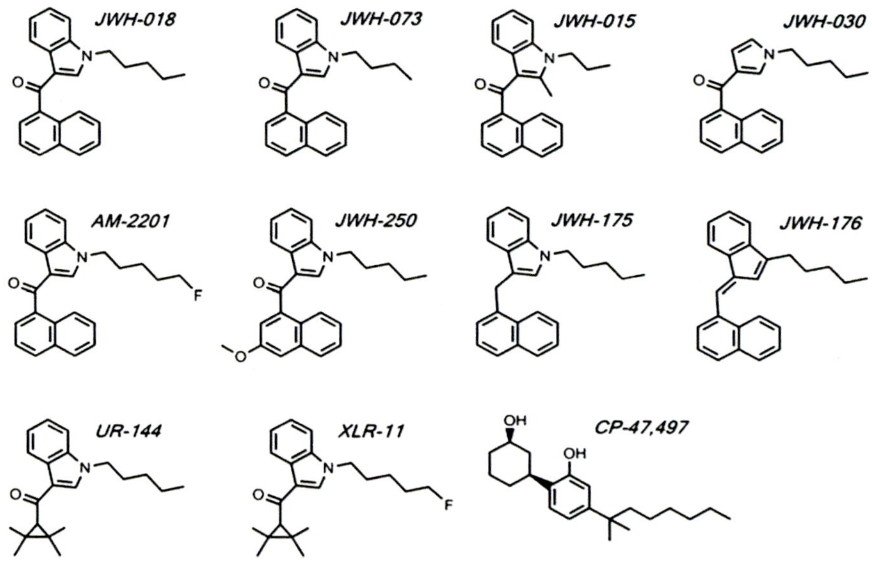

Figure 1.2. Chemical structures of synthetic cannabinoids.

Source: https://www.ncbi.nlm.nih.gov/pmc/articles/PMC5392241/

However, Δ^9-THC's frequently shown low in vitro efficacy does not always correspond to partial agonism in vivo; in fact, Δ^9-THC frequently exhibits in vivo efficacy on par with completely effective agonists. Furthermore, sudden cessation of long-term marijuana use or administration of Δ^9-THC causes a withdrawal syndrome in both humans and rodents, which is correlated with a localized downregulation and desensitization of CB1Rs in the brain. Therefore, compared to Δ9-THC, it's possible that commercial SCB products that contain highly effective agonists will exacerbate the negative effects of tolerance, dependence, and withdrawal from SCB abuse. For example, the commercial SCB product "Spice Gold" caused humans to experience a dependence syndrome and withdrawal phenomenon following an abrupt cessation of use (Moran et al., 2011). This syndrome included intense cravings for the drug, high blood pressure, nausea, tremors, excessive sweating, and nightmares. While concurrent laboratory studies found that a combination of the SCBs JWH-018 and CP-47,497 was present in this commercial smoking blend at the time and in the region where the aforementioned case occurred, the active ingredients of this product were not forensically determined in the product itself or in fluids or tissue from the case subject.

When Δ^9-THC is broken down, only one active metabolite, 11-hydroxy-Δ^9-THC, is produced, and it has a lower affinity for CB1 receptors than the original drug. However, unlike their carboxylated metabolites, which neither bind to nor activate CB1Rs, the metabolism of commercial SCBs, such as JWH-018, JWH-073, and AM-2201, results in a number of major mono-hydroxylated metabolites that maintain nanomolar binding affinity for CB1Rs.

Apart from maintaining a high affinity for CB1 receptors, in vitro functional tests (G-protein activation) reveal that the primary mono-hydroxylated metabolites of JWH-018, JWH-073, and AM-2201 display partial to complete effectiveness at CB1 receptors, akin to the fully effective CP-55,940. Significantly, the in vivo cannabimimetic actions of mono-hydroxylated metabolites JWH-018 and JWH-073 induced significant hypothermic and locomotor depressant responses in mice. CB1R antagonist/inverse agonist 1-(2,4-dichlorophenyl)-5-(4-iodophenyl)-4-methyl-N-(1-piperidyl)pyrazole-3-carboxamide (AM-251) attenuates these effects, indicating that these metabolites, like their parent ligands, are mediating their effects through the CB1R. Furthermore, there's a chance that the negative effects of using SCBs are linked to the effects of metabolites. For example, it has been demonstrated that a number of JWH-018, JWH-073, and AM-2201's mono-hydroxylated metabolites maintain high CB1R activity and affinity and may interact additively or synergistically with other SCBs.

Additional contributing factors to the adverse effects of SCB use can be:

(1) Drug effects of non-cannabinoid-like ligands found in commercial SCB products,

(2) Variations in batch-to-batch preparations with differences in the concentration and content found in commercial SCB products, and

(3) An exacerbation of SCB adverse effects in drug users with preexisting conditions.

Certain oxidized metabolites of SCBs may act as antagonists at CB1Rs, despite evidence suggesting that mono-hydroxylated metabolites of JWH-018, JWH-073, and AM-2201 are active at CB1Rs in both in vitro and in vivo assays. The 7-hydroxyindole derivative of JWH-073 has been demonstrated to bind to CB1Rs with nanomolar affinity at pharmacologically relevant concentrations of up to 10 μM, without causing any G-protein activation, despite the fact that it has not been found in human urine (Moran et al., 2011). Additionally, JWH-073's 7-hydroxyindole derivative has been demonstrated by Schild analysis to competitively oppose G-protein activation in vitro. This oxidized derivative of JWH-073 was given to mice beforehand to lessen the effects of JWH-018-induced hypothermia. On the other hand, this metabolite did not affect the analgesia, catalepsy, or locomotor activity that JWH-018 induced. Overall, these in vitro and in vivo results, in addition to the fact that the 7-hydroxyindole derivative of JWH-073 was not found in human urine, indicate that it is possible that humans do not form this oxidized derivative of JWH-073 or that it does not easily pass through the blood–brain barrier.

Apart from the fact that a major human glucuronidated metabolite of JWH-018 (5-hydroxypentyl-β-D-glucuronide) exhibits CB1R antagonism in vitro, there is also evidence that a human oxidation product of JWH-018 functions as a CB1R antagonist. Fascinatingly, this investigation also revealed that 11-nor-9-carboxy-THC-β-D-glucuronide, a significant structurally similar glucuronidated THC metabolite, lacked CB1R activity and affinity. Together, these data show that SCB hydroxylated and glucuronidated metabolites may both maintain a sizable affinity for CB1Rs even in the absence of intrinsic activity, suggesting that certain SCB metabolites may cause physiologically meaningful antagonistic effects on CB1Rs.

The main focus of discussions regarding the pharmacological and toxicological effects of SCBs has been on comprehending the responses that are induced by CB1R. Many SCBs exhibit comparable binding and functional activity at the second major CBR subtype, CB2R, in addition to their high affinity and notable intrinsic activity at the CB1R. While CB2Rs are most commonly found on immune cells in peripheral regions and are linked to immune functions, inflammation, and bone formation, CB1Rs are primarily found within the central nervous system. More recent research has shown that the CNS's low levels of CB2R activation can modify the qualities of alcohol, nicotine, and cocaine abuse. Furthermore, it has been demonstrated that JWH-018 and JWH-073's mono-hydroxylated metabolites still have strong CB2R efficacy and affinity.

Remarkably, research has suggested that endocannabinoid signaling plays a role in controlling the serotonin system. For example, it has been demonstrated that long-term CB2R activation causes 5-HT2A receptors in the mouse prefrontal cortex to be upregulated. Mental illnesses like anxiety and psychosis can result from abnormalities in the central nervous system's 5-HT2A function. Furthermore, a key mechanism of action for hallucinogenic substances is 5-HT2A receptor signaling. Anxiety and psychosis, two common side effects of SCB use, are not frequently seen with Δ^9-THC. The upregulation of 5-HT2A receptors induced by SCBs or SCB metabolites, which is mediated through CB2R activation, may be a factor in the anxiety and psychosis that are reported following exposure to SCBs, which are present in commercially available abuse-ready formulations. Regarding this, a case study described four patients who smoked a product containing the SCB AM-2201 while in the clinic and were hospitalized for psychosis (Sobolevsky, 2012). The authors reported the onset of new psychotic symptoms and a significant worsening of mood and anxiety symptoms in four patients. Despite the fact that all patients took the same medication, each patient's clinical picture was significantly different, which may indicate that different people's metabolisms of AM-2201 contributed to the range of effects seen. Future research on CB1R and CB2R signaling in relation to the pharmacological and toxicological effects of SCBs and their metabolites is therefore obviously crucial. Future research should also take into account these medications' ability to alter the expression and functionality of other, non-CBR systems.

1.5.3 Synthetic Cannabinoid Drug–Drug Interactions

Commercial SCB preparations frequently combine several medications, and the concentrations of these particular SCBs differ significantly between products or even between batches of the same product. Drug-drug interactions may therefore occur both within and between these various mixtures of SCBs, which may add to the negative effects and abuse-related aspects of using these medications. As previously mentioned, according to mouse studies, depending on the exact endpoint being studied and the drug dose ratio used, co-administration of JWH-018 and JWH-073 resulted in additive, synergistic, or antagonistic interactions compared to administration of either drug alone. In vitro and in vivo assays using mice for Δ^9-THC discrimination and analgesia, as well as cellular model displacement of radioligand binding from CB1Rs, provided evidence of the synergistic effects of these two SCBs. Blended mixtures of SCBs can affect the relative potency of both their beneficial and negative effects, in addition to their synergistic effects. Furthermore, abusing multiple substances can result in unpredictable SCB effects, which could exacerbate the negative effects of abuse. Future research is required to comprehend the interactions between SCBs and other drugs of abuse, as well as the co-exposure to these interactions (Sobolevsky, 2012).

When SCBs are used in conjunction with different prescription medications, there is a chance that negative drug-drug interactions could occur due to their shared metabolism via P450 isoforms. CYP2C9 is potently inhibited by commonly prescribed medications like sertraline, an antidepressant, and valproic acid, an anticonvulsant and mood stabilizer; CYP1A2 is strongly inhibited by medications like fluvoxamine, an antidepressant, and ciprofloxacin. Major polymorphic enzyme CYP2C9 is also in charge of the metabolism of several clinically significant medications, including the blood thinner warfarin, the anticonvulsant phenytoin, the antidiabetic tolbutamide, the antihypertensive losartan, and the nonsteroidal anti-inflammatory drug ibuprofen. Two "loss of function" variants (CYP2C9*4 and CYP2C9*5) are among the more than five allelic variants of CYP2D6 that have been found. Likewise, CYP1A2 is in charge of the metabolism of many psychiatric drugs, such as cholinesterase inhibitors used to treat Alzheimer's disease (tacrine), antidepressants (imipramine, clomipramine, and fluvoxamine), and antipsychotics (olanzapine, clozapine, haloperidol, and thioridazine). However, this enzyme is highly conserved and does not share any common functional polymorphisms. Because SCBs also function as substrates for these P450 isoforms, using SCBs raises the risk of drug-drug interactions (Hutter, 2012).

1.6 The Challenge of Fentanyl, Meth, and Other Synthetic Drugs

You would probably have assumed that the overdose crisis in the United States was finally coming to an end if someone had told you in 2015 that by 2021, the number of overdose deaths caused solely by the two most historically lethal drugs—heroin and cocaine—would have dropped by more than half. Rather, the emergence of synthetic drugs caused drug overdose deaths to skyrocket to over 100,000 annually—a truly disruptive innovation that US drug policy is only now starting to address.

To define the crucial phrase, synthetic drugs are compounds that are not derived from plants but rather can be made in a lab. In the U.S. and Canada. Synthetic fentanyl and its derivatives are outcompeting heroin, which is derived from the poppy plant, in the black market for opioids. In 2021, these synthetics alone or in combination with other drugs took the lives of over 70,000 Americans (or 66% of the 106,699 drug-related overdose deaths). Cocaine, which is derived from coca leaves, has lost market share to another synthetic stimulant, methamphetamine. Synthetic tranquilizers, like xylazine and benzodiazepines, have become increasingly popular, which has led to an increase in addiction and fatalities, especially when combined with opioids. The U.S. is also dealing with a plethora of so-called NPS, like mephedrone and MDMA, which combined draw more users than more traditional, "minor" drugs like PCP, GHB, and LSD.

To define the crucial phrase, synthetic drugs are compounds that are not derived from plants but rather can be made in a lab. Synthetic fentanyl and its derivatives are surpassing heroin, which is derived from the poppy plant, in the illicit opioid markets of the U.S. and Canada. In 2021, these synthetics alone or in combination with other drugs took the lives of over 70,000 Americans (or 66% of the 106,699 drug-related overdose deaths). Cocaine, which is derived from coca leaves, has lost market share to another synthetic stimulant, methamphetamine. Synthetic tranquilizers, like xylazine and benzodiazepines, have become increasingly popular, which has led to an increase in addiction and fatalities, especially when combined with opioids. Additionally, the U.S. is dealing with a plethora of so-called NPS, like mephedrone and MDMA, which combined draw more users than more traditional, "minor" drugs like PCP, GHB, and LSD. Parents, activists, legislators, and clinicians in desperate search of answers to the synthetic drug crisis frequently approach drug policy analysts, including the writers of this brief. This is our brief response. Unfortunately, it's not a very positive one. The market for synthetic drugs cannot be solved easily, and the four main pillars of drug policy—enforcement, treatment, harm reduction, and prevention—all have limitations. However, the country should cease doing some harmful things and improve upon others.

Policymakers must:

- Maintain prohibition of the production and sale of synthetic drugs
- Expect law enforcement to shrink market-related harms, such as violence, but not necessarily to shrink the supply of the drugs themselves
- Keep expanding medication-assisted treatment and access to naloxone
- Embrace the shunning of illegal drugs as a cultural norm
- Be generous toward those who are struggling, including those suffering from drug addiction

Sadly, overdose deaths will likely continue to be higher than historical averages due to the easy access to potentially fatal temptations in the U.S.A. Such realism is honest—and sincerity is the best basis for policy—but it is also depressing.

Synthetics Are Different—and Difficult

Synthetic drug production is quick, affordable, and feasible practically anywhere. The internet has made it possible for nearly anyone to learn how to make simpler "recipes" and the chemical ingredients that go into making them. This implies that illicit supply networks have a greater ability to substitute confiscated synthetic drugs than they do for substances like heroin or cocaine. Similarly, trafficking organizations can be quickly replaced if they are shut down.

Farmland for opium poppies or coca plants is needed to produce heroin or cocaine, and peasant labor is needed to tend the crops. There is always a risk of political unrest, droughts, crop infestation, and eradication efforts. Keeping inventories is necessary to protect against crop failures, seizures, and other disruptions; however, inventories are susceptible to raids by law enforcement or other criminals. These expenses are eliminated from traffickers' ledgers by synthetic drugs. Moreover, drug traffickers don't have to wait patiently for a crop to finish growing because they can synthesize drugs whenever they want. Because of this, it is more difficult for law enforcement to stop the supply from being supplied, even though in the past, restrictions on precursor chemicals have led to some (brief) successes, especially for methamphetamine, until traffickers discovered other ways to synthesize the drug.

For traffickers, the cost benefits of synthetic drugs are greatest for fentanyl. Producing fentanyl is up to 100 times less expensive per dose at higher market levels than heroin. This economic reasoning never stops.

The cost-benefit of meth is also significant. It frequently retails for less than half as much per unit weight as cocaine (for example, $100–$200 per ounce vs. Almost $1,000 for cocaine in Los Angeles), and the meth high lasts longer even with similar dose sizes. Because of the ensuing fundamental challenge to drug policy, now is a good time to reconsider its four established pillars—enforcement, treatment, harm reduction, and prevention—and consider whether four is enough.

First Pillar: Law Enforcement

Rejecting drug legalization does not imply blind faith in drug law enforcement's abilities, but a sober analysis reveals that law enforcement can accomplish a lot. Law enforcement occasionally succeeds in limiting availability. The first synthetic fentanyl was created in 1959, and by the 1970s, it was evident that it was more cost-effective than heroin. However, because law enforcement quickly contained multiple prior outbreaks, illegally produced fentanyl did not become a serious problem until about 2015. Similar to how methamphetamine took decades to spread throughout the nation, enticing, affordable goods with legitimate corporations supporting them don't sit in isolated areas.

It is appropriate to attribute the delayed spread of methamphetamine and fentanyl to enforcement and prohibition. Over a generation of Americans went through their peak drug-using years when methamphetamine was only available in certain areas of the country and illegal fentanyl was virtually nonexistent.

Unfortunately, it is very difficult to remove a drug market once it has gained traction. Though the Taliban has suppressed approximately 90% of the opioid production in Afghanistan, the Communist Party of China virtually eradicated opium addiction after 1949, and free societies would rightfully find it intolerable that their civil liberties be violated in such cases.

In a free society, forcing traffickers to operate in inefficient ways is frequently the best that law enforcement can do. Due to higher prices and less accessibility, drug use has historically decreased as a result. Due to their low cost of production, law enforcement may now have to settle for depending more on the latter.

For the same reasons that cause some people who eat healthily at home to struggle with self-control at all-you-can-eat buffets, there is value in keeping drugs hidden and away from Madison Avenue marketing budgets and expertise. Stated differently, law enforcement can assist someone who wishes to abstain from drugs in avoiding daily temptations, but it typically cannot prevent someone who is determined to obtain drugs from discovering them (Seely, 2011).

Additionally, it is important to note that lower prices do not always have negative consequences. While they may attract individuals with low income, such as teenagers, to drug use, lower prices can also potentially reduce the financial burden on those who are already struggling with addiction and decrease profits for drug dealers.

Law enforcement can retreat from pointless and ineffective actions when it is liberated from irrational expectations, such as those to seal the borders or establish drug-free zones. Long prison terms are unnecessary for retail salespeople and other easily replaceable employees of higher-ups in the organization. Furthermore, Americans shouldn't depend on uncooperative foreign nations to stop the production of synthetic drugs, which can be done in numerous other locations. Because fentanyl is so powerful, the U.S. consumes less than ten metric tons of it annually; it could easily fit inside any of the seven million trucks or cargo containers that cross the southern border every year. A single pure pound can be used to create 200,000 fentanyl-laced pills, which can then be shipped from Mexico, China, or any other location to the United States.

Just as public health can concentrate on minimizing the harms from drug use, police should concentrate on lessening the negative effects of drug sales. For instance, shut down the outdoor drug markets that are causing harm to communities in Portland, Boston, San Francisco, Seattle, Philadelphia, and other cities. Although driving drug markets underground does not stop sales, it does lessen the chaos, tension, and criminality that surrounding neighborhoods and communities experience from open-air markets.

In the words of CUNY criminologist David Kennedy, there are open-air markets in many American neighborhoods, but drug use and sales occur in many other neighborhoods as well. We refer to them as suburbs. All Americans should be entitled to the freedom from being harassed or intimidated by blatant retail drug sellers; this should not only be a privilege enjoyed by the wealthy.

Efforts to deter drug sales at street corners, like the High Point (North Carolina) strategy and Operation Ceasefire in Boston, were among the more effective methods of dealing with these illegal markets. Similar reasoning can be used at all market levels by giving priority to the most harmful groups (such as the most violent), strategies (such as smuggling by successfully infiltrating border agents rather than using stealth), and goods (such as pills that are mistakenly labeled Adderall or Ativan but actually contain fentanyl). While not all drug dealers are good people, there are those who are, and they almost all pay attention when law enforcement makes it known which offenses will receive more attention than others.

A significant contribution can be made by placing the truly horrible at a competitive disadvantage in comparison to the merely bad. Law enforcement is aware of these differences, of course, but other considerations, like quantity possessed, are given too much weight in sentencing guidelines and case prioritization. To physically transport their drugs, kingpins employ readily replaceable underlings, and it is these underlings who are frequently the targets of quantity-based sentencing programs.

Second Pillar: Drug Treatment

Methamphetamine and fentanyl, being synthetic drugs, have some production and market economic similarities, but their effects on users and available treatment options are very different.

In spite of forty years of efforts by the National Institute on Drug Abuse and pharmaceutical companies, there are currently no FDA-approved pharmacotherapies for treating stimulant addiction, such as cocaine and methamphetamine addiction. This is problematic because "talk therapy" by itself is not a very effective means of combating highly addictive substances.

On the other hand, there are a number of FDA-approved drugs for treating opioid-use disorder (OUD, the official name for the condition that was formerly known as opioid addiction). For OUD, medication-assisted treatment is one of the most well-studied and economical medical interventions available. People's lives can be significantly improved by stabilizing them on opioid agonists (like methadone) or partial agonists (like buprenorphine) that are supplied lawfully and are less harmful. Some patients respond favorably to naltrexone, an opioid-blocking drug; this is especially true of the injectable form, which lasts for a month. These drugs ought to be available in all medical and jail settings, be covered by all insurance policies, both public and private.

Yet MAT isn't a treatment. Even with excellent treatment, the majority of OUD patients who are admitted will relapse, sometimes repeatedly, and each relapse increases the chance of a lethal overdose. The yearly death rates of individuals already in MAT are actually five to fifteen times higher than those of age-matched peers without OUD, according to multiple long-term follow-up studies. Compare blindness and broken arm medical care to grasp that seeming contradiction. The medical system can "mold" broken arms and restore people to nearly new conditions. In contrast, medical care is rarely able to restore the vision of those who have lost it, despite the fact that we can do a lot to help them live better.

In this sense, OUD is not as difficult as blindness, but it is more akin to blindness than to broken arms under a range of difficult circumstances. While some people do recover completely, many do not, and even those who do may require multiple rounds of treatment before they can fully recover. The adage "treatment works" is true for OUD in that it is unquestionably superior to no treatment overall, but it can also inflate expectations for those who are directly impacted by addiction and policymakers.

Furthermore, many people with active OUD are ambivalent about quitting illicit drug use, despite the fact it is difficult to imagine anyone being ambivalent about giving up blindness. According to data from a national survey, people with substance use disorders typically avoid treatment because they do not want it. London Breed, the mayor of San Francisco, provided a recent example of this phenomenon. She stated on "X" in July that none of the 115 persons who were cited or arrested for public drug use during a two-week period as part of a new enforcement initiative accepted a treatment offer.

By offering treatment as an alternative to incarceration, policymakers can increase the demand for it from people who have been arrested for drug possession or other nonviolent offenses. This idea has been used in many different effective programs; the most well-known of these is probably the drug courts, which provide continuous, close supervision.

While there is disagreement over the morality of "coerced treatment," there shouldn't be any concerning its efficacy. Over 2,000 patients were tracked for five years in the largest long-term prospective study, which revealed similar treatment satisfaction and outcomes for patients who were mandated as well as those who were voluntary. In the event that equally effective voluntary and mandatory treatment programs are available, the voluntary option is preferable due to the desire for freedom. However, if forced treatment or not seeking treatment are the only options available, forced treatment is preferable for both the person and the community.

Another strategy is to monitor compliance through regular testing and provide incentives for voluntary treatment or mandatory treatment for drug abuse, but to leave it up to the individual how they become abstinent. Some of these strategies include contingency management, which is essentially paying users for abstinence and other health behavior changes; programs for professionals such as doctors, airline pilots, and flight attendants that link returning to work to abstinence; and so-called swift, certain, and fair consequences for closely monitored use or nonuse. These methods have been used not only with opioids but with all drugs, including alcohol and stimulants like methamphetamine, and they have a remarkable track record of success with many of them. They do not, however, have the same level of support from medical professionals as pharmacotherapies. This may be due in part to the fact that they are uncomfortable with the idea that addiction is a chronic, relapsing illness and that they justify the involvement of law enforcement in treating addiction.

Third Pillar: Harm Reduction

Historically, harm reduction has been a public health initiative that aims to lessen drug use's risk factor without necessarily lowering drug usage overall. Certain places, especially cities along the Pacific coast, define it more liberally as endorsing an individual's unrestricted right to use drugs without regard for the effects on other people and without being stigmatized for doing so.

Harm reduction has achieved significant successes, including the implementation of syringe exchange programs that have lowered the transmission of HIV/AIDS and other blood-borne diseases. Naloxone, an overdose rescue drug, has also been instrumental in preventing numerous opioid overdose deaths. While the need for syringe exchange programs may have decreased due to advances in the treatment of HIV/AIDS, they are still vital and should continue to receive support, with 43 states currently having these programs in place. Universal access to naloxone is essential, and 33 states, regardless of political affiliation, have issued standing-order prescriptions so that pharmacies can provide the medication promptly to those in need. Similar to fire extinguishers and AEDs, naloxone should be readily available in high-risk settings such as bars, public libraries, and schools. These products are like safety nets that no one wishes to use but are essential to have nearby in case of emergencies.

In some places, notably the Canadian province of British Columbia and US cities like Portland and San Francisco, the public health and libertarian strands of harm reduction converge extensively. Other steps that fall under the category of harm reduction include drug testing services that assist individuals buying illegal drugs in knowing exactly what they are buying and supervised consumption sites that offer a safe environment for individuals to use drugs that they have bought from dealers. However, it's unclear if these additional harm-reduction efforts scale effectively enough to have an effect on the general public.

All drugs are no longer illegal in British Columbia, which also offers free healthcare services, including a clinic where patients can obtain heroin on-site. To lessen reliance on the "toxic" supply of illegal opioids, it expanded the prescribed "safer supply" during the pandemic, allowing participants to bring home substantial amounts of legally supplied opioids. However, its annual overdose death rate (44 per 100,000) in 2021 is higher than the U.S.A. The Deep South has a rate of 37 cases per 100,000 people, which is significantly higher than the rate in British Columbia.

Fourth Pillar: Prevention through Programing and Culture

In conclusion, ending epidemics involves preventing new cases rather than just providing health services to those affected. Prevention, which is often undervalued in drug policies, is actually the fourth crucial element. Despite receiving minimal resources and recognition, prevention is cost-effective and can greatly benefit the population, even if its impact on individuals is minimal.

Critics dismiss prevention because some well-known programs, such as D.A.R.E., fell short. But the original D.A.R.E. is a 40-year-old program. It was created during the competition between the IBM PC/XT and the DEC Rainbow 100, Apple Lisa, and ACT Apricot for the title of best personal computer. Since then, preventive techniques have advanced significantly. Research indicates that nearly half a million teenagers were spared from starting to smoke thanks to the national "truth" anti-tobacco campaign. Initiatives like Communities That Care and Big Brothers Big Sisters have been shown to be beneficial in reducing teen drug and alcohol use as well as mental health issues. All schools must have consistent funding for these programs (Griffin, 1998).

Prevention is not limited to children. Public service campaigns that emphasize prevention, such as informing parents to store or discard extra prescription opioids or outlining the availability of naloxone, may also be beneficial. The healthcare system, which distributes more addictive drugs than the black markets, is a critical additional target for campaigns and education initiatives. These medications are necessary for effective treatment, but they also carry a risk. For this reason, cautious prescribing procedures are essential. Furthermore, drug prevention goes beyond government-run initiatives, which may have little impact on people's behavior in comparison to the cultural influence of factors like how much friends, family, and neighbors support or oppose drug use. The baby-boom generation was raised on horror tales involving marijuana. The belief that conservative warnings about drug use are unfounded and ineffective was internalized by the baby boomer generation, in part because the marijuana they grew up with was much less potent than what is currently legally sold in stores.

But times have changed, and a pill laced with fentanyl can actually kill you now. It makes sense and is compassionate to try to move the U.S. culture to be less accepting of the use of illicit drugs. The easy counterargument is that nothing ought to be stigmatized. While it is possible that no one should be stigmatized, certain actions, such as driving while intoxicated, hitting one's spouse, and purchasing and reselling drugs on the streets, are undoubtedly wrong. One of the biggest achievements of public health is the demonization of cigarette smoking. A lower death toll could result from polite society treating illegal drugs with the same contempt.

A Closer Look

Pharmacology and Demand-related Factors of Synthetic Drug

The pharmacology of synthetic drugs may appeal to certain drug users and provide benefits to illicit suppliers. Many synthetic medications have significantly higher potencies than the plant-based counterparts they imitate. This is particularly true for heroin and fentanyl. Maybe 25–50 times as potent as heroin is fentanyl. Because traffickers can more easily conceal smaller quantities of pure fentanyl instead of larger volumes of heroin, this translates into reduced legal risk and, consequently, costs. Compared to roughly metric tons of heroin, it has been estimated that as little as a few tons of pure fentanyl would be required to meet the yearly consumption of opioids sourced illegally in the United States. Smuggling risks can be mitigated by smaller quantities, though occasionally, legal routes are used to transport synthetic drugs with high potencies and purity. For instance, prior to 2019, law enforcement in the United States regularly reported high-purity seizures of fentanyl in the international postal and courier systems, sometimes amounting to as little as one gram.

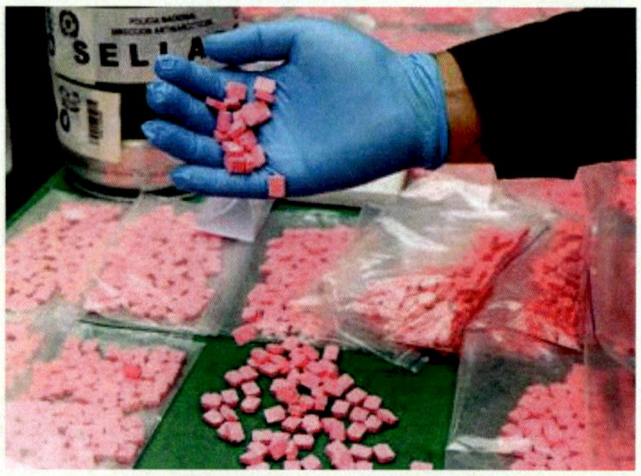

Because of its potency compared to heroin, even small amounts of low-purity fentanyl can be smuggled through various methods to meet demand. The potential for a higher-potency product allows trafficking organizations to distribute the risk of interception across numerous individuals or vehicles, making synthetic drugs more difficult to stop and leading to lower retail prices. This trend is evident in the US, where the purity-adjusted wholesale price of illicitly produced fentanyl powder dropped over 50% between 2016 and 2021.

Methamphetamine acts more slowly than cocaine in a similar manner. This may result in less frequent redoing, which certain buyers may find appealing. Methamphetamine has additional pharmacological properties that draw some people in. Methamphetamine produces a stronger stimulant effect by increasing dopamine release and inhibiting its reuptake, in contrast to cocaine, which only blocks dopamine reuptake.

Methamphetamine's increased potency and reduced cost per dose, along with more fruitful sources of production, as documented in North America, South-East Asia, and Western and Central

Europe, indicate that the drug's prevalence is rising. Early warning and drug services monitoring systems indicate that methamphetamine supply is rising in Western and Central Europe, where amphetamine has historically been more prevalent.

A combination of supply and demand factors determines the single-drug market dynamics. Purer or less expensive drugs are usually sought after by users, particularly price-sensitive heavy users. If inexpensive drugs appear in tablet form and don't require injection, snorting, or smoking, novice users might be less reluctant to try them. This is especially true if the drugs seem to have been taken out of the pharmaceutical system. Drugs that are synthetic can be produced and supplied at a lower cost per dosage and can be designed in a way that accommodates current user preferences and behaviors, like taking tablets.

Summary

- Synthetic drugs refer to substances that are artificially modified from naturally occurring drugs and can exhibit both therapeutic and psychoactive effects.
- The compounds on which the development is based are now known as lead compounds, while the synthetic compounds developed from lead are called its analogues.
- The focus on the development of new synthetic drug compounds has resulted in the incorporation of many other disciplines, such as biochemistry and molecular biology, into medicinal chemistry.
- There are seven major structural groups, which are naphthoylindoles, naphthylmethylindoles, naphthoypyrroles, naphthylmethylindenes, phenylacetylindoles, cyclohexylphenols, and classical cannabinoids respectively.
- The adverse effects of synthetic drugs are hard to determine as they usually contain other chemicals with variable concentrations, and human studies are limited.
- Synthetic cannabinoids act asSCRA by binding to cannabinoid receptors CB_1 and CB_2. Its binding towards CB_1 receptor will lead to receptor phosphorylation that recruits β-arrestin 1 and β-arrestin 2, resulting in a loss of responsiveness and internalization (endocytosis of molecules by the cell).
- Drug detection in body fluids requires specific reference data from the target drug. A common pitfall in the detection of NPS is the lack of reference data available for spectrometers to identify the presence of structurally modified illicit substances.
- In the pharmaceutical and chemical industries, SARs have long been used to design drugs and chemicals with commercially desirable properties. This has particularly been the case in the area of drug design, where chemicals with desired pharmacologic and therapeutic activities are sought.
- Trends in drug abuse frequently follow a cycle whereby individual drugs or consumption patterns re-emerge at different times and/or in different regions.
- The international drug control system is guided by the need to strike a balance between ensuring the availability of substances used for legitimate medical purposes and preventing their diversion into illicit markets.
- The range of drugs which provide the effects favored by current 'youth cultures' and which are frequently used simultaneously extends from ecstasy and related substances to stimulants and hallucinogens.
- In geographical terms, the demand for performance-enhancing and dance drugs can be expected to spread along with improvements in the standard of living, stronger buying power, and free-market economies.
- Several of the substances and substance classes that are attractive to consumers in the recreational drug scene are equally attractive for clandestine manufacturers in terms of level of risk and financial returns.

References

1. Walsh, Kenneth B.; Andersen, Haley K. (2020-08-25). "Molecular Pharmacology of Synthetic Cannabinoids: Delineating CB1 Receptor-Mediated Cell Signaling". International Journal of Molecular Sciences. 21 (17): 6115.
2. Janssen, Paul A. J.; Leysen, Josée E.; Megens, Anton A. H. P.; Awouters, Frans H. L. (1999-09-01). "Does phenylethylamine act as an endogenous amphetamine in some patients?". The International Journal of Neuropsychopharmacology. 2 (3): 229–240.
3. Khan, JaVed I.; Kennedy, Thomas J.; Christian, Donnell R. (2012), "Phenethylamines", Basic Principles of Forensic Chemistry, Totowa, NJ: Humana Press, pp. 157–176.
4. Valento, Matthew; Lebin, Jacob (2017-07-06). "Emerging Drugs of Abuse: Synthetic Cannabinoids, Phenylethylamines (2C Drugs), and Synthetic Cathinones". Clinical Pediatric Emergency Medicine. 18 (3): 203–211.
5. Evans-Brown, Michael; Sedefov, Roumen (2018), "Responding to New Psychoactive Substances in the European Union: Early Warning, Risk Assessment, and Control Measures", New Psychoactive Substances, vol. 252, Cham: Springer International Publishing, pp. 3–49.
6. Wiley JL, Marusich JA, Huffman JW, Balster RL, Thomas BF. Hijacking of basic research: the case of synthetic cannabinoids. Methods Rep RTI Press. 2011;2011:17971.
7. Brents LK, Reichard EE, Zimmerman SM, Moran JH, Fantegrossi WE, Prather PL. Phase I hydroxylated metabolites of the K2 synthetic cannabinoid JWH-018 retain in vitro and in vivo cannabinoid 1 receptor affinity and activity. PLoS One. 2011;6:e21917.
8. Chin CN, Murphy JW, Huffman JW, Kendall DA. The third transmembrane helix of the cannabinoid receptor plays a role in the selectivity of aminoalkylindoles for CB2, peripheral cannabinoid receptor. J Pharmacol Exp Ther. 1999;291:837–844.
9. Rajasekaran M, Brents LK, Franks LN, Moran JH, Prather PL. Human metabolites of synthetic cannabinoids JWH-018 and JWH-073 bind with high affinity and act as potent agonists at cannabinoid type-2 receptors. Toxicol Appl Pharmacol. 2013;269:100–108.
10. Atwood BK, Huffman J, Straiker A, Mackie K. JWH018, a common constituent of 'Spice' herbal blends, is a potent and efficacious cannabinoid CB receptor agonist. Br J Pharmacol. 2010;160:585–593.
11. Huestis MA. Pharmacokinetics and metabolism of the plant cannabinoids, delta9-tetrahydrocannabinol, cannabidiol and cannabinol. Handb Exp Pharmacol. 2005;(168):657–690.
12. Watanabe K, Yamaori S, Funahashi T, Kimura T, Yamamoto I. Cytochrome P450 enzymes involved in the metabolism of tetrahydrocannabinols and cannabinol by human hepatic microsomes. Life Sci. 2007;80:1415–1419.
13. Zhang Q, Ma P, Iszard M, Cole RB, Wang W, Wang G. In vitro metabolism of R(+)-[2,3-dihydro-5-methyl-3-[(morpholinyl)methyl]pyrrolo [1,2,3-de]1,4-benzoxazinyl]-(1-naphtha-lenyl) methanone mesylate, a cannabinoid receptor agonist. Drug Metab Dispos. 2002;30:1077–1086.
14. Zhang Q, Ma P, Wang W, Cole RB, Wang G. Characterization of rat liver microso-mal metabolites of AM-630, a potent cannabinoid receptor antagonist, by high-performance liquid chromatography/electrospray ionization tandem mass spectrometry. J Mass Spectrom. 2004;39:672–681.

15. Chimalakonda KC, Bratton SM, Le VH, Yiew KH, Dineva A, Moran CL, James LP, Moran JH, Radominska-Pandya A. Conjugation of synthetic cannabinoids JWH-018 and JWH-073, metabolites by human UDP-glucuronosyltransferases. Drug Metab Dispos. 2011;39:1967–1976.
16. Moran CL, Le VH, Chimalakonda KC, Smedley AL, Lackey FD, Owen SN, Kennedy PD, Endres GW, Ciske FL, Kramer JB, Kornilov AM, Bratton LD, Dobrowolski PJ, Wessinger WD, Fantegrossi WE, Prather PL, James LP, Radominska-Pandya A, Moran JH. Quantitative measurement of JWH-018 and JWH-073 metabolites excreted in human urine. Anal Chem. 2011;83:4228–4236.
17. Hutter M, Broecker S, Kneisel S, Auwarter V. Identification of the major urinary metabolites in man of seven synthetic cannabinoids of the aminoalkylindole type present as adulterants in 'herbal mixtures' using LC-MS/MS techniques. J Mass Spectrom. 2012;47:54–65.
18. Sobolevsky T, Prasolov I, Rodchenkov G. Detection of urinary metabolites of AM-2201 and UR-144, two novel synthetic cannabinoids. Drug Test Anal. 2012;4:745–753.
19. Seely KA, Prather PL, James LP, Moran JH. Marijuana-based drugs: innovative therapeutics or designer drugs of abuse? Mol Interv. 2011;11:36–51.
20. Griffin G, Atkinson PJ, Showalter VM, Martin BR, Abood ME. Evaluation of canna-binoid receptor agonists and antagonists using the guanosine-5′-O-(3-[35S]thio)-triphosphate binding assay in rat cerebellar membranes. J Pharmacol Exp Ther. 1998;285:553–560.

Chapter

CHEMISTRY OF SYNTHETIC DRUGS

2

Contents

Introduction

The goal of synthetic drugs, also known as new psychoactive substances (NPS), is to replicate the effects of popular illegal substances like cocaine, cannabis, MDMA, and lysergic acid diethylamide (LSD). The chemical structures of synthetic drugs differ from those of the illegal substances they are intended to replace. To try and stay ahead of the law, producers of synthetic drugs alter their chemical structures regularly.

Certain synthetic drugs may be promoted as "safe," "legal," and acceptable substitutes for illegal drugs. This does not imply that they are safe or lawful, though. A synthetic drug packet does not specify a dosage. Additionally, the chemicals may vary from packet to packet. There are differences between the effects of two packets from the same batch. There are questions about what is actually in synthetic drugs because they are not regulated or quality controlled. It is difficult to determine how dangerous synthetic drugs are at any given dosage because they appear so frequently. The short- and long-term effects of these substances have not been thoroughly studied. On the other hand, synthetic cannabis is said to cause more severe adverse effects than actual cannabis.

Orientation and Directional Terms

Term	Definition	Illustration
Synthetic cannabinoids (SCBs)	SCBs refer to a class of lab-made substances that are chemically similar to chemicals found in the cannabis plant, though they often produce very different effects. Some SCBs have potential or current medical uses but many are illicitly manufactured and sold.	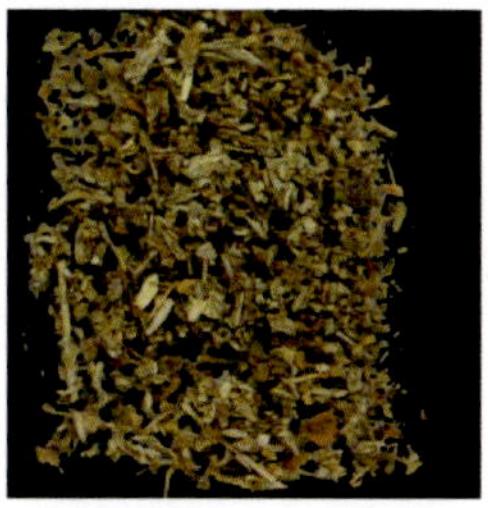
Phenethylamines	Phenethylamine (PEA) is an organic compound, natural monoamine alkaloid, and trace amine, which acts as a central nervous system stimulant in humans.	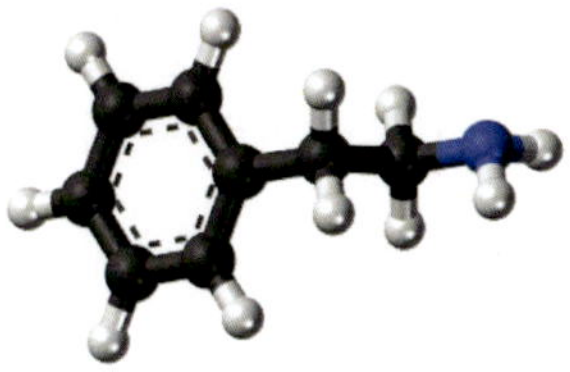
Synthetic cathinones	Synthetic cathinones are a class of lab-made stimulants chemically related to substances found in the khat plant.	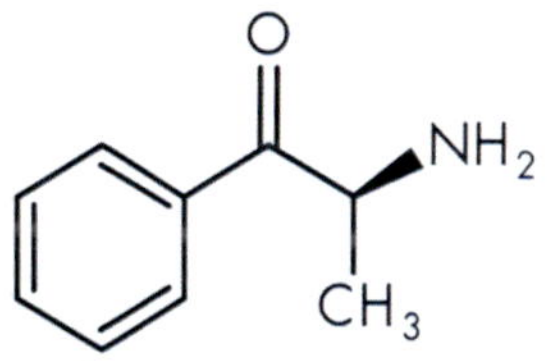
Tryptamines	Tryptamines are naturally occurring alkaloids found in a variety of plants and life forms around the world and exist in > 1500 natural varieties.	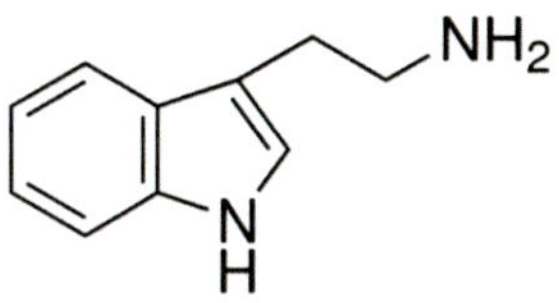
Piperazines	Piperazine is an organic compound that consists of a six-membered ring containing two nitrogen atoms at opposite positions in the ring. Piperazine exists as small alkaline deliquescent crystals with a saline taste.	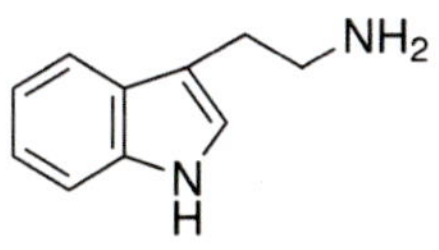

2.1 History and Development of Synthetic Drugs

Drugs classified as synthetics are those that have been artificially created from naturally occurring substances and have the ability to have both therapeutic and psychoactive effects (Rinaldi et al., 2020). In a medical context, synthetic medications with psychotropic properties can treat insomnia. The pharmacology and side effects of the majority of synthetic drugs are unknown since there are few human studies and clinical trials. It is important to seek professional advice before using synthetic drugs, as misuse can be fatal. NPS are substances that have the latter effect. Their goal is to change the original drug's structure in order to mimic the effects of illegal substances. The "synthesized drug" can enter the market in this way and go undetected. Nonetheless, the public's health is at risk due to the lack of clarity surrounding these substances' harmful effects. These medications are currently under Early Warning System (EWS) surveillance. Synthetic stimulants, SCBs, and synthetic depressants are the three main types of NPS. Benzodiazepines, cannabinoids, and phenethylamines are common examples of these categories (Arora et al., 2020). Certain receptors, such as dopamine, serotonin, and cannabinoid receptors, are either stimulated or inhibited to produce the psychoactive effect.

2.1.1 The First Synthetic Medicines

Unlike "inorganic" compounds derived from other sources, "organic" compounds are those that are extracted from plants or animals. It was thought that "only God" could create the former. However, in 1836, the German chemist Friedrich Wohler created urea—which was previously only isolated from urine—by heating ammonium cyanate, an inorganic substance. This groundbreaking synthesis paved the way for attempts to create other carbon-based compounds that were previously limited to being derived from living things. The first synthetic dye, "mauvine," was unintentionally discovered in 1856 by William Henry Perkin, a young English chemistry student. This discovery was crucial for the development of the pharmaceutical industry. This finding inspired German and Swiss dye manufacturers to create new artificial colors and learn about the new chemistry (Khan et al., 2012). At the age of 21, Perkin took out a family loan to establish his own dyestuffs company, which would later combine with other chemical manufacturers in the UK to become Imperial Chemical Industries (ICI).

The development of medicine was greatly impacted by synthetic dyes. By greatly expanding the variety of biological stains, they hastened the advancement of histology and bacteriology. The quest for novel colors sparked interest in organic chemistry, which in turn sparked the hunt for fresh pharmaceuticals. The first synthetic medication was acetophenetidine, which Bayer first sold as a pain reliever in 1885 in Leverkusen, Germany, under the Phenacetin brand (Banister et al., 2015). It is the source of the common household remedy paracetamol today. Acetylsalicylic acid, which went on sale in 1897, was the second significant synthetic medication. Dr. Felix Hoffmann, who worked in Bayer's research lab, created the medication, which was marketed as aspirin and sold all over the world as a novel and practical treatment for "rheumatic pains." From these modest beginnings, Bayer developed into the enormous corporation known as IG Farbenindustrie.

2.1.2 The Development of The Industry

The various endeavors that produced the materials used in medicine gave rise to the pharmaceutical industry. Apothecaries, chemists, druggists, and herbalists were able to obtain dried parts of different plants during the early 19th century, either through local harvesting or importation. The former were bought from spice traders who primarily imported spices, but they also occasionally carried medicines such as opium from Persia and cinchona and ipecacuanha bark from South America. Similar purchases were made from dry-salters (dealers in items like gums, oils, pickles, and so forth) for basic chemicals and minerals. These products were used by pharmacists, chemists, and apothecaries to make a variety of preparations, such as extracts, tinctures, mixtures, lotions, ointments, and tablets. Some practitioners produced more of these than they needed for their own use and sold them in large quantities to their peers (Shafi et al., 2020).

Certain medicines had actual value, but their effectiveness varied greatly. Examples of these include preparations made from cinchona bark, deadly nightshade, foxglove (digitalis), ergot of rye (*Claviceps purpurea*), and opium (dried latex from *Papeverum somniferum*). Quinine was the name given to the active alkaloid of cinchona bark by French chemist Joseph Pelletier in 1820. After this achievement, he went on to isolate a number of other alkaloids, such as strychnine from nux vomica and atropine from belladonna. The standardization of many medications and the subsequent commercial extraction of their active ingredients were made possible by his efforts and those of other researchers.

One of the first firms to extract pure alkaloids in commercial quantities was the Edinburgh pharmacy of T. H. Smith Ltd. Manufacturers were forced to establish their own laboratories when pharmacopeias began to include information about chemical assays. Pharmaceutical chemistry is the study of the molecular and mechanistic aspects of pharmaceuticals, and the discipline emphasizes the chemistry of drug design and development, drug action, drug transport, drug delivery, and targeting or Pharmaceutical chemistry is a science that makes use of the general laws of chemistry to study drug, i.e, their preparation, chemical nature, composition, structure, influence on an organism and studies the physical and chemical properties of drugs, the methods of quality control and the conditions of their usage.

Understanding biological processes and drug action mechanisms at the molecular level is essential to the development of new pharmaceuticals. The word "drug" comes from the French word "drogue," which denotes a dry herb. Any chemical that, when absorbed into the body of a living organism, modifies normal bodily function is generally considered a drug. A material used for disease diagnosis, prevention, treatment, or palliation is another definition of a drug. There isn't a single accurate definition because there are various interpretations in the fields of medicine, law, and common usage (Shafi et al., 2020).

According to the World Health Organization, a drug is a chemical or biological product that is meant to be used for the benefit of the user to alter or investigate physiological systems or pathological states. A medication can change (increase or decrease) an existing function, but it cannot produce a new one. Not all chemicals are drugs, but all drugs are chemicals. Certain governments have legal definitions for drugs. "Articles intended for use in the diagnosis, cure, mitigation, treatment or prevention of disease in man or other animals" and "articles (other than food) intended to affect the structure or any function of the body of man or other animals" are included in the Federal Food, Drug and Cosmetic Act definition of "drug" in the United States. There are four primary sources of drugs: plants, animals, minerals, and man-made chemicals. Medications can be easily separated into two categories: non-prescription drugs, which are available "over the counter" (OTC), and prescription drugs, which are thought to be dangerous to use unless under a doctor's supervision. Each medication has three names: i.e., chemical name, trade name (registered proprietary brand), and approved name (non-proprietary). The drug's chemical makeup is revealed by its chemical name. There are two types of non-proprietary names: the approved name, which is the same as the adopted or generic name (a name that may or may not be included in the pharmacopeia), and the official name, which may be the same as the generic name. The pharmaceutical company that sells the drugs owns the exclusive right to the proprietary name, even though it may not have created the medication itself. Consequently, a medicine may be marketed under numerous proprietary names by various companies, but each nation has a single official or generic name. A medication in dosage form is one that can be given to a patient in a variety of ways for the purpose of diagnosing or treating a medical condition. Pharmacopoeias and other official and unofficial compendias recognize pharmaceutical preparations. The pharmaceutical preparation is being replaced with dosage form. They offer precise and safe drug dosages for the treatment of illnesses.

A dosage form is a physical form of medication, like an injection or capsule. The dosage form of a particular medication determines the administration route. The same compound may be available in different dosage forms because different medical conditions may call for different administration routes. In cases where oral dosage forms are difficult to administer due to persistent vomiting, it may be more prudent to use a suppository or an injection. Additionally, some medications may need to be taken in particular dosage forms. Solid, liquid, and semisolid dosage forms are the three primary types of dosage forms (Khan et al., 2012).

Among the different oral solid dosage forms, tablets are the most acceptable due to their advantage over other dosage forms. The word "Quality" with reference to a dosage form is comprehensive and refers to characteristics like potency, uniformity, purity, pharmacological action, stability etc. Pharmaceutical companies have a legal as well as a moral obligation to create dosage forms that are safe, effective, and non-toxic. The term "total quality control" describes an organized effort by the entire organization to prevent or eliminate errors at every stage of production to produce a flawless product through a series of measures (Evans-Brown et al., 2018).

A drug product's quality must be considered throughout the product and process design phase. Physical plant layout, space, ventilation, cleanliness, and sanitation all impact quality during regular production. A lot of businesses make use of statistical process control. In manufacturing operations, traditional statistical process controls typically involve randomly selecting and evaluating a portion of the output. Before defective parts can be produced, manufacturing process variances of critical tolerances are continuously tracked and corrected.

Pharmacopoeias and other official and unofficial compendia are used to maintain the quality of the drug. The Greek words pharmakon, which means drug, and poiein, which means make, are the origin of the word pharmacopeia. The book of drug standards in Bergame, Italy, is credited with coining the term in 1580. The main body of the Pharmacopoeias, a class of drug compendia, consists of monographs on drugs and auxiliary substances. The structural and chemical formula, information, description, identification, purity data, and instructions for dosage and storage are all included in a monograph. A pharmacopeia is updated and revised on a regular basis. There are two types of drugs on the market: i.e., medications, both generic and brand. The equivalent of name-brand medications is a generic drug. Generic drugs have the same chemical components.

The FDA (Food and Drug Administration) states that generic medications are bioequivalent to brand-name medications. Therefore, when compared to brand-name medications, generics are just as effective and have the same dosage, method of administration, and mode of action. Generally speaking, generic medications are created and produced after the patent on their brand-name equivalent has expired. The United States is approving generic drugs. FDA prior to going on sale. Every manufacturer of generic medications must demonstrate that their product is bioequivalent to the brand-name medications. There has always been a misunderstanding among patients and their families regarding the distinctions between branded and generic medications. Contrary to popular belief, generic medications are not inferior to brand-name medications. Both branded and generic medications have the same names for dosage, quality, strength, and safety. Their price and appearance are the only things that separate the two. Generally speaking, generic medications are far less costly than name-brand ones. Sometimes the forms of generic and brand-name medications differ; for example, a generic tablet may not look like a brand-name capsule.

2.2 Drug

2.2.1 Tablet Role in Therapy

The most crucial route of administration for drugs intended to have systemic effects is oral. The parenteral route is not commonly used for self-administration of medication, except insulin therapy. Only recently has the topical route of administration been used to administer medications to the body for systemic effects. Two classes of marketed products are nitroglycerin, used to treat angina, and scopolamine, used to treat motion sickness.

Parenteral administration is useful for treating medical emergencies when the patient is unconscious or unable to swallow, as well as for administering different kinds of maintenance therapy to hospitalized patients. However, it is likely that at least 90% of all medications intended to cause systemic effects are taken orally. Whether a drug can be taken orally to achieve the desired result is one of the first things a pharmaceutical company looks into when a new drug is discovered. In the event that it cannot, the medication is mainly administered in a hospital or doctor's office. Solid oral dosage forms are the preferred class of product for drugs administered orally; if a patient cannot self-administer, the drug's sales represent only a small portion of what the market would otherwise be. These are the justifications for this preference.

Tablets and capsules are examples of unit dosage forms, where a single standard dosage of the medication has been precisely measured. Liquid oral dosage forms, including syrups, suspensions, emulsions, solutions, and elixirs, are typically made with one medication dosage per 5 to 30 mL. Then, using a teaspoon, tablespoon, or other measuring tool, the patient is instructed to measure their own medication. When a patient administers their own medication, such dosage measurements are usually inaccurate by a factor of 20 to 50%.

Advantages

The advantages of tablets include the following:

- Unit dosage forms are the most effective because they provide the least variability in content and the highest level of dose precision among all oral dosage forms.

- Their cost is the lowest of all oral dosage forms.
- They are the lightest & most compact of all oral dosage forms.
- They are, in general, the easiest & cheapest to package & ship of all oral dosage forms.
- Product identification, with an embossed or monogrammed punch face, maybe the easiest and least expensive option. It doesn't require any extra processing steps.
- If tablet disintegration is not too rapid, they might offer the most ease of swallowing with the least tendency to "hang up" above the stomach, especially when coated.
- They lend themselves to certain special-release profile products, such as enteric or delayed-release products.
- They have the best-combined properties of chemical, mechanical & microbiologic stability of all the oral forms.
- They are better suited to large-scale production thane other unit oral forms.

Disadvantage

The disadvantages of tablets include the following:

- Certain medications exhibit flocculent low-density characteristics or are amorphous, making them resistant to compression into dense compacts.
- Medication with low wetting, slow dissolving qualities, optimal absorption in the gastrointestinal tract at high dosages, or any combination of these characteristics may be hard or impossible to formulate and produce as a tablet that will still offer sufficient or complete drug bioavailability.
- It may be necessary to coat the tablets or, if practical, encapsulate or entrap the drugs before compressing them if they have an unpleasant taste, an unpleasant smell or are sensitive to air moisture or oxygen. In these situations, the capsule might be the most effective and economical course of action.

Types & Classes of Tablets

Tablets are categorized according to their form and manufacturing process, their function or administration route, and the kind of drug delivery system they represent within that route.

Oral Tablets for Ingestion:

- Compressed tablets or standard compressed tablets (CT)
- Multiple compressed tablets (MCT)
    a. Layered tablets.
    b. Compression-coated tablets
- Repeat - action tablets
- Delayed – action & enteric coated tablets.
- Sugar & chocolate-coated tablets.
- Film-coated tablets.
- Chewable tablets.

Tablets Used in the Oral Cavity:

- Buccal tablets
- Sublingual tablets
- Troches & lozenges
- Dental cones

Tablets Administered by Other Routes:

- Implantation tablets
- Vaginal tablets

Tablets Used to Prepare Solutions:

- Effervescent tablets.
- Dispensing tablets (DT)
- Hypodermic tablets (HT)
- Tablet triturates (TT)

2.2.2 Analgesic

Any medication used to relieve pain falls into the broad category of analgesics, sometimes referred to as painkillers. Greek words an- ("without") and algos ("pain") are the roots of the English word analgesic. Analgesic medications affect the central and peripheral nervous systems in a variety of ways. There are medications used to treat aches and swelling, and people have always looked for substances or therapies that can lessen pain. Salicin, a chemical found in the leaves and bark of willow trees, was used as an analgesic in the past. An analgesic is sometimes defined as a medication that merely masks pain without addressing its underlying causes. This definition is not correct. Certain medications, like many opiate painkillers and over-the-counter medications like acetaminophen, do relieve pain without treating or removing its cause. The WHO pain ladder, which was initially created to treat pain associated with cancer, is frequently used to find appropriate medications in a step-by-step fashion. When selecting analgesics, the severity and response to other medication determine the choice of agent. The type of pain also influences the choice of analgesic: traditional analgesics are less effective for neuropathic pain, and drug classes like tricyclic antidepressants and anticonvulsants, which are not typically classified as analgesics, can often be beneficial. There are two main classes of analgesics:

- Non-narcotic analgesic
- Narcotic analgesic.

Non-narcotic analgesiccs further classified into two major classes

- Nonsteroidal anti-inflammatory drug (NSAIDs)
- Acetaminophen (Paracetamol).

2.2.3 Nonsteroidal Anti-Inflammatory Drugs

NSAIDs, or non-steroidal anti-inflammatory drugs, are what they are commonly referred to as. These medications are referred to as "non-steroidal" to differentiate them from steroids, which have a similar depressant and anti-inflammatory effect in addition to a wide range of other effects. Most NSAIDs have a pKa of 3-5, making them weak acids. The mucosa of the stomach and intestines effectively absorbs them. They have a high protein binding (usually greater than 95 %) to albumin in plasma, which limits their distribution volume, usually close to the plasma volume.Although some medications are partially excreted in bile, the majority of NSAIDs are metabolized in the liver by oxidation and conjugation to inactive metabolites that are normally eliminated in urine. In some disease states, metabolism may be abnormal, and accumulation may happen even at normal dosages. NSAIDs, or non-steroidal anti-inflammatory drugs, decrease prostaglandin levels throughout the body by inhibiting the ids (COX) enzymes.

Thus, persistent pain, inflammation, and fever are decreased. Cyclooxygenase (COX) is an enzyme that the body's cells use to produce prostaglandins. COX-1 and COX-2 are the two COX enzymes. Both enzymes convert arachidonic acid—which is itself obtained from the cellular phospholipid bilayer by phospholipase A2—into prostaglandins and thromboxane, which are known to induce fever, pain, and inflammation. Prostaglandins, which shield the stomach and support platelets, are only produced by COX-1. NSAIDs can lead to stomach ulcers and increase bleeding because they decrease prostaglandins, which shield the stomach and aid in blood clotting and platelets. The body's local reaction to an infection or injury is inflammation. Numerous harmful agents, such as heat, cold, trauma, microbial invasion, etc., can cause it. Inflammation serves to either eliminate or neutralize foreign invaders and/or prepare the body for tissue healing. Long-term use of almost all NSAIDs inhibits prostaglandin synthesis and the enzyme COX.

Aspirin, indomethacin, diclofenac, piroxicam, ibuprofen, naproxen, and mefenamic acid are examples of non-COX selective drugs. Nimesulide, meloxicame, nabumetone, and aceclofenac are examples of preferential COX-2 inhibitors. Celecoxib, rofecoxib, valdecoxib, parecoxib, etoricoxib, and lumiracoxib are examples of highly selective COX-2 inhibitors. Despite its anti-inflammatory properties, paracetamol lacks significant effects. This could be because it primarily inhibits COX in the central nervous system. Additionally, some people theorize that paracetamol works by inhibiting the recently identified COX-3 isoform. NSAID side effects that occur most frequently include nausea, vomiting, diarrhea, constipation, decreased appetite, rash, headache, dizziness, and sleepiness. NSAIDs may also result in edema by causing fluid retention. The most dangerous side effects are prolonged bleeding following an injury or surgery, ulcers, liver failure, and kidney failure. NSAIDs are typically prescribed to treat the following conditions symptomatically: osteoarthritis, rheumatoid arthritis, and inflammatory arthropathies (e.g., acute gout, dysmenorrhea, metastatic bone pain, headaches and migraines, ankylosing spondylitis, psoriatic arthritis, reiter's syndrome, mild-to-moderate pain from inflammation and tissue damage, pyrexia, and renal colic. Since aspirin is the only NSAID that can permanently inhibit COX-1, it is also recommended for the inhibition of platelet aggregation, which helps prevent adverse cardiovascular events and manage arterial thrombosis.

2.2.4 Antibiotics

Antibiotics were developed by Vuillemin in 1889 and are used to stop and eradicate microbial growth. Antibiotics are substances that are made to hinder and even destroy the growth of microorganisms, including bacteria, fungi, viruses, and molds. Between the 1940s and 1960s, the terms "antibiotic" and "chemotherapeutic drug" were used interchangeably. Antibiotics were naturally occurring medications that were made by a variety of bacteria or fungi. From this perspective, the creation of the first sulfonamide in 1932 marked the beginning of the history of antibiotics. The preparation of the first semisynthetic antibiotics from the penicillin molecule, methicillin, and ampicillin, in 1960 marked a significant advancement in medical science. These drugs were active against staphylococci and common gram-negative bacteria like *E. coli*, *H. influenzae* or *S. enterica* (including *S. typhi abdominalis*). Many more semisynthetic antibiotics were developed later on. Numerous novel antibiotics that are highly compatible with patients have also been introduced to treat community infections. Among these contemporary—and occasionally trendy—drugs are oral cephalosporins, novel macrolides, doxycyclin, and fluoroquinolones. That being said, the development of readily absorbed, reasonably safe antibiotics frequently resulted in overuse and a sharp increase in bacterial resistance (Pintori et al., 2017). Antibiotic agents can be categorized into the following groups.

- β-Lactam antibiotics
- Aminoglycoside antibiotics
- Tetracyclines antibiotics
- Chloramphenical antibiotics
- Macrolides & other drugs

Macrolides Drugs

These antibiotics are static and reversibly inhibit ribosomal protein synthesis. Macrolide is the class name because the structure is derived from a 14–16-member macrocyclic lactone ring. The evolution of macrolides has been remarkable. At first, they were effective against both gram-positive and gram-negative bacteria, as well as anaerobes, spirochetes, and obligatory intracellular pathogens like chlamydiae and mycoplasmata. Macrolides have anti-inflammatory as well as anti-bacterial properties; at the time, erythromycin was the most significant medication. Its frequent, unpleasant side effects, such as nausea and vomiting, limited its use.

Paracetamol

Acetaminophen, sometimes referred to as paracetamol, is a well-known, over-the-counter, peripherally-acting antipyretic analgesic medication. As a result, it is frequently found in over-the-counter analgesics and medications for the flu and cold. One common over-the-counter analgesic (pain reliever) and antipyretic (fever reducer) is paracetamol, also known as acetaminophen. It is a main component of many cold and flu remedies and is frequently used to treat fever, headaches, and other mild aches and pains. When combined with opioid analgesics or NSAIDs, paracetamol is also used to treat more severe pain (such as pain from cancer). The first aniline derivative to be discovered to have both analgesic and antipyretic effects was acetanilide, which A. swiftly marketed as Antifebrin and used in medicine. Cahn and P. Hepp in the year 1886. However, its intolerable harmful effects—the most concerning of which is cyanosis brought on by methemoglobinemia—led to a search for less hazardous derivatives of aniline.

Clinical pharmacologist Joseph von Mering didn't try paracetamol on patients until 1887, despite the fact that Harmon Northrop Morse had already synthesized it at John Hopkins University in 1877 by reducing p-nitrophenol with tin in glacial acetic acid. The "rediscovery" of paracetamol occurred when Brodie and Axelrod (1949) demonstrated that phenacetin could also be converted to the painkiller paracetamol. Sterling-Winthrop Co. introduced the medicine to the American market for the first time in 1953. which argued that because it was safe for kids and those with ulcers to take, it was better than aspirin. Since it was included in the British Pharmacopoeia in 1963, paracetamol has grown in popularity as a relatively safe analgesic that doesn't interfere much with other medications (Valento et al., 2017). Until the 1970s, paracetamol was not widely accepted due to safety concerns; however, in many countries, including the UK, sales of paracetamol surpassed those of aspirin in the 1980s. Phenacetin's commercial collapse coincided with this, as it was attributed to hematological toxicity, analgesic nephropathy, and abuse potential because of its psychotropic effects.

Discovery

About a century ago, a patient's prescription for acetanilide, a similar molecule, was accidentally found to have painkilling properties, leading to the discovery of paracetamol's therapeutic effects. However, because acetanilide is toxic in moderation, chemists changed its chemical structure to create a less dangerous substance that still had analgesic effects. N-acetyl-para-aminophenol, or acetaminophen in the US, and paracetamol (derived from para-acetyl-aminophenol) in the UK, was one of these compounds. The body partially transforms the original substance, acetanilide, into a combination of paracetamol and aniline. Aniline is toxic, but paracetamol acts as an analgesic (Walsh and Anderson, 2020).

Theory of Paracetamol

Molecular Formula: C8H9

Structure: 1

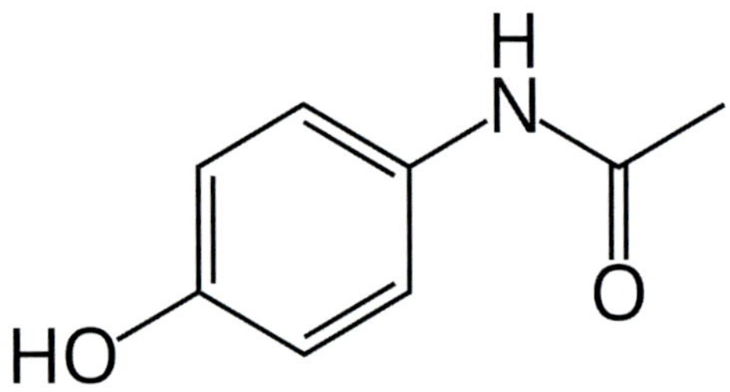

Figure 2.1: Paracetamol.

Source: By Benjah-bmm27 - Own work, Public Domain, https://commons.wikimedia.org/w/index.php?curid=826823

Molecular Weight: 151.16

Chemical name: 4-hydroxyacetanilide

Category: Analgesic, antipyretic

Dose: 500 mg to lg every 4 to 6 h, up to 4g daily, divided doses.

Description: White crystals or white crystalline powder

Solubility: Freely soluble in ethanol (95%) and in acetone, sparingly soluble in Water, very slightly soluble in dichloromethane and in ether

Storage: Store in well-closed, light-resistant containers.

Standards: Paracetamol contains not less than 99.0 %% and not more than 101.0 % of $C_8H_9NO_2$

Synthesis

One of the most widely used medications in the world, paracetamol, is produced in large quantities. Morse created it for the first time in 1878 by reducing para-nitro phenol in glacial acetic acid with tin. The acetic acid acetylated the para-aminophenol that the reducing action of the tin had produced in-situ. Subsequently, by starting with para-aminophenol and acetylating with acetic acid, this manufacturing process was made simpler. Since then, this process has undergone numerous modifications.

Commercial manufacture

There are currently several commercial manufacturing techniques in use worldwide. The most typical beginning material is phenol, which is nitrated to produce a blend of para- and ortho-nitro phenol. To synthesize a paracetamol, the para-nitro phenol is reduced to para-aminophenol and then acetylated with acetic anhydride.

Other commercial processes include: Parcacetamol comprises an amide group in the para (1, 4) pattern and one hydroxyl group in place of the benzene ring core. Acetamide (ethanamide) is the amide group.

The lone pair on the hydroxyl oxygen, the benzene pi cloud, the nitrogen lone pair, the p orbital on the carbonyl carbon, and the lone pair on the carbonyl oxygen are all conjugated, making it an extensively conjugated system. The benzene ring is also extremely reactive due to the presence of two activating groups.

Towards electrophilic aromatic substitution. All of the ring's positions are essentially equally activated because the substituents are ortho, para directing, and para with regard to one another. Additionally, the conjugation significantly lessens the basicity of the nitrogen and oxygen while delocalizing the charge developed on the phenoxide anion to make the hydroxyl acidic. The single-step synthesis from nitrobenzene to para-aminophenol is conversion of phenol to para-nitrosophenol, followed by reduction and acetylation. Monochlorobenzene is filtered, hydrolyzed, and then acetylated.

Mechanism of Action

The fact that paracetamol lowers the synthesis of prostaglandins, or proinflammatory chemicals, casts doubt on the mechanism by which it lowers fever and pain. Paracetamol has less anti-inflammatory properties than aspirin, but both drugs block the synthesis of prostaglandins. Similarly, paracetamol does not prevent the synthesis of thromboxanes, a chemical that promotes blood clotting, while aspirin does. Since aspirin is known to inhibit the COX family of enzymes, a lot of research has focused on whether paracetamol also inhibits COX because of the partial similarities between the two drugs' actions. It is now evident that paracetamol works through a minimum of two channels. By lowering the COX enzyme's oxidized form, parcetamol stops it from forming pro-inflammatory compounds. Moreover, the endogenous cannabinoid system is modulated by paracetamol.

Paracetamol is metabolized into AM404, a compound that has various actions, including inhibiting the uptake of the endogenous cannabinoid/anandamide by neurons. This prevents the activation of the main pain receptor in the body, the TRPV1 receptor. Additionally, AM404 inhibits sodium channels similar to the anesthetics lidocaine and procaine (Broadley, 2009). It has been shown that these actions individually reduce pain, suggesting a possible mechanism for the pain-relieving effects of paracetamol. Recent studies have demonstrated that when cannabinoid receptors are blocked, paracetamol loses its analgesic effect, indicating that its pain-relieving properties are mediated by the endogenous cannabinoid system. There are theories that suggest paracetamol works by inhibiting the COX-3 isoform of the COX enzyme family, which produces pro-inflammatory chemicals. However, research has shown that the COX-3 enzyme may not have inflammatory actions in humans and mice. Another theory proposes that paracetamol blocks COX, like aspirin, but in an inflammatory environment where there is a high concentration of peroxides, the oxidation state of paracetamol may prevent its actions. This suggests that paracetamol may not directly affect inflammation but instead acts in the central nervous system to reduce temperature where the environment is less oxidative. The exact mechanism of how paracetamol affects COX-3 is still a subject of debate.

Pharmacokinetics

Paracetamol has a plasma half-life of 1-4 hours. It is present in the majority of bodily fluids and is mostly metabolized in the liver. Most metabolic products appear in the urine within 24 hours, but very little unchanged drug is eliminated in the urine. Since it is only absorbed after it has left the stomach and entered the duodenum, its onset of action is typically slower than that of other mild analgesics, like aspirin.

Efficacy

Adults with osteoarthritis who experience chronic pain responded similarly well to ibuprofen and paracetamol in a randomized controlled trial. Nonetheless, the standard OTC dose of ibuprofen provides more pain relief than the standard dose of paracetamol in a randomized controlled trial of children with acute musculoskeletal pain.

Nimesulide

A non-steroidal anti-inflammatory drug (NSAID) called nemesulide is prescribed to treat a number of inflammatory and painful conditions, including painful osteoarthritis, primary dysmenorrhea, and post-operative pain. During its 19 years on the market, mesulide has been sold in more than 50 countries, and during that time, 346 million treatment courses have been given out.

Because of its distinct COX-1/COX-2 selectivity ratio, proven safety, and effectiveness, mesulide has become more popular due to recent worries about the safety of selective COX-2 inhibitors. Research conducted by Drs. George (GGI) Moore, Bob Scherrer, Karl F. Swingle, and their associates at Riker Laboratories Inc. led to the development of nemesulide. They reasoned that as evidence began to emerge in the late 1960s linking free radicals to chronic inflammatory diseases, medications that scavenge these radicals may have unique anti-inflammatory properties that could be used to manage chronic inflammation. They conducted a thorough structure-activity analysis to ascertain the sulphonamides' pharmacological characteristics (Smith et al., 2015). Due to their antibiotic effect, Svartz and her colleagues at Pharmacia in Sweden had previously believed that this class of agents had antirheumatic activity in the 1940s. This was demonstrated by their "Comparative Analysis of the Combination (Paracetamol I. P. as well as Nimesulide B. P. Tablets 9 led to the creation of sulphasalazine, a conjugate of sulphonamide and salicylate. Moore and colleagues discovered through their structure-activity analyses that the strong lipophilic characteristics of the CF3SO2 group—which acts as a potent electron attractor (Hammet coefficient, s = 1.3)—and the acidic properties of trifluoro-alkane-sulphonamides are linked to the anti-inflammatory properties of these compounds.

When nemesulide, also known as R-805, was synthesized in the beginning of 1971, it surprisingly had the best acute therapeutic ratio. Nimesulide (R-805) was developed as a result of the nitro group's acidic characteristics being recognized. The nitro group is situated at the para-position of the methyl-sulfonamide moiety. R-805 was studied for clinical efficacy and safety in rheumatoid arthritis patients after its initial discovery and subsequent pharmacological and toxicological investigations. These investigations demonstrated the medication's ability to effectively reduce pain and inflammation.

Theory of Nimesulide

Molecular Formula: $C_{13}H_{12}N_2O_5S$

Structure: 2

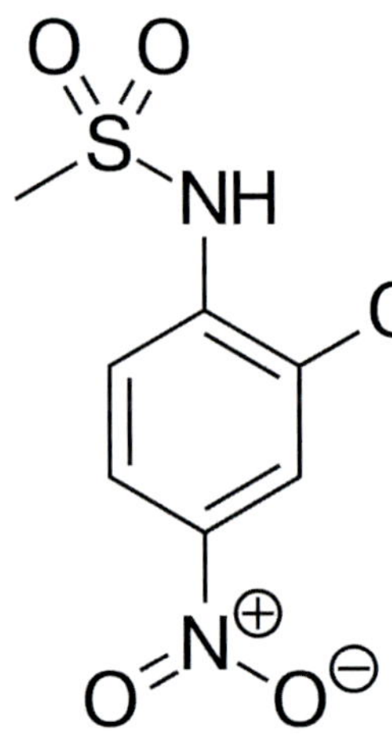

Figure 2.2: Nimesulide.

Source: By The original uploader was ZeframCochrane81 at English Wikipedia. Later versions were uploaded by Rifleman 82 at en.wikipedia., Public Domain, https://commons.wikimedia.org/w/index.php?curid=20791895

Molecular Weight: 308.31

Chemical name: N- 4'-nitro-2'-phenoxyphenyl methane sulfonamide

Category: Analgesic, Anti-inflammatory

Dose: Adults: 100 mg twice daily

Children: 5mg/kg of body weight in 2 or 3 divided doses

Description: Pale white - yellowish white crystalline powder

Solubility: Poor aqueous solubility and soluble in acetone, chloroform and ethyl acetate and is slightly soluble in ethanol

Storage: Store in well-closed, light-resistant containers.

Standards: Nimesulide contains not less than 98.5 % and not more than 101.5 % of $C_{13}H_{12}N_2O_5S$

Mechanism of Action

Prostaglandin synthetase is irreversibly inhibited by nemesulide, which also inhibits the production of PGE2 and PGF2. At much lower doses than those linked to gastrointestinal toxicity, mesulide exhibits anti-inflammatory activity. Nimesulide has no effect on the arachidonic acid metabolism in organs like the stomach, kidneys, and lungs that are typically affected by other NSAIDs at doses that inhibit acute inflammation. Furthermore, mesulide has a greater effect at inflammatory sites. Nimesulide also functions through a number of other non-prostaglandin pathways, such as the scavenging of free radicals, the impact on histamine release and activity, the influence on neutrophil peroxidase, the breakdown of cartilage and the synthesis of metalloprotease, the inhibition of phosphodiesterase type IV, the aggregation of platelets, and the synthesis of platelet-activating factor. Nimesulide also reduces the release of cytokines by blocking the release of tumor necrosis factor. This has an anti-inflammatory effect (Favretto et al., 2013). Nimesulide's antipyretic effect was initially shown in test subjects. Nimesulide's therapeutic antipyretic efficacy has now been clinically demonstrated in a number of double-blind studies involving both adults and children.

Pharmacokinetics

Following oral ingestion, the medication is fully absorbed. It is dispersed throughout the tissue and heavily (90%) bound to serum proteins. It goes through multiple mechanisms of rapid and extensive biotransformation. Urine is the primary metabolite, which is its hydroxy derivative (OH-nimesulide) conjugated with glucuronic acid. Compared to adults, children absorb it more quickly and thoroughly. Compared to adults, children have a shorter terminal half-life (2:03 hours) (3:02 hours). The accumulation of hydroxy-nimesulide is caused by an increased terminal elimination half-life in patients with moderate renal failure.

Therapeutic Uses

When treating osteoarthritis, rheumatoid arthritis, acute and chronic respiratory tract inflammation, dysmenorrhea, and thrombophlebitis, nimesulide is a useful anti-inflammatory and analgesic medication. By scavenging the free radicals that cause tissue damage and causing a rapid recovery of the respiratory mucosa's vital functions, it can regulate the inflammatory process. By doing this, complications like bronchopulmonary diseases or chronic sinusitis may not arise. Nimesulide has been shown to have superior antipyretic properties than aspirin, mefenamic acid, and naproxen, and it requires fewer doses to completely resolve fevers. Nimesulide inhibits the production of superoxide anion and phosphodiesterase type IV at therapeutic concentrations. Chronic asthma can be effectively treated by inhibiting this enzyme, which suppresses the release of histamine from basophils (Patel et al., 2021).

Azithromycin

These are some of the characteristics of the macrolides antibiotic medication known as azithromycin (AZM), which is made by streptomycin species. They are called macrolides because they typically contain 12 to 17 atoms (the Greek word macros means large). A dimehylamino moiety on the sugar residue, a ketone group, and two amino sugars glycosidically attached to the nucleus. When compared to other macrolides, they are more potent. It works well against both cocci and bacilli that are Gram positive bacteria as well as helpful Gram negative cocci. Azithromycin, a semi-synthetic derivative of Erythromycin, is the source of the drug flurithromycin, clarithromycin, and the most recent medication, AZM. Orally administration is used. 10% of it is excreted by the kidneys. Erythromycin's AZM Beckman rearrangement into a 9-oxime produced a 15-member intermediate that, when reduced by 7 N-methylation, produced AZM basic nitrogen atoms that were positioned inside glycone. AZM is active mostly against tuberculosis and other problems; its terminal half (t1/2) is 50 hours, and its distribution volume is 30 liters per kilogram. It has a prolonged half-life of 68 hours and is very stable in acidic conditions. It is less active than erythromycin and more active than respiratory infections caused by homophiles influenza (Cooper et al., 2016). Its bioavailability is reduced by 43% when food is consumed. The FDA has approved AZM for the treatment of infections and tuberculosis.

Theory of Azithromycin

Molecular Formula: $C_{38}H_{72}N_2O_{12}$

Structure: 3

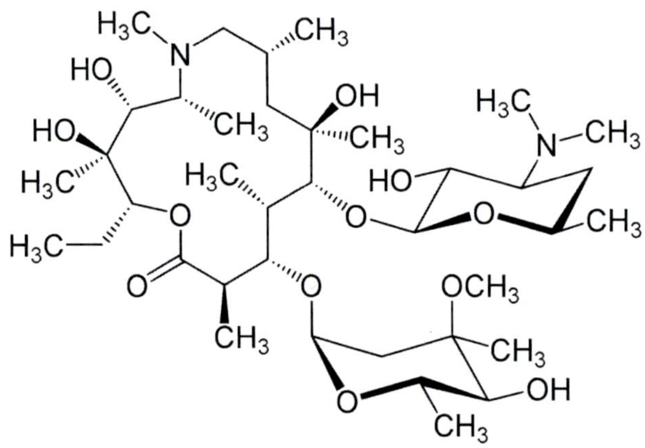

Figure 2.3: Azithromycin.

Source: By Yikrazuul - Own work, Public Domain, https://commons.wikimedia.org/w/index.php?curid=4938127

Molecular Weight: 749.00

Chemical name: (2R, 3S, 4R, 5R, 8R, 10R, 11R, 12S, 13S,14S)-11- ((2S,3R,4S,6R)-4 (dimethylamino)-3-hydroxy-6- methyltetrahydro-2Hpyran-2- yloxy)-2-ethyl-3,4,10- trihydroxy-13-((2S,4R,5S)-5-hydroxy-4-methoxy4hyltetrahydro-2H-Pyran-2-yloxy)-3,5,6,8,10,12,14-heptamethyl-1-oxa 6cyclopentade-can-5-one.

Category: Antibiotics and Antibacterial

Dose: Adults: 2 gm as a single dose.

Children: 60 mg/kg as a single dose, up to a maximum of 2 gm.

Description: White crystalline powder.

Solubility: In case of suspension form, there is no aqueous solubility and tablet form is low water soluble and slightly soluble in ethanol.

Storage: Store in well-closed, light-resistant containers.

Standards: Azithromycin contains not less than 98.5 % and not more than 101.5 % of $C_{38}H_{72}N_2O_{12}$.

Mechanism of Action

First available for oral administration, azithromycin belongs to a new class of antibiotics known chemically as azalides, a subclass of macrolides. By attaching itself to the 50S ribosomal subunit of vulnerable organisms, azithromycin prevents microbes from synthesizing proteins. The synthesis of nucleic acids is unaffected. AZM is a class of macrolide antibiotics that inhibit the synthesis of bacterial proteins. After giving AZM orally in a single dose of 500 mg to subjects who had fasted, the subjects' mean maximum serum concentration (Cmax) increased from 0 to 87 µg/mL in approximately 0 to 3 hours, with a mean area under the curve (AUC0–24) of 3 to 5 µg/mL. Azithromycin has an absolute bioavailability of 37%. When antacids are taken together, the amount of absorption remains unchanged. However, Cmax is lowered by as much as 30%. Azithromycin absorption was unaffected by the administration of cimetidine (800 mg) two hours before azithromycin. Azithromycin's binding to serum proteins varies within a concentration range that approximates human exposure, falling from 51% at 0.02 µg/mL to 7% at 2 µg/mL (Isbar et al., 2013).

Pharmacokinetics

The number of members in each lactone ring determines the division of the macrolide family. Although the 14-chain macrolides have a higher frequency of adverse reactions, they have a stronger antibacterial effect. The gastrointestinal tract absorbs the medications fairly well. Antibiotics called macrolides are extremely safe and non-toxic. However, gastrointestinal problems can happen, particularly when taking 14-chain macrolides like azithromycin. There have been numerous reports of interactions between macrolide and other medications. Their basis lies in either deactivating the hepatic cytochrome P-450 enzyme system or altering bioavailability by influencing the gut flora. For gravid women, macrolides are typically prescribed. Macrolides are used to treat respiratory infections, particularly legionellosis and "atypical pneumonia." Although they function somewhat less than 14-chain macrolides, members of the 16-chain lactone subgroup have fewer side effects (Cooper et al., 2016). Azithromycin is a representative of those medications. This medication has unique pharmacokinetic characteristics and is marginally more effective against sensitive gram-negative bacteria.

A Closer Look

Benzodiazepine

The term "benzos" refers to benzodiazepines (BZD, BDZ, or BZs), a class of depressant medications whose primary chemical structure is the combination of a benzene and a diazepine ring. For the treatment of ailments like anxiety disorders, sleeplessness, and seizures, they are prescribed. Leo Sternbach made the initial benzodiazepine discovery by accident in 1955 with chlordiazepoxide (Librium), which Hoffmann-La Roche commercialized in 1960. In 1963, diazepam (Valium) was introduced. Benzodiazepines were the most prescribed drugs in the world by 1977; however, their use is still commonplace due to a number of factors, including the introduction of selective serotonin reuptake inhibitors, which reduced prescription rates.

Benzodiazepines are depressants that exert a sedative, hypnotic (sleep-inducing), anxiolytic (anti-anxiety), muscle relaxant, and anticonvulsant effect by amplifying the action of the neurotransmitter gamma-aminobutyric acid (GABA) at the GABAA receptor. Anterograde amnesia and dissociation can also be brought on by high dosages of several shorter-acting benzodiazepines. Withdrawal from alcohol, agitation, seizures, insomnia, anxiety, panic disorder, muscle spasms, and premedication for dental or medical procedures are among the conditions for which benzodiazepines are beneficial. There are three types of benzodiazepines: short-, intermediate-, and long-acting. For the treatment of insomnia, short- and intermediate-acting benzodiazepines are preferred; longer-acting benzodiazepines are advised for the treatment of anxiety.

For brief periods of time—two to four weeks—benzodiazepines are thought to be safe and effective, though they can have paradoxical side effects like aggression or behavioral disinhibition as well as cognitive impairment. Long-term use may result in "impaired thinking or memory loss," according to the Department of Health (Victoria). Depression and anxiety. agitation, hostility, paranoia, etc. A small percentage of people experience paradoxical side effects from benzodiazepines, like increased anxiety or agitation. Because of their negative withdrawal effects, impulsivity, and aggression, benzodiazepines are linked to an increased risk of suicide. Because of worries about physical dependence, benzodiazepine withdrawal syndrome, declining effectiveness, and an elevated risk of dementia and cancer, long-term use of these drugs is controversial. Because older adults are more likely to experience negative side effects in the short and long term, benzodiazepines are all included in the Beers List of drugs that are not appropriate for older adults. The safety of benzodiazepines during pregnancy is a topic of debate. Although they are not considered major teratogens, there is still some doubt as to whether they can result in cleft palate in a small percentage of babies and whether prenatal exposure can have neurobehavioural effects; withdrawal symptoms in the newborn are known to occur.

Although benzodiazepines are less toxic than their predecessors, the barbiturates, when taken in excess, can still result in dangerous deep unconsciousness, and fatalities are rare when benzodiazepines are used alone. When combined with other depressants of the central nervous system (CNS), like alcohol and opioids, there is a greater chance of toxicity and lethal overdose. Benzodiazepines are regulated in the majority of nations and are frequently used recreationally. They are also frequently taken in conjunction with other addictive substances.

Summary

- Synthetic drugs refer to substances that are artificially modified from naturally-occurring drugs and are capable of exhibiting both therapeutic and psychoactive effects.
- The chemicals extracted from plants or animals were known as "organic" as opposed to "inorganic" compounds made from other sources.
- The oral route of administration is the most important method of administering drugs for systemic effects. Except in cases of insulin therapy, the parenteral route is not routinely used for self - administration of medication. The topical route of administration has only recently been employed to deliver drugs to the body for systemic effects, with two classes of marketed products; nitroglycerin for the treatment of angina & scopolamine for the treatment of motion sickness.
- An analgesic (also known as a painkiller) is any member of the diverse group of drugs used to relieve pain.
- The non-steroidal anti-inflammatory drugs, usually abbreviated to NSAIDs or NAIDs. The term "non-steroidal" is used to distinguish these drugs from steroids, which (among a broad range of other effects) have a similar depressing, anti-inflammatory action.
- Antibiotics was developed by Vuillemin in 1889. These are used to inhibit and destroy the growth of the microorganism.
- Macrolide drugs are static antibiotics that reversibly inhibit protein synthesis on the ribosomal level. The structure is derived from a 14- to 16-member macrocyclic lactone ring, therefore the class name "macrolide".
- Paracetamol, also known as acetaminophen, is a long-established, nonprescription, peripherally-acting antipyretic analgesic drug. As such, it is a common ingredient in over-the-counter analgesics and cold and flu remedies.
- Nimesulide is a non-steroidal anti-inflammatory drug (NSAID) indicated for the management of a variety of painful and inflammatory conditions like post-operative pain, primary dysmenorrhea, and painful osteoarthritis.
- Azithromycin AZM is a macrolide antibiotic drug produced by the streptomycin species. It has various features. Macrolides usually have 12 to 17 atoms, hence the name.

References

1. Arora, Nidhi; Dhiman, Prashant; Kumar, Shubham; Singh, Gurpreet; Monga, Vikramdeep (2020-02-17). "Recent advances in synthesis and medicinal chemistry of benzodiazepines". Bioorganic Chemistry. 97: 103668. doi:10.1016/j.bioorg.2020.103668. ISSN 0045-2068. PMID 32106040. S2CID 211556193.
2. Banister, Samuel D.; Stuart, Jordyn; Kevin, Richard C.; Edington, Amelia; Longworth, Mitchell; Wilkinson, Shane M.; Beinat, Corinne; Buchanan, Alexandra S.; Hibbs, David E.; Glass, Michelle; Connor, Mark (2015-05-08). "Effects of Bioisosteric Fluorine in Synthetic Cannabinoid Designer Drugs JWH-018, AM-2201, UR-144, XLR-11, PB-22, 5F-PB-22, APICA, and STS-135".

ACS Chemical Neuroscience. 6 (8): 1445–1458. doi:10.1021/acschemneuro.5b00107. ISSN 1948-7193. PMID 25921407.

3. Broadley, Kenneth J. (2009-12-04). "The vascular effects of trace amines and amphetamines". Pharmacology & Therapeutics. 125 (3): 363–375. doi:10.1016/j.pharmthera.2009.11.005. ISSN 1879-016X. PMID 19948186.

4. CE, Smith, JP Sutcliffe, OB Banks (2015-06-02). An overview of recent developments in the analytical detection of new psychoactive substances (NPSs). Royal Society of ChemistryLondon. OCLC 1269494147.

5. Cooper, Ziva D. (2016-06-28). "Adverse Effects of Synthetic Cannabinoids: Management of Acute Toxicity and Withdrawal". Current Psychiatry Reports. 18 (5): 52. doi:10.1007/s11920-016-0694-1. ISSN 1523-3812. PMC 4923337. PMID 27074934.

6. E, Isberg, Vignir Paine, James Leth-Petersen, Sebastian Kristensen, Jesper Langgaard Gloriam, David (2013). Structure-activity relationships of constrained phenylethylamine ligands for the serotonin 5-ht2 receptors. OCLC 1035205954.

7. Evans-Brown, Michael; Sedefov, Roumen (2018), "Responding to New Psychoactive Substances in the European Union: Early Warning, Risk Assessment, and Control Measures", New Psychoactive Substances, vol. 252, Cham: Springer International Publishing, pp. 3–49, doi:10.1007/164_2018_160, ISBN 978-3-030-10560-0, PMID 30194542, retrieved 2022-03-16

8. Favretto, Donata; Pascali, Jennifer P.; Tagliaro, Franco (2013-04-23). "New challenges and innovation in forensic toxicology: Focus on the "New Psychoactive Substances"". Journal of Chromatography A. 1287: 84–95. doi:10.1016/j.chroma.2012.12.049. ISSN 0021-9673. PMID 23332303.

9. Khan, JaVed I.; Kennedy, Thomas J.; Christian, Donnell R. (2012), "Phenethylamines", Basic Principles of Forensic Chemistry, Totowa, NJ: Humana Press, pp. 157–176, doi:10.1007/978-1-59745-437-7_13, ISBN 978-1-934115-06-0, retrieved 2022-03-16

10. Patel, Monica; Finlay, David B.; Glass, Michelle (2021-11-26). "Biased agonism at the cannabinoid receptors – Evidence from synthetic cannabinoid receptor agonists". Cellular Signalling. 78: 109865. doi:10.1016/j.cellsig.2020.109865. ISSN 0898-6568. PMID 33259937. S2CID 227254963.

11. Pintori, Nicholas; Loi, Barbara; Mereu, Maddalena (2017-05-14). "Synthetic cannabinoids: the hidden side of Spice drugs". Behavioural Pharmacology. 28 (6): 409–419. doi:10.1097/fbp.0000000000000323. ISSN 0955-8810. PMID 28692429. S2CID 4913772.

12. Rinaldi, Raffaella; Bersani, Giuseppe; Marinelli, Enrico; Zaami, Simona (2020-03-07). "The rise of new psychoactive substances and psychiatric implications: A wide-ranging, multifaceted challenge that needs far-reaching common legislative strategies". Human Psychopharmacology: Clinical and Experimental. 35 (3): e2727. doi:10.1002/hup.2727. ISSN 0885-6222. PMID 32144953. S2CID 212621941.

13. Shafi, Abu; Berry, Alex J.; Sumnall, Harry; Wood, David M.; Tracy, Derek K. (2020-09-26). "New psychoactive substances: a review and updates". Therapeutic Advances in Psychopharmacology. 10: 204512532096719. doi:10.1177/2045125320967197. ISSN 2045-1253. PMC 7750892. PMID 33414905.

14. Valento, Matthew; Lebin, Jacob (2017-07-06). "Emerging Drugs of Abuse: Synthetic Cannabinoids, Phenylethylamines (2C Drugs), and Synthetic Cathinones". Clinical Pediatric Emergency Medicine. 18 (3): 203–211. doi:10.1016/j.cpem.2017.07.009. ISSN 1522-8401.

15. Walsh, Kenneth B.; Andersen, Haley K. (2020-08-25). "Molecular Pharmacology of Synthetic Cannabinoids: Delineating CB1 Receptor-Mediated Cell Signaling". International Journal of Molecular Sciences. 21 (17): 6115. doi:10.3390/ijms21176115. ISSN 1422-0067. PMC 7503917. PMID 32854313.

Chapter 3

DESIGNER DRUGS: HISTORY AND EVOLUTION

Contents

Introduction

A designer drug is a structural or functional analog of a controlled substance that is intended to resemble the original drug's pharmacological effects without being detected by standard drug tests, being classified as illegal, or both. Designer drugs encompass psychoactive substances that have been classified as NPS by the European Union, in addition to analogs of performance-enhancing drugs like designer steroids. Initially created by academic or industrial researchers, some of these were co-opted for recreational use after they were found to have more potent derivatives with fewer side effects and shorter duration (possibly also because it is easier to apply for patents for new molecules). Secret laboratories were used to create other designer drugs for the first time. Some of these medications may cause unanticipated side effects because their safety and efficacy have not been fully assessed in trials on humans and animals. One could classify the creation of designer drugs as a branch of drug design. Examining changes to well-known active pharmaceuticals, such as their structural analogs, stereoisomers, and derivatives, produces new medications with potentially very different effects from the original (e.g., demonstrating enhanced potency or diminished side effects). Sometimes, despite having entirely different chemical structures, designer drugs have effects that are comparable to those of other well-known drugs (e.g., THC versus JWH-018). Although the term "synthetic drug" is very broad and can refer to almost any synthetic drug, it is frequently used to refer to recreational synthetic drugs, sometimes even meaningless drugs (e.g., LSD, whose psychedelic side effects were inadvertently discovered) (King and Kicman, 2011).

Regardless of a drug's legal status or even whether its structurally similar analog has similar pharmacological effects, certain jurisdictions forbid the trading of drugs that bear a striking structural resemblance to a prohibited drug. Due to legal ambiguity, their trade is considered a gray market item in other jurisdictions. Designer drugs may be illegal regardless of the legal status of structurally similar drugs; in both situations, their trade may occur on the black market. Some jurisdictions may have analogous laws that forbid drugs that are similar in chemical structure to other prohibited drugs.

Orientation and Directional Terms

Term	Definition	Illustration
New psychoactive substances (NPS)	NPS are a complex and diverse group of substances often known as either designer or synthetic drugs, or by the more popular but misleading colloquial term of 'legal highs'.	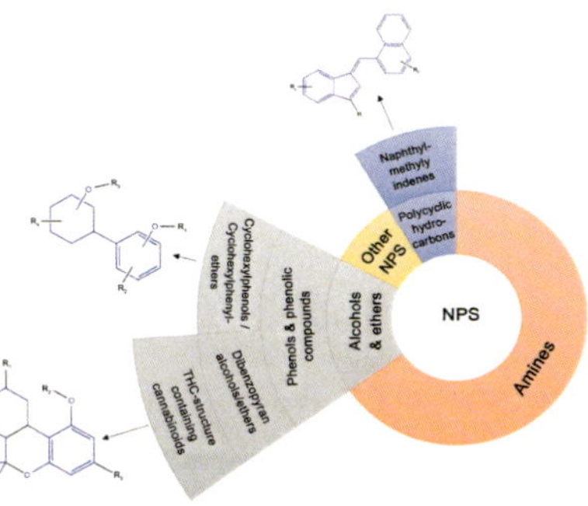
Synthetic drug	Synthetic drugs refer to substances that are artificially modified from naturally-occurring drugs and are capable of exhibiting both therapeutic and psychoactive effects.	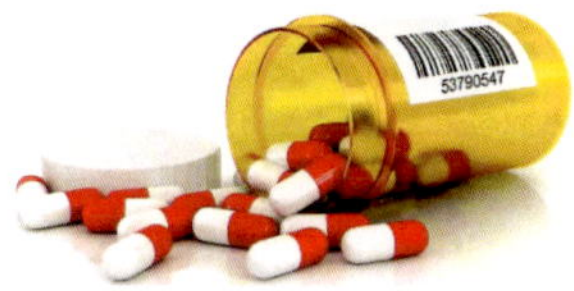
Phencyclidine	An infamous hallucinogenic sought for its ability to induce the illusion of euphoria, omnipotence, superhuman strength, and social and sexual prowess.	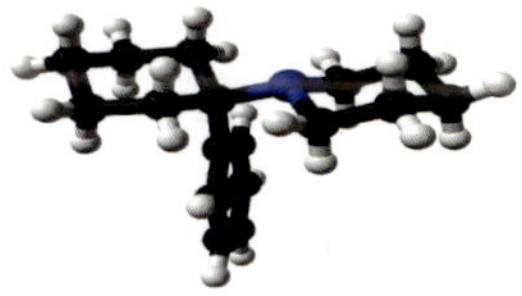
Micrograms	A microgram or microgramme is a unit of mass equal to one millionth (1×10^{-6}) of a gram.	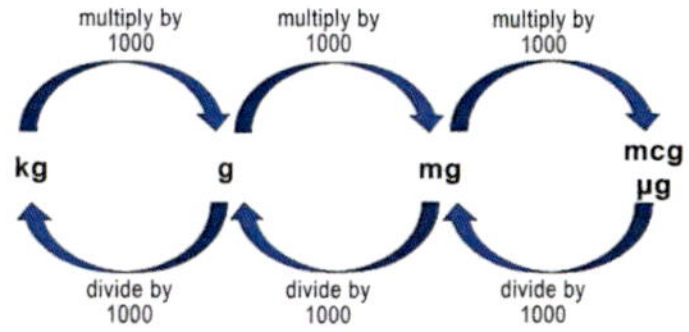
Tetrahydrogestrinone	A synthetic and orally active anabolic–androgenic steroid which was never marketed for medical use. It was developed by Patrick Arnold and used by several high-profile athletes such as Marion Jones, Barry Bonds, and Dwain Chambers.	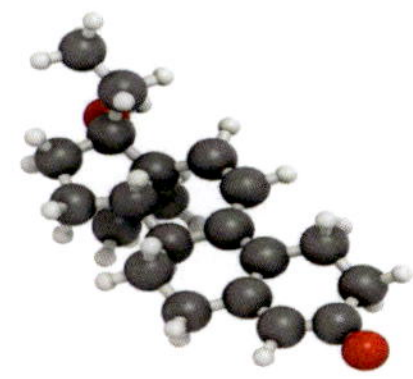

3.1 Designer Drugs: Fundamental Concept and Development

Designer drugs are made of synthetic materials intended to resemble the physiological effects of other drugs that are abused. Although many designer drugs are altered to avoid being categorized as illegal, they share chemical similarities with other drugs that are abused. Furthermore, they are frequently changed in ways that make them imperceptible to traditional drug screening methods. The majority of designer drugs attempt to mimic stimulants such as cocaine, ecstasy, and opiates. Regrettably, overdosing on designer drugs can also occur. Users of these synthetic drugs run the risk of experiencing severe side effects, such as overdose and death, due to their unpredictable pharmacology. The fact that designer drugs are created covertly makes them one of the most difficult substances to detect (Jhonson et al., 2013). As a result, there is little information available about the drugs' composition, chemistry, and effectiveness. Cannabinoids, phenethylamines, phencyclidines (or arylcyclohexamines), tryptamines, piperazines, pipradrols, and N-ring systems are the seven categories of designer drugs recognized by the FBI. Liquid chromatography–tandem mass spectrometry (LC-MS/MS) is primarily used by labs to test for established drugs; it is not designed to identify or measure drugs that have undergone synthetic modification.

Utilizing more advanced analytical techniques like time of flight (TOF) or orbitrap mass spectrometry, these designer drugs can be found in urine. Compared to conclusive techniques like LC-MS/MS, these technologies are more labor-intensive and require more advanced equipment. The Current Procedural Terminology (CPT) code used for drug screening currently only reimburses $60. This reimbursement was set up for the older ToxiLab thin-layer chromatography technique and the historical immunoassay screens. The more recent technologies detect more than a thousand potential drugs, including designer drugs, but the method of drug testing is labor-intensive. The present reimbursement is so low that using more sophisticated technologies for drug detection would not be financially feasible for a hospital or commercial laboratory. In order to fairly compensate laboratories that want to include designer drugs in their drug testing panels, a CPT code for the use of the more modern technologies for toxicological analysis needs to be developed. We think there is enough information on designer drug overdose deaths to justify testing for them in certain patient populations, like those in drug rehab centers.

Reimbursement would require medical necessity, and we propose the following guidelines:

- Patient is in a pain clinic or drug rehabilitation facility
- Clinical signs of impairment
- Positive immunoassay screen, but negative by the usually targeted LC-MS/MS analysis of common drugs
- Suspicion of designer drug use
- Physician (provider) requests further testing

For example, a significant fraction of current opioid deaths are related to fentanyl, and there are multiple fentanyl derivatives available to patients that we are unable to identify with our current targeted testing. Better designer drug use detection would be possible with the application of TOF-based analytical techniques. This is not feasible with current reimbursement (Kelly, 2011).

3.1.1 History and Development

Designer drugs are, as they are commonly

used, illicit chemicals created in laboratories. The term "methamphetamine" is used to refer to amphetamine derivatives like Ecstasy (3,4, methylenedioxymethamphetamine; MDMA) and methamphetamine, as well as frequently abused drugs like fentanyl, ketamine, lysergic acid diethylamide (LSD), phencyclidine (PCP), quaaludes, and GHB (gammahydroxy butyrate). Designer drugs make up a sizable share of the illicit drug trade. The goal of designer drug synthesis is typically to produce a novel analog of a well-known chemical. Pharmaceutical companies have created analogsof some legal drugs in an effort to improve their safety, efficacy, or accessibility for the general public. In fact, the term "designer drug" was first used to describe legal pharmaceuticals. When US authorities started to worry about the use of synthetic heroin like fentanyl, it was first applied to illegal substances in the 1980s. Either way, the phrase evoked designer jeans commercials and suggested the faddishness and affluent status associated with high-end merchandise. The production of illegal designer drugs in covert laboratories impeded efforts to control them through more conventional means, like import restrictions, and they were believed to pose serious physical and psychological risks to users, which raised alarm (Kelly, 2011). Overdosing was more likely because some designer drugs were much stronger than the drugs they were meant to replace in popular culture. Furthermore, small mistakes made during the synthesis process could produce substances that are far more lethal than the intended outcome and very different from it.

The potential for producing distinct designer versions of the same medication occasionally made designer drug regulation challenging. Sometimes, after lawmakers passed legislation outlawing a substance used in designer drugs, a slightly modified version would emerge that used ingredients not included in the original legislation. The Controlled Substance Analogue Enforcement Act, also known as the Designer Drug Act, was included in the Anti-Drug Abuse Act of 1986 in the United States to address this issue. It forbade the production of "substantially similar" substitutes for illegal substances. In the mid-1980s, when crack cocaine was seen as a serious issue, American concerns about designer drugs began to wane. Fears about synthetic drugs, particularly Ecstasy and methamphetamine, were rekindled in the 1990s (Brandt, 2010). Young people's consumption of ecstasy during "rave" dances led to its integration into youth subcultures. Concern over the so-called "date-rape drugs"—synthetic chemicals like gamma hydroxybutyrate, or GHB—that were used to knock out potential victims arose again in the late 1990s.

1920s–1930s

Many substitute morphine esters were soon produced and distributed after the second International Opium Convention was passed in 1925, which expressly outlawed morphine and heroin, the diacetyl ester of morphine. The most prominent of these were acetylpropionylmorphine and dibenzoylmorphine, which are not covered by the Opium Convention despite having effects that are almost exactly the same as heroin. This prompted the League of Nations Health Committee to adopt a number of resolutions in an effort to regulate these novel drugs, which finally resulted in the adoption of the first comprehensive analogs laws in 1930, which extended legal control to all morphine, oxycodone, and hydromorphone esters. Diethyl ether was marketed and used as an alternative to illicit alcoholic beverages in several countries during the Prohibition era in the 1930s, providing another early example of what could be loosely called designer drug use (Weigand et al., 2012).

1960s–1970s

Many new synthetic hallucinogens were developed in the 1960s and 1970s; one famous instance is the 1967 sale of extremely strong DOM tablets in San Francisco. Recently, new compounds were added to the controlled drug schedules one by one as they became problematic, leaving little room for prosecution over drug analogs. During this time, two notable legal cases included the prosecution of Tim Scully and Nicholas Sand in 1973 for producing ALD-52, or the acetyl amide of LSD. ALD-52 was not a controlled substance at the time of their conviction, but they were found guilty because they had to have been in possession of illegal LSD in order to manufacture ALD-52. Several phencyclidine (PCP) analogs were also introduced to the black market in the late 1970s (Weigand et al., 2012).

1980s–early 1990s

In the 1980s, the term "designer drug" was introduced to describe a range of synthetic opioid drugs, primarily derived from the fentanyl molecule, including α-methylfentanyl. The term became well-known when MDMA (ecstasy) saw a surge in popularity in the middle of the 1980s. Many drugs were being sold on the black market, such as heroin, in the 1980s, when the term was first used. A lot of them relied on meperidine or fentanyl. One, MPPP, was discovered in certain instances to contain an impurity known as MPTP, which, from just one dosage, caused brain damage that could result in a syndrome akin to late-stage Parkinson's disease. Highly potent fentanyl analogs that frequently resulted in unintentional overdoses were another issue. Laws were passed to give the DEA the authority to emergency schedule chemicals for a year, with an optional 6-month extension, while gathering evidence to justify permanent scheduling, in addition to the previously mentioned analog laws, because the government was unable to prosecute individuals for these drugs until after they had been successfully marketed. For MDMA, emergency scheduling power was utilized for the first time. Even though their own judge determined that MDMA should be classified as a Schedule III drug due to its proven medical uses, the DEA, in this case, scheduled MDMA as a Schedule I drug and kept this classification after review. This emergency scheduling power has since been applied to several other medications, such as 2C-B, AMT, and BZP (Weigand et al., 2012). The first medicine to be denied permanent scheduling and return to legal status after being emergency-scheduled was TFMPP, a piperazine medication, in 2004.

Methamphetamine resurfaced as a major public health concern in the United States in the late 1980s and early 1990s, prompting tighter regulations on precursor chemicals in an effort to reduce the amount of the drug produced domestically. This resulted in the emergence of a number of substitute stimulant drugs, the most prominent of which were methcathinone and 4-methylaminorex. However, despite receiving enough attention from authorities to prompt the legal scheduling of these substances, their distribution was comparatively restricted, and methamphetamine remained the market leader for illicit synthetic stimulants overall.

Late 1990s–2004

The amount of designer drugs being sold online skyrocketed in the late 1990s and early 2000s. Certain marketers of designer drugs, specifically psychedelic drugs belonging to the tryptamine and phenethylamine family, are credited with coining the term and idea of research chemicals. The theory was that by marketing the compounds as being intended for use in science rather than for human consumption, the intent clause of the U.S.A. There would be no analog drug laws. Still, a few years later, during Operation Web Tryp, the DEA raided numerous vendors (including RAC Research) and JLF Primary Materials, among other suppliers. This procedure was substantially expedited when suppliers started using search engines like Google for advertising, connecting their websites to queries on terms like chemical names and phrases like psychedelic or hallucinogenic. The media and authorities became interested in the topics of consumptive use and the sources of the chemicals when they were discussed widely in public forums. The US Drug Enforcement Administration conducted an operation known as Web Tryp in 2004, raiding and closing down multiple online vendors of research chemicals. Two manufacturers of chemicals were shut down with assistance from Chinese and Indian authorities. Even though their products were still legal in most parts of the world, many other online retailers quickly stopped operating. Hallucinogens with chemical similarities to drugs like psilocybin and mescaline make up the majority of substances that were sold as research chemicals during this time. Similar to other hallucinogens, these drugs are frequently used to promote introspection, spiritual growth, or leisure (Winstock et al., 2011). Certain research chemicals that are available in the market can serve as building blocks for the synthesis of other substances that may have psychoactive properties. For instance, 2C-H can be utilized to create 2C-B and 2C-I, among other substances. Over the past century, pharmaceutical companies, academic institutions, and independent researchers have conducted numerous investigations into structural variations. These studies have produced some of the research chemicals that are currently in use. Alexander Shulgin is a renowned researcher who, in addition to co-authoring the books TiHKAL and PiHKAL (in which he presented syntheses and pharmacological explorations of hundreds of substances), testified as an expert witness on behalf of the defense in multiple court cases against producers of psychoactive drugs.

Since selling research chemicals in pill form would undermine the claims that they were being sold for non-consumptive research, most chemical suppliers sold their products in bulk as powder rather than pills. The active dosages of various substances can range from micrograms to hundreds of milligrams. It is important for the end user to weigh doses using a precision scale rather than estimating or eyeballing them. However, many users failed to do this, which resulted in numerous ER visits and fatalities. This was a major contributing factor to the emergency scheduling of various substances and ultimately, Operation Web Tryp. Certain compounds, like 5-Meo-DiPT and 2C-B, did eventually gain enough traction to be marketed as pills in order to reach a larger market. These pills were given the street names Nexus and Foxy, respectively. When a chemical becomes this well-known, it usually doesn't take long for it to be added to the list of scheduled (i.e., illicit) substances. The first widespread use of novel anabolic steroids by competitive athletes occurred in the late 1990s and early 2000s. The International Olympic Committee has prohibited steroids since 1976, but because there are so many anabolic agents available for use in humans and animals, laboratory testing for all of the drugs has always been unable to keep up with athletes' discovery of new compounds to use. It became much harder for athletes to use these drugs covertly after more formalized testing procedures were implemented, particularly with the establishment of the World Anti-Doping Agency in 1999. This led to the development of new and powerful anabolic steroid drugs like tetrahydrogestrinone (THG), which were not picked up by the usual tests.

2005–2021

In recent years, there has been a significant expansion in the variety of compounds sold as designer drugs. While traditionally, designer drugs were opioids, hallucinogens, or anabolic steroids, the possibilities are now only limited by scientific and patent literature. Designer stimulants like geranamine, mephedrone, MDPV, and desoxypipradrol, designer sedatives like methylmethaqualone and premazepam, and designer analogs of sildenafil have become popular choices. In addition, designer cannabinoids like JWH-018 and (C8)-CP 47,497 have emerged as active components of "herbal smoking blends." Synthetic cannabinoid agonists and research ligands for cosmetic purposes, such as melanotan peptides, have also become more prevalent in the designer drug market (Winstock et al., 2011).

"...what is new is the wide range of substances now being explored, the aggressive marketing of products that have been intentionally mislabelled, the growing use of the internet, and the speed at which the market reacts to control measures."

—EMCDDA director Wolfgang Goetz (November 2009).

The emergence of Mephedrone and other cathinones marked a significant shift in the world of designer drugs. These substances went from being relatively unknown and ineffective products sold in head shops to powerful drugs that could rival traditional substances on the black market. Mephedrone, in particular, saw a rapid increase in popularity in 2009, leading to widespread media attention and eventual prohibition in multiple countries.

This sudden rise in demand for cathinones prompted the development of new substances attempting to replicate the effects of Mephedrone. With a growing customer base and ample financial incentives, innovation in the designer drug market soared. As a result, the market expanded rapidly, with an increasing number of new substances being discovered each year.

Between 2009 and 2013, the European Monitoring Centre for Drugs and Drug Addiction (EMCDDA) identified a total of 268 new drugs, including not only cathinones but also cannabinoids, stimulants, benzodiazepines, psychedelics, dissociatives, and other drug classes. Synthetic cannabinoids (SCBs), in particular, accounted for a significant portion of these new drugs, with 209 different variations reported between 2008 and 2021.

Overall, the designer drug market has seen a proliferation of new and diverse substances in recent years, with SCBs being the most prevalent among the substances monitored by the EMCDDA. The constant influx of new drugs poses a challenge for drug enforcement agencies trying to keep up with evolving trends in the illicit drug trade.

2022–present

The rise of grey-market suppliers of synthetic peptide hormones in the early 2020s was fueled by the perceived (though unproven) safety of peptides and the legal challenges associated with regulating them. These websites offer peptide medications that are primarily intended for non-recreational use and promoted for their alleged ability to improve performance, prevent aging, and improve appearance. To ensure the legal ambiguity of their operations, some vendors hire medical professionals and implement stringent measures. The development and sale of increasingly legally contentious research chemicals persisted online, but the market for these chemicals became much more accessible when peptide "research chemical" vendors began to emerge in the early 2020s (Spiller et al., 2011).

3.1.2 Performance-Enhancing Designer Drugs

Anabolic steroids, peptide hormones, growth factor mimetics, and hormone and metabolic modulators are examples of designer doping agents that are becoming more and more common outside of the professional sports world. These drugs primarily target performance and appearance, acting on the hormone system via a variety of varied mechanisms. Renal failure, gynecomastia, secondary hypogonadism, hypertension, ischemic stroke, cardiotoxicity, and hepatotoxicity are among the side effects linked to performance-enhancing designer drugs. Designer drugs used to increase sexual performance have also emerged; examples include phosphodiesterase-5 inhibitors, which have no established safety profile, and substances used to improve athletic performance and appearance. These drugs may cause serious drug-drug interactions or visual disturbances.

3.1.3 Treatment of Designer Drug Addiction

When patients are admitted to the hospital due to the harmful effects of designer drugs, this presents a great chance to counsel them to cut back on their substance use and get them started on treatment. Patient education and healthcare provider awareness are the cornerstones of public health initiatives to address the new challenges posed by designer drugs. If the diagnosis is made early, simple reminders to stop can be helpful, but they are usually insufficient. It is common for patients who use designer drugs to have mixed feelings about altering their behavior (Spiller et al., 2011). As a sign of respect for the patient's autonomy, the clinician should demonstrate empathy without being confrontational. Patients can make the most informed decisions about altering their behavior by being given relevant and accurate information about the possible risks associated with designer drugs and being encouraged to make healthy choices. While reminding the patient that they are responsible for everything they do, doctors should actively involve the patient in the problem-solving process. Rather than placing the blame for the patient's lack of motivation to change on them, the practitioner should encourage the patient to pursue recovery from designer drug use. Precise knowledge regarding the relative dangers and unidentified side effects of these products aids in a patient's decision-making regarding whether to stick with a specific product, try to quit using it or seek out more specialized addiction treatment.

Acute and long-term treatment is probably required once a designer drug use disorder is diagnosed, despite the paucity of prospective treatment data. In general, one can recovered from substance use disorders (SUDs), and people who receive treatment are less disabled than those who do not. The components of long-term treatment for designer drug use disorders are probably similar to those of other forms of addiction treatment, including behavioral components like motivational enhancement therapy, individual and group counseling with cognitive-behavioral therapy, and 12-step self-help group facilitation. Family members ought to be taken into account when designing a treatment plan, especially for young adults or adolescents. Regretfully, there are no pharmacologic treatment data available to direct the management of individuals with designer drug use disorders. Information directing them to nearby community resources for addiction treatment should be given to patients diagnosed with SUD in the ED or during hospital inpatient stays. You can locate doctors in the US who are certified to treat addictive disorders by visiting the websites of the American Academy of Addiction Psychiatry or the American Society of Addiction Medicine. Referring the patient to a nonphysician counselor—who can be located via the website of the National Association for Alcohol and Drug Abuse Counselors—may occasionally be more practical and economical (Carhart-Harris et al., 2011).

Treating designer drug SUD is a complex task for various reasons. Designer drugs encompass a wide range of substances with different effects on the mind and body, making treatment challenging. Additionally, users are often young and may engage in polysubstance use, complicating the treatment process. The sporadic use of these drugs in social settings may downplay the seriousness of the issue. Healthcare providers must be well-informed and prepared to address the diverse combinations of substances used, particularly in cases involving club drugs. A supportive treatment environment is crucial for success. Despite the need for multiple treatment sessions, the cost-effectiveness of addiction treatment is evident. Helping patients recover from addiction and resume normal life is a fulfilling experience for healthcare professionals.

3.2 Trends in Designer Drug Development and Usage

Advances in synthetic chemistry and shifts in societal attitudes toward recreational substances have led to significant changes in the landscape of designer drug development and usage in recent years. Designer drugs are synthetic substances that are created to mimic the effects of traditional drugs like cannabis, cocaine, or MDMA while avoiding legal restrictions. They are also referred to as novel psychoactive substances (NPS). One notable development is the rise of SCBs, which are substances made to bind to the same brain receptors as the naturally occurring cannabinoids found in marijuana. Despite being linked to serious side effects like psychosis, seizures, and even death, these substances—which are frequently sold as herbal incense or legal highs—have become more and more popular because they are easily accessible and thought to be legal. Synthetic cathinones, also referred to as bath salts, are becoming increasingly popular. They function as stimulants akin to amphetamines or cocaine. Due to their involvement in several widely reported events involving severe agitation, hallucinations, and violent conduct, these drugs became well-known. The development of designer drugs is marked by a persistent alteration of chemical structures to evade legal restrictions, which presents formidable obstacles for law enforcement and public health authorities in terms of identifying and managing their dissemination.

In addition, the emergence of virtual markets and the dark web has made it easier for designer drugs to be distributed internationally, allowing people to buy these substances covertly and without identification. This accessibility has led to the widespread use of designer drugs among some demographics, especially young adults and partygoers, along with the attraction of new experiences and the desire to avoid drug testing. The covert character of these transactions, however, raises questions regarding the quality, purity, and possible adulteration of the products, raising the possibility of unforeseen consequences and negative reactions. Furthermore, the phenomenon of drug analogs highlights the adaptability of designer drug manufacturers in eluding legislative efforts to curb their proliferation. Here, existing controlled substances are given slight structural modifications to create new variants with similar pharmacological effects. A game of cat and mouse between regulators and covert laboratories is perpetuated by the rapid pace of innovation in synthetic chemistry, which allows manufacturers to produce new analogs faster than laws can be enacted, despite legislative efforts to ban specific compounds. To tackle the issue of designer drug use, various approaches have been employed, including harm reduction strategies, public awareness campaigns, law enforcement initiatives, and legislative measures. These include focused legislation that forbids the use of specific classes of compounds rather than single substances, increased internet marketplace surveillance, and educational initiatives to increase public knowledge of the dangers of designer drug use. Furthermore, harm reduction strategies like drug-checking services and overdose prevention initiatives work to lessen the negative effects of designer drugs and stop related harms from happening in communities that are already at risk (Hu et al., 2011).

3.2.1 Chemical Composition and Pharmacology of Designer Drugs

Designer drugs that are frequently used have a variety of chemical structures and modes of action that contribute to their psychoactive effects on the central nervous system. Examples of these drugs are SCBs, cathinones, and hallucinogens. For example, SCBs are structurally varied substances that are made to bind to cannabinoid receptors in the brain and resemble the effects of delta-9-tetrahydrocannabinol (THC), the primary psychoactive ingredient in cannabis. These substances frequently have chemical structures that are very different from those of THC, but they are designed to interact with cannabinoid receptors highly selectively, producing strong psychoactive effects. SCBs are generally composed of an aromatic ring-based core scaffold, which is frequently replaced with different functional groups like halogens, alkyl chains, or heterocyclic moieties. These changes have the potential to dramatically change the compound's pharmacological characteristics, including potency, selectivity, and duration of action. The mechanism by which SCBs work is to bind to cannabinoid receptors (CB1 and CB2) in the brain and other peripheral tissues. This modulates the release of neurotransmitters and signaling pathways linked to mood, perception, and cognition. However, a number of negative effects, such as anxiety, paranoia, hallucinations, and cardiovascular problems, are brought on by the ' high potency and unpredictable pharmacokinetics of SCBs.

A beta-keto group sets cathinones apart from other stimulants, but they all have a phenethylamine backbone, like amphetamines and methamphetamines. Cathinones are a different class of designer drugs. Increased synaptic concentrations of these neurotransmitters result from this structural modification, which also increases their potency and affinity for monoamine transporters, specifically the dopamine and norepinephrine transporters. In terms of structure, cathinones can be substituted at different points along the phenethylamine scaffold. More potency and selectivity for the dopamine transporter are frequently obtained by substituting at the alpha carbon. The pharmacokinetic characteristics of cathinones and receptor binding affinity can also be affected by substituents like halogens or alkyl chains. Cathinones work mechanistically to produce increased neurotransmitter signaling and arousal by encouraging the release of dopamine, norepinephrine, and serotonin from presynaptic neurons and blocking their reuptake. But using cathinones is linked to a number of negative side effects, such as agitation, tachycardia, hypertension, hyperthermia, and psychosis. These side effects can be made worse by inconsistent potency between formulations and a lack of quality control (Carhart-Harris et al., 2011).

A wide range of drugs known as hallucinogens can cause profound changes in sensory experiences and altered states of consciousness. They can also cause changes in mood, perception, and cognition. Hallucinogens can be structurally categorized into a number of chemical families, such as phenethylamines (e.g., mescaline), attemptstamines (e.g, DMT), psilocybin, and ergolines (e.g., LSD). Notwithstanding their structural variations, hallucinogens all work by activating serotonin receptors, specifically the 5-HT2A subtype, which are found in brain areas related to mood regulation and sensory processing. Hallucinogens alter perception, thought processes, and emotional reactions by activating these receptors, which change neuronal activity and neurotransmitter release. Numerous factors, including dosage, mode of administration, set (user expectations, mindset), and setting (environmental context), can affect the subjective effects of hallucinogens. Although hallucinogens are generally thought to have a low potential for toxicity and dependence, they can have acute negative effects such as anxiety, panic attacks, and psychosis, especially in people who are prone to mental health issues.

3.2.2 Legislative Responses to Designer Drugs

The effectiveness of legislation intended to regulate the manufacture, distribution, and use of designer drugs is impacted by the difficulty in keeping up with the quickly changing chemical formulations. Legislative initiatives have been helpful in addressing particular designer drug compounds or classes, but regulatory control is difficult to uphold due to the dynamic nature of synthetic chemistry. Conventional legislative methods usually schedule specific substances or classes of substances as controlled substances, making it illegal to manufacture, distribute, or possess them.

This reactive strategy, though, might not be sufficient to deal with the steady stream of new designer drugs that hit the market, since covert labs can readily alter chemical structures to create analogs that have comparable pharmacological effects but are unique enough to get around legal restrictions. Enforcement actions are further complicated by the worldwide nature of designer drug production and distribution since producers can easily adjust to changes in legislation by moving their operations to countries with less stringent laws or by taking advantage of legal loopholes. Because online marketplaces and the dark web provide anonymity, it becomes more difficult to enforce laws because designer drugs can be discreetly sold and distributed internationally without the need for physical middlemen. Additionally, law enforcement's capacity to identify and bring to justice those involved in the trafficking of designer drugs is hampered by the absence of forensic techniques and standard testing protocols for identifying novel compounds. Legislative control efforts are further complicated by the widespread adulteration and mislabeling in the designer drug market. Manufacturers frequently conceal the true nature of their goods from regulatory scrutiny by using legal loopholes to pass off their products as plant food, research chemicals, or unfit for human consumption. Authorities find it challenging to distinguish between legitimate and illegal substances due to this obfuscation, which causes delays in the scheduling of new compounds and hinders efforts to stop their use and distribution. Some jurisdictions have responded to these challenges by enacting proactive legislative strategies that, instead of focusing only on specific substances, aim to preemptively ban entire classes of compounds or structural analogs.

The goal of lawmakers' broader language is to prevent manufacturers from trying to circumvent regulations by making small changes to already-existing compounds. This allows for a wider range of chemical structures with similar pharmacological properties to be included. Nevertheless, the challenge of precisely characterizing and classifying heterogeneous chemical structures in the quickly changing designer drug landscape may restrict the efficacy of this strategy (Carhart-Harris et al., 2011). To further address the underlying causes of designer drug use and lessen related harms, strong public health initiatives, such as education, prevention, and harm reduction tactics, must be implemented in tandem with legislative efforts. Policymakers, law enforcement, medical professionals, and community stakeholders can work together to develop comprehensive strategies that address the many issues that designer drugs present. Furthermore, coordinating regulatory responses and stopping the cross-border spread of designer drugs depend on international cooperation and information-sharing mechanisms.

3.2.3 Health Risks and Adverse Effects of Designer Drugs

Designer drugs are a vast category of artificial substances that are made to resemble conventional illegal substances. Depending on the particular substance, dosage, mode of administration, and individual factors, users may experience a wide range of physiological and psychological effects from these substances. For instance, SCBs—often sold as synthetic marijuana or spice—have been shown to bind to cannabinoid receptors in the brain, altering mood, perception, and thought processes. SCBs can have euphoric, calming, altered sensory perception, and impaired coordination short-term effects. More severe negative effects, such as anxiety, paranoia, hallucinations, fast heartbeat, elevated blood pressure, and seizures, can also be brought on by these drugs. SCBs have also been linked to a number of acute toxicities that can cause hospitalization or even death, such as acute kidney injury, myocardial infarction, ischemic stroke, and respiratory depression. Similarly, synthetic cathinones, also referred to as bath salts, increase the release and decrease the reuptake of neurotransmitters like serotonin, norepinephrine, and dopamine to produce stimulant effects. Synthetic cathinones may cause short-term euphoria, decreased appetite, increased energy, and alertness. However, these substances can also induce severe agitation, paranoia, hallucinations, delusions, psychosis, and violent behavior, often requiring medical intervention or psychiatric care. Furthermore, synthetic cathinones have been implicated in cases of serotonin syndrome, a potentially life-threatening condition characterized by hyperthermia, agitation, muscle rigidity, and autonomic dysfunction, particularly when used in combination with other serotonergic drugs.

Hallucinogens like LSD, psilocybin, and NBOMe compounds can cause intense changes in perception, thinking, and emotions by interacting with serotonin receptors in the brain. These substances can lead to visual and auditory hallucinations, distorted senses, altered time perception, introspective experiences, and increased empathy. While hallucinogens are generally seen as having low toxicity and addiction potential, they can still trigger adverse reactions such as anxiety, panic attacks, and psychosis, especially in people with pre-existing mental health conditions or in uncontrolled environments (Johnston et al., 2014). Some users may also experience hallucinogen-induced persisting perception disorder, which involves recurring visual disturbances or flashbacks; though the exact prevalence and long-term effects are not well understood. The proliferation of new designer drugs with unknown effects poses even greater risks. Cases of toxicity and overdose have been linked to synthetic opioids, dissociatives, and potent SCBs, which can cause serious health issues like respiratory depression, heart failure, coma, and death, requiring immediate medical attention. The lack of regulation and inconsistencies in potency among different versions of these substances heighten the danger of accidental overdoses and negative reactions, particularly when users are unaware of what they are ingesting.

3.2.4 Social and Cultural Factors Influencing Designer Drug Use

A complex interplay of socio-cultural factors, such as peer pressure, media portrayals, and perceptions of safety and legality, influences the use of designer drugs. Peer pressure is a major factor in determining how people feel and act when it comes to drug use because peer groups and social networks can act as channels for the sharing of knowledge, customs, and behaviors around substance use. Designer drug use may be seen in many social circles as a way to rebel against societal norms, fit in, or socialize, especially among adolescents and young adults. People who use designer drugs to feel validated and like they belong in their social circles may do so as a result of peer pressure and social acceptance in these groups. The way that designer drugs are portrayed in the media is also very important in influencing how the general public views these drugs. Popular media portrayals of drug use in films, TV series, music videos, and online platforms have the power to normalize or glamorize substance use, which can affect how viewers view the advantages and disadvantages of various drugs. Furthermore, erroneous or sensationalized media portrayals of designer drugs may exacerbate misunderstandings and disinformation regarding their effects, safety, and legality, which may encourage more experimentation or use among particular groups motivated by curiosity. On the other hand, by disseminating accurate information and encouraging people to make educated decisions for themselves and their communities, media campaigns and public health initiatives that seek to increase awareness about the risks associated with designer drugs can help offset these influences.

Perceptions of legality and safety also play a significant role in shaping patterns of designer drug use. The perceived legality of designer drugs, particularly those marketed as "legal highs" or "research chemicals," can influence individuals' willingness to experiment with these substances, as they may perceive them as safer or less stigmatized than traditional illicit drugs. Moreover, the availability of designer drugs through head shops and internet marketplaces, frequently with deceptive labels or disclaimers, may contribute to users' beliefs about their safety and legality (Kronstrand et al., 2014). Designer drugs, however, may not go through stringent testing or quality control procedures, which leaves room for unknown safety profiles and unpredictable effects, including the possibility of toxicity or overdose. In addition, despite evidence to the contrary, people may mistakenly believe that a drug's legal status indicates its acceptability or harmlessness, which could lead to a perception of its safety or legitimacy being bolstered by legislative attempts to regulate designer drugs.

3.2.5 Harm Reduction Strategies for Designer Drug Users

A variety of tactics geared toward lessening harm to people individually, in groups, and throughout society are included in harm reduction approaches, which are intended to minimize the risks connected with the use of designer drugs. These strategies recognize that some people may still use drugs in spite of efforts to stop or discourage them from doing so, and they use practical interventions to lessen the possible negative effects of drug use. A number of harm reduction tactics, such as drug-checking services, education about overdose prevention, and access to treatment and support services, have been put into place to address the unique risks connected to the use of designer drugs.

People can examine the purity and makeup of the substances they plan to take by using drug-checking services, commonly referred to as drug testing or pill testing. In order to determine whether particular compounds are present in a sample, these services often entail the use of analytical techniques like mass spectrometry or high-performance liquid chromatography (HPLC). Drug-checking services enable people to make better-informed decisions about whether or not to use drugs by giving them information about the composition and potency of the drugs they are using. Furthermore, drug testing services can detect unforeseen impurities or adulterants in drug samples, assisting in the avoidance of unintentional overdoses or negative reactions. The risk of fatal or non-fatal overdoses linked to the use of designer drugs is significantly decreased by overdose prevention education. Information on identifying the telltale signs and symptoms of an opioid overdose, how to reverse an opioid overdose with naloxone, an opioid antagonist, and how to seek emergency medical attention in the event of an overdose are all possible topics covered in this education (Krotulski et al., 2018). Overdose prevention education can prevent fatal overdoses and lessen the demand for emergency medical services by giving people the information and abilities they need to react appropriately in such circumstances. In addition, community members can be better equipped to intervene in overdose situations by participating in outreach programs that provide naloxone kits to populations that are considered at-risk, such as those who use stimulants or opioids.

For those who use designer drugs and struggle with SUDs, access to treatment and support services is crucial. Peer support groups, medication-assisted treatment (MAT), residential rehabilitation programs, and outpatient counseling are a few possible treatment options. Treatment and support services can help people cut back or stop using drugs, enhance their general health and well-being, and address underlying factors that contribute to substance use by offering evidence-based interventions catered to the needs of people with SUDs. Additionally, harm reduction programs can lessen the negative effects of continued drug use, such as infectious diseases, overdose, and social marginalization, by offering nonjudgmental support, resources, and referrals to people who are unable or unwilling to stop using drugs.

3.2.6 Pharmacological Innovations in Designer Drug Development

Modern synthetic chemistry and pharmacology have accelerated the creation of new designer drugs, which have resulted in a proliferation of compounds made to mimic the effects of conventional illegal drugs while avoiding legal constraints. These developments are the result of multiple factors, such as improvements in pharmacological research, easier access to precursor chemicals, and advances in synthetic methodologies. Utilizing computational modeling and structure-activity relationship (SAR) studies to guide the design of analogs with desired effects and predict the pharmacological properties of novel compounds is one noteworthy trend. Researchers can logically design molecules that target particular receptors or neurotransmitter systems, improving potency, selectivity, and pharmacokinetic properties by utilizing computational tools and bioassay data. One of the main tactics used to get around the law's prohibitions on designer drugs is the use of chemical modifications and analogs. Through minor modifications to the chemical structure of currently available compounds, scientists can produce analogs that have comparable pharmacological effects but are sufficiently different to not be classified as controlled substances under the law. Changing functional groups, adjusting the stereochemistry, or adding structural motifs that provide resistance to metabolic degradation are examples of common modifications (Krotulski et al., 2018). Additionally, researchers can explore unexplored chemical space and find new pharmacophores with desired activity profiles by synthesizing novel scaffolds or hybrid structures inspired by known psychoactive compounds.

The development of designer drugs has also accelerated due to the advent of new synthetic methodologies that allow for the quick synthesis and assessment of large compound libraries, such as flow chemistry, microwave-assisted synthesis, and high-throughput screening techniques. By using these methods, lead compounds can be optimized more quickly for the desired pharmacological properties, and a wider range of chemical spaces can be explored. Additionally, researchers can now more accurately and sensitively characterize the chemical structures and mechanisms of action of novel designer drugs thanks to advancements in analytical techniques like mass spectrometry, nuclear magnetic resonance spectroscopy, and high-resolution imaging methods. However, the quick development of designer drugs poses difficulties for law enforcement and regulatory bodies in identifying and limiting their spread. A game of cat and mouse between regulators and covert laboratories results from legislative attempts to outlaw particular compounds or classes of substances, which frequently react reactively and follow the development of new analogs. Furthermore, the worldwide reach of the designer drug trade, enabled by virtual marketplaces and anonymous transactions, adds another layer of complexity to the management of regulations and enforcement actions. Detecting and prosecuting offenders involved in the trafficking of designer drugs is further complicated by the absence of forensic techniques and standardized testing protocols for the identification of novel compounds.

3.3 Designer Drugs: Mechanism of Action and Adverse Effects

Originally, the term "designer drugs" was used to refer to novel compounds that are created by secretly altering popular drugs of abuse to maintain or improve their pharmacologic effects while eluding legal restrictions. These days, the term is used more broadly to refer to substances that come from academic or industrial research but are never approved by medical authorities. Certain substances that are referred to as designer drugs may not meet the traditional definition of a designer drug because they are approved for medical use in other countries. The dissemination of designer drugs and the gathering of information about them are greatly aided by the Internet. Designer drug availability is continuously rising, and usage trends and patterns vary over time. Drug control authorities are faced with a challenge because of this, which may endanger public health. The same categories that classify traditional drugs of abuse—stimulants, sedatives, dissociatives, cannabinoids, and psychedelics—also apply to designer drugs. Nevertheless, unlike conventional drugs of abuse, newly developed drugs can evade detection through regular drug testing, and there is frequently little information available regarding their negative consequences. For healthcare professionals who treat patients who are intoxicated, understanding the mechanism of action and potential clinical complications of designer drugs is essential (Krueger et al., 2014).

3.3.1 Stimulants

Amphetamine, cocaine, and MDMA are examples of monoaminergic stimulants that are commonly abused drugs. Additional stimulants, like dextroamphetamine and methylphenidate, are frequently administered to treat attention-deficit/hyperactivity disorder (ADHD). Prescription drug research is currently being conducted on MDMA for the treatment of posttraumatic stress disorder. In addition to interacting with monoaminergic receptors and other targets, stimulants primarily modulate monoaminergic neurotransmission by interacting with the transporters of norepinephrine, dopamine, and serotonin (5-hydroxytryptamine [5-HT]) (NET, DAT, and SERT, respectively). Monoaminergic stimulants mediate non-exocytotic monoamine efflux at monoamine transporters by acting as substrates or transporter inhibitors. Variations in selectivity (Figure 3.1) and strength (Figure 3.2) at the various transporters produce various pharmacological outcomes, various clinical potencies (i.e., the required dosage to produce a psychoactive effect), and various abuse risks. Chemicals that are specific for DAT versus SERT indicates a high potential for abuse by facilitating dose-dependent and abuse-related intracranial self-stimulation. On the other hand, drugs that are specific for the SERT vs. DAT reduce intracranial self-stimulation that is dose-dependent, suggesting a decreased risk of abuse. A higher abuse potential may arise from repeated exposure to substances with similar activity at the DAT and SERT, as this could maintain the expression of DAT-mediated abuse-related effects while fostering tolerance to SERT-mediated abuse-limiting effects. Designer stimulants are becoming more and more accessible, and using them can lead to a range of physiological issues and mood disorders, which are covered in the sections that follow for each class of designer stimulant (Krueger et al., 2014).

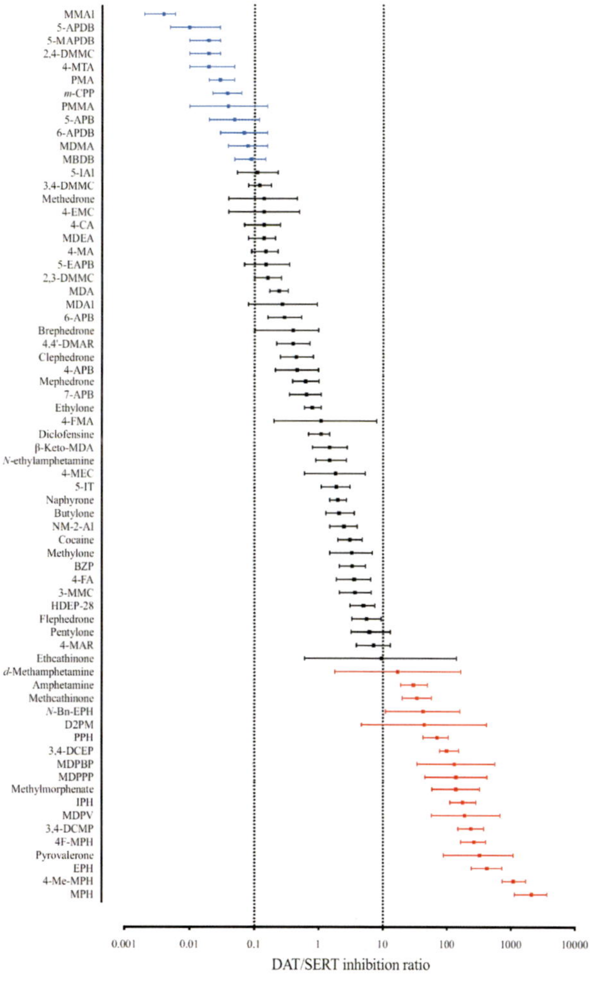

Figure 3.1. Dopamine transporter (DAT) vs. serotonin transporter (SERT) selectivity of a variety of stimulants. Stimulants with low (< 0.1) DAT/SERT ratios are likely to induce entactogenic MDMA-like effects, while substances with a high (> 10) DAT/SERT ratio are associated with distinct psychostimulant effects and a high abuse potential. The DAT/SERT ratio is expressed as 1/DAT IC_{50}: 1/SERT IC_{50}. Full names of the substances and source of pharmacological data are provided in the supplementary information

Source: https://www.ncbi.nlm.nih.gov/pmc/articles/PMC7225206/bin/204_2020_2693_Fig1_HTML.jpg

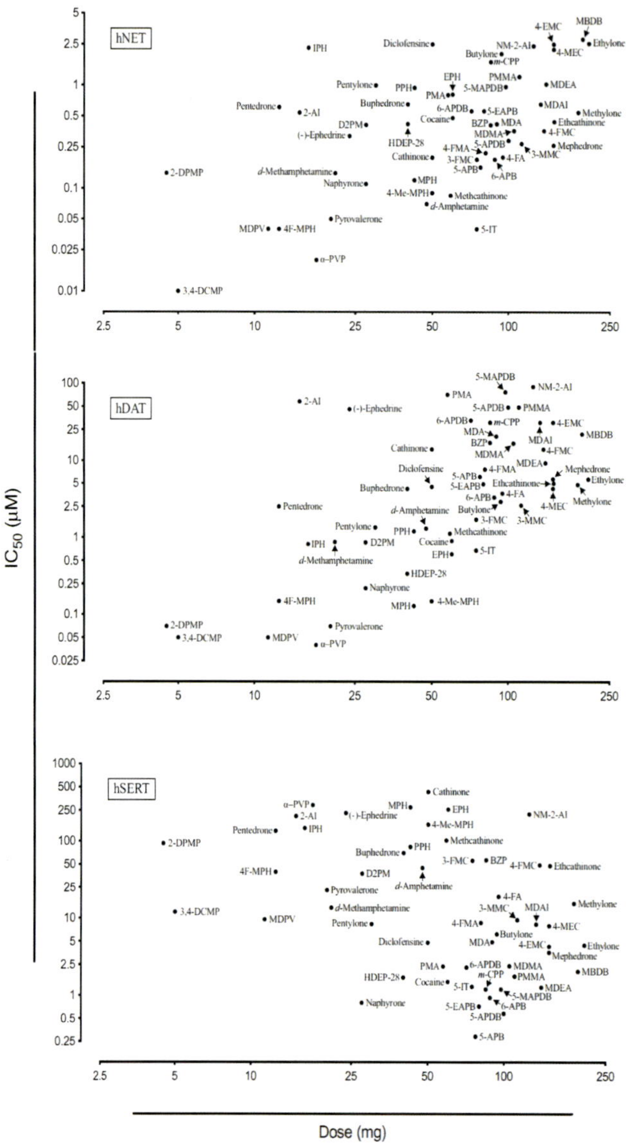

Figure 3.2. Correlation between reported clinical potencies and in vitro monoamine transporter inhibition of a variety of stimulants.

Source: https://www.ncbi.nlm.nih.gov/pmc/articles/PMC7225206/bin/204_2020_2693_Fig2_HTML.jpg

Amphetamines

Apart from the conventional amphetamines used for medical and recreational purposes, a number of amphetamine designer drugs that have no approved medical use have also become accessible. The most widely used amphetamine designer drug is without a doubt MDMA. It wasn't until many years later that Merck synthesized it for the first time in 1912 as a precursor in a novel chemical pathway. Following its introduction into psychotherapy in the 1980s, MDMA gained popularity as a recreational drug known by the street name "ecstasy," which quickly resulted in its outlawing in the majority of nations. Reintroduced gradually, MDMA shows promise as a treatment for posttraumatic stress disorder in psychotherapy. Lately, a range of additional amphetamine derivatives, frequently with ring substitutions (Figure 3.3), have become more and more well-known as designer drugs, many of which were first made available lawfully.

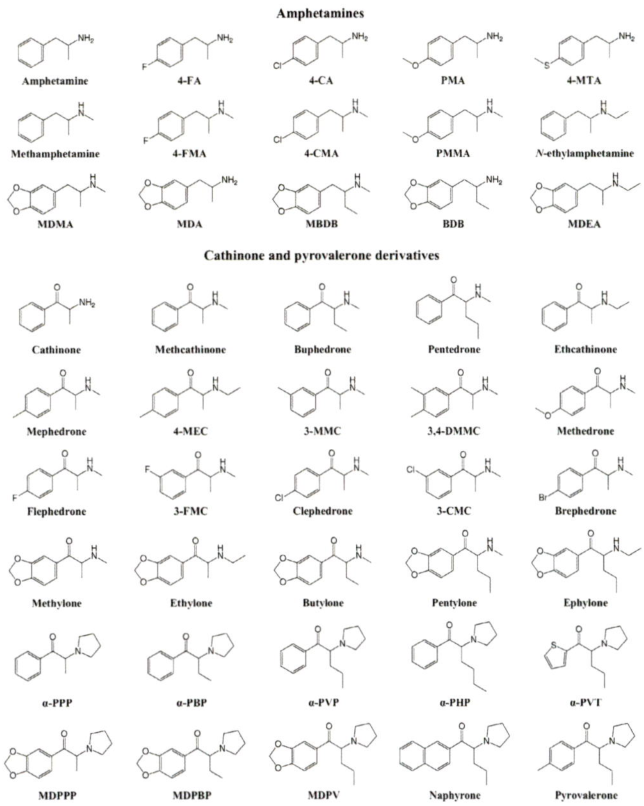

Figure 3.3. Examples of amphetamine, cathinone, and pyrovalerone derivatives. Full names of the substances are provided in the supplementary information.

Source: https://www.ncbi.nlm.nih.gov/pmc/articles/PMC7225206/bin/204_2020_2693_Fig3_HTML.jpg

Cathinone and Pyrovalerone Derivatives

Designer drugs containing cathinone are derived from the alkaloid cathinone (β-keto-amphetamine) present in the leaves of the Catha edulis plant. While some of the compounds have long been known, the widespread recreational use of synthetic cathinones is a relatively recent development. A number of other synthetic cathinones have been studied for their medicinal uses, primarily as anorectic or antidepressant drugs, but only a small number were ever put on the market due to abuse concerns. Based on the structure of pyrovalerone, a synthetic cathinone that was created in the 1960s as a treatment for obesity, exhaustion, and lethargy, pyrovalerone derivatives are a subgroup of cathinones. The term "bath salts" is still frequently used to refer to synthetic cathinones due to their initial deceptive marketing (Kudo et al., 2015). At the moment, artificial cathinones (Figure 3.3). The European Monitoring Center for Drugs and Drug Addiction (EMCDDA) keeps an eye on the majority of designer stimulants.

Benzofuran and indole derivatives

Several designer drugs have been developed that are analogs of MDMA and its metabolite 3,4-methylenedioxyamphetamine (MDA). In these analogs, the benzodioxole group is substituted with a dihydrobenzofuran, benzofuran, or indole group (Figure 3.4).

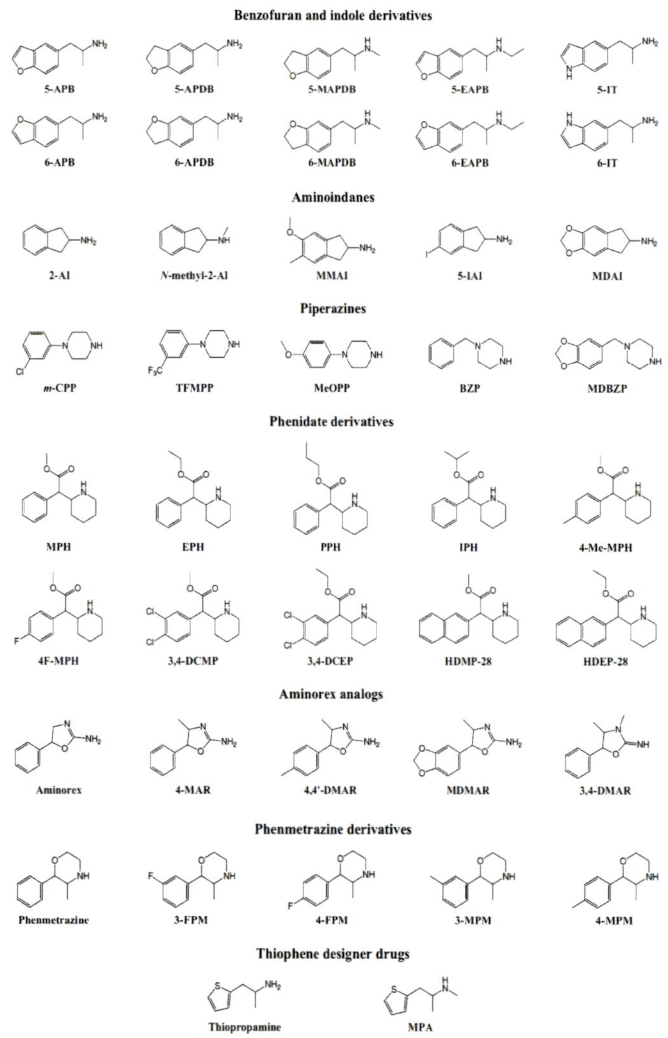

Figure 3.4. Examples of stimulant designer drugs and reference substances. Full names of the substances are provided in the supplementary information.

Source: https://www.ncbi.nlm.nih.gov/pmc/articles/PMC7225206/bin/204_2020_2693_Fig4_HTML.jpg

A study that looked at the function of ring oxygen atoms in interactions between MDA and monoamine transporters initially included an investigation into certain benzofuran designer drugs. The positional isomers of the psychedelic tryptamine α-methyltryptamine (αMT) are 5-(2-aminopropyl)indole (5-IT, 5-API) and 6-(2-aminopropyl)indole (6-IT, 6-API), which are indole designer drugs that originated from industrial research.

Aminoindanes

Designer pharmaceuticals containing aminoindane (Figure 3.4) have become extensively accessible since the first-generation designer stimulants—such as mephedrone—were eventually subject to regulatory oversight. Aminoindanes, which are conformationally restricted analogs of amphetamine, were first studied for their potential as bronchodilatory, analgesic, and anti-Parkinson drugs. Later, they were found to have potential therapeutic benefits. Compared to entactogens that do not contain aminoindane, certain aminoindane designer drugs have been found to have reduced serotonergic neurotoxicity. The intended psychoactive effects of designer drugs containing aminoindanes include euphoria, a slight distorting of time, space, and vision, intensified color perception, empathy, and arousal.

Piperazines

Designer drugs with piperazine (Figure 3.4), due to their somewhat MDMA-like pharmacological profile, either alone or in combination, have been sold extensively as legal party pills or powders and have shown up as pure substances or adulterants in pills that are sold as "ecstasy." The piperazine moiety is present in many therapeutic medications, and certain piperazine-designer drugs have been used in medicine in the past (Kudo et al., 2015). For instance, meta-chlorophenylpiperazine (m-CPP), an active metabolite of several antidepressants, and 1-benzylpiperazine (BZP), which has been studied as an antihelmintic and antidepressant. Trifluoromethylphenylpiperazine (TFMPP), 1-(3,4-methylenedioxybenzyl)piperazine (MDBZP), and 4-methoxyphenylpiperazine (MeOPP) are other commonly used piperazine designer drugs.

Phenidate derivatives

Designer drugs have emerged that are variations of the piperidine prescription medication methylphenidate (Figure 3.4), with phenyl ring substitutions and varying carbon side chain lengths. Phenidate derivatives, like methylphenidate, have the potential to produce euphoria and improve cognition. Many methylphenidate-based designer drugs were developed as part of drug development projects and later made their way onto the recreational drug market either as pure compounds or as branded goods. Since methylphenidate has a similar pharmacological and subjective effect profile to cocaine when inhaled, phenidate derivatives can be used as cocaine replacements.

Aminorex analogs

As designer drugs, several analogs of the anorectic agent aminorex are now accessible (Figure 3.4). In certain regions of Europe, aminorex was initially sold as an over-the-counter appetite suppressant in the 1960s. However, it was taken off the market a few years later due to an epidemic of chronic pulmonary hypertension that was linked to numerous fatalities.

4-methylaminorex (4-MAR) and 4,4′-dimethylaminorex (4,4′-DMAR) are two examples of aminorex analogs that have made their way onto the designer drug market. These compounds have been linked to euphoria, physical and mental stimulation, sociability, empathy, arousal, and changes in visual perception. A thorough analysis of the development of designer drug analogs to aminorex and its usage history was just released.

Phenmetrazine derivatives

The reinforcing stimulant phenmetrazine was taken off the market after it was found to be ineffective as an appetite suppressant. Phenmetrazine-derived designer drugs (Figure 3.4) constitute a comparatively unexplored class of pharmaceuticals, with 3-fluorophenmetrazine (3-FPM) usage appearing to be the most common. Phenmetrazine derivatives with ring fluorination, like the parent compound, exhibit minor substrate activity at the SERT but are substrates at the NET and DAT. It has been reported that ring-methylated phenmetrazine derivatives exhibit increased potency at the SERT, as well as activity at the NET and DAT. Like ring-substituted amphetamine and cathinone designer drugs, para-substituted compounds were shown to have the strongest serotonergic effects among the phenmetrazine derivatives (Kueppers and Cooke, 2015).

A stimulatory toxicity akin to amphetamines is anticipated from designer drugs containing phenmetrazine, based on their mechanism of action. Within the framework of the Swedish STRIDA project, a number of non-fatal intoxications involving 3-FPM were documented, the majority of which had adverse sympathomimetic reactions (Krueger et al., 2014).

Yet, polydrug intoxication made it impossible to attribute the effects that were seen to 3-FPM, as evidenced by the clinical features' inclusion of certain opposing effects (however, because one-third of patients experienced severe adverse events, including both miotic and dilated pupils, hypertension, and hypotension), the authors of this case series concluded that 3-FPM is a dangerous substance. There have been reports of severe kidney damage and limb ischemia linked to intravenous 3-FPM use, in addition to other polydrug intoxications involving the drug. In the case report that was published later, the authors postulated that the intravenous administration of 3-FPM caused widespread ischemia and severe vasoconstriction, potentially along with concurrent infection.

Thiophene designer drugs

Designer drugs have emerged in the form of several amphetamine and cathinone analogs that have a thiophene group in place of the phenyl ring (Figure 3.4).

When thiophene designer drugs were initially introduced in the 1940s, they were said to produce effects similar to those of their phenyl ring analogs. To date, methiopropamine, a thiophene analog of methamphetamine, has been the subject of the majority of pharmacological investigations and toxicological reports.

3.4 Designer Drugs: Assessment and Management

Concern over synthetic analogs of controlled substances being produced and sold to get around drug laws and avoid interdiction is spreading globally. Referred to as "designer drugs" or "legal highs," these substances are (see Table 3.1).

These are drugs that have psychotropic effects and are purposefully sold and distributed for recreational use by taking advantage of gaps in the law governing controlled substances. Nonchemists can directly obtain the synthetic compounds or easily synthesize those using easily accessible raw materials. Chemicals are frequently packaged with labels that misrepresent the contents of the product, which can differ greatly in terms of concentration and chemical content. In an effort to reduce legal risk, labels frequently state, "not for human consumption." The use of designer drugs has increased over the past ten years, particularly among young adults, and for some users, this has resulted in serious issues.

Table 3.1. Designer drugs

Drug class	Chemical name	Chemical origin	Slang names
Stimulant	Mephedrone	Cathinone	Bath salts (Ivory Wave, Vanilla Sky), meow-meow, M-Cat
	Methylone		
	Methylenedioxypyrovalerone (MDPV)		Sextacy
	Naphyrone		NRG-1
Cannabinoid	JWH-018; JWH-073; JWH-250	Laboratory of J.W. Huffman	Spice, K2, K9, Aroma, herbal highs, Scooby Snax
	CP 47,497; CP 47,497-C8; CP 59,540; cannabicyclohexanol	Pfizer laboratory	
	HU-210	Hebrew University laboratory	
	UR-144	CB2 receptor agonist	
	Oleamide	Fatty acid	
	XLR-11, AKB-48		
	AM-2201, AM-694		
Hallucinogen	25I-NBOMe	Free University of Berlin	N-bomb, Solaris, Smiles, Cimbi-5
	25B-NBOMe		
	25C-NBOMe		

Source: https://www.ncbi.nlm.nih.gov/pmc/articles/PMC4422150/

Epidemiology of Emerging Designer Drugs

The majority of young adults who use designer drugs are men in their mid-to late-20s, though the age range for this group includes teens and adults 40 years of age. Designer drug users are typically unmarried, with lower incomes and educational levels. Certain subpopulations, like regular cannabis users, college students, and nightclub-goers, may use synthetic cannabinoids (SC) products more frequently. In 2011 and 2012, the annual prevalence of SC consumption among seniors in high school was 11%. With the exception of cannabis, which has constant yearly use, annual prevalence rates among high school seniors fell to 8% in 2013. Despite this decline, the drug remained more common than all other illicit substances. Bath salt use, at 1% in the same sample, seems to be somewhat less common than SC. The epidemiology of synthetic hallucinogens is not currently included in national surveys, and overall hallucinogen use in the US is still very low.

The rising acceptance of designer drugs can be attributed to various factors, including novelty, accessibility, and marketing. Designer drug packaging is eye-catching and colorful, and the product names are meant to entice younger people to try them. Because designer drugs are sold without age restrictions, younger people find them appealing as well. Widespread accessibility, including online shopping, has led to increased use. Marketing designer drug products as "legal high" substitutes could help create the impression that they are safer or purer than traditional illegal drugs, which could lead to a rise in usage. Teens involved in foster care or the criminal justice system are also at risk. Risk factors for teenage experimentation with and problems stemming from designer drug use include parents with SUDs, poor family relationships, poor discipline, or high family conflict. A number of state and federal initiatives that forbid the production, distribution, and ownership of numerous designer compounds have been implemented in recent years in response to the growing use of designer drugs and their associated consequences. Despite regulatory efforts, the use of designer drugs has continued, but there may be a national trend toward lower consumption of some of these drugs. In certain groups, such as the US military, use seems to be increasing; this could be due to a desire to avoid being caught by urine drug tests. The use of designer drugs is particularly common among substance-abusing military personnel (Kueppers and Cooke, 2015). Many times, patients who come in to see the consequences of designer drug use use more than one drug.

3.4.1 Bath salts

Pharmacology

The active ingredient in most designer stimulants is cathinone, which is the main alkaloid found in the herbal stimulant khat (Catha edulis). Mephedrone, methylenedioxypyrovalerone (MDPV), and methylone are three of the main substituted cathinones marketed as bath salts. A larger family of stimulants that includes amphetamine, methamphetamine, and (MDMA, or "ecstasy") includes the designer-substituted cathinones. Through the facilitation of extracellular release and reuptake inhibition, substituted cathinones appear to increase extracellular levels of the monoamine neurotransmitters serotonin, norepinephrine, and dopamine. Similar sympathomimetic, subjective, and reinforcing effects of the substituted cathinones are probably explained by these neurochemical effects. Similar to stimulants like amphetamines and cocaine, the pharmacology and product effects (like tachycardia, increased alertness, and potential for psychosis) seem to be present.

Acute clinical effects

The majority of designer stimulants are administered intravenously, though they can also be taken orally, intramuscularly, or intravenously. Smoking mephedrone is not recommended. Anecdotally, the effects seem to peak 45-90 minutes after dosing, begin to wear off after 2-3 hours, and then gradually diminish over the next 6–12 hours. To extend the desired effects of a session, users may take more than one dose. Increased energy, alertness, concentration, sexual stimulation, empathy, talkativeness, mood enhancement, euphoria, and decreased appetite are popularly reported effects that overlap with cocaine, amphetamine, and MDMA.

Adverse psychiatric effects

The majority of users report sporadic negative effects. Acute toxicity has been linked to higher binge eating and multiple substance exposure. Acute agitation is a defining feature of poisoning. Patients may have severe psychosis, characterized by delusions, hallucinations (mainly visual), and paranoia. Tolerance to substituted cathinone is probably brought on by repeated dosing, as suggested by the correlation between increased amount and frequency of use. Mephedrone binges involving large consecutive doses have been documented. Chronic users have reported experiencing tiredness, insomnia, agitation, depression, and congestion in their nasal passages as withdrawal symptoms. Some users develop compulsive use and cravings associated with the dependence syndrome. The risk of developing a severe, diagnosable SUD from long-term substitution use of cathinone is relatively high (Krueger et al., 2014).

Adverse physiologic effects

The number of stimulant/sympathomimetic-related toxicology cases reported annually doubled from 6% in 2010 to 12% in 2011, with bath salts playing a major role in this increase. Effects like diaphoresis, palpitations, tense or spasming muscles, and bruxism (clenching of the jaw) are frequently reported. The majority of people display autonomic hyperactivity during exams (e.g., tachycardia, high blood pressure). Nasal side effects include sore throats, mouths, and nasal passages, as well as epistaxis. Clinical signs of sympathomimetic toxicity include neurological and cardiovascular symptoms. Bath salt use has been linked to myocarditis and cardiac arrhythmias. Similar to MDMA, significant hyponatremia has been linked to mephedrone use. This is probably because of a combination of sweating, electrolyte loss, and antidiuretic hormone secretion. More severe renal impairments include rhabdomyolysis-associated acute renal failure and acidosis. Mephedrone and MDPV have been linked to fatalities in reports.

Contaminants may have negative effects in addition to those caused by cathinones. Studies on product analysis have shown that substances like cocaine, amphetamine, ketamine, lidocaine, procaine, caffeine, and even piperazine compounds are adulterated. Stimulant-containing adulterants may intensify the effects of bath salts and increase the risk of toxicity by boosting the sympathetic nervous system's effects or the likelihood of cardiac arrhythmias. There is a paucity of empirical or prospective data on the long-term detrimental physiological effects of using substituted cathinones. Nonetheless, neurotoxicity makes sense (e.g., neuronal degeneration, monoamine depletion), as well as the emergence of physiological dependence in frequent users, which is characterized by tolerance and withdrawal symptoms.

3.4.2 Synthetic Cannabinoids

Pharmacology

The principal cannabinoid found in cannabis is delta-9-tetrahydrocannabinol (THC), which functions as a partial agonist at the CB1 receptor found in all parts of the body, particularly the central nervous system. Full or partial CB1 agonists, which are used recreationally, were first created in various university laboratories for research purposes. Many times, single or combinations of distinct SC compounds are sprayed onto virtually unknown amounts of psychoactively inert ground plant matter to mimic incense or potpourri. These products are used recreationally. Currently, regardless of branding, all products containing SC are referred to as "Spice.". In comparison to THC, SCs are frequently more effective and potent CB1 agonists, and they may also have a longer half-life, all of which could increase the toxicity of cannabinomimetics. The wide concentration ranges and significant compositional variability of SC in products can further increase the risk of toxicity.

Acute clinical effects

Intranasally or orally ingested, SCs are usually smoked using a joint, bowl, or water pipe. Acute effects such as tachycardia, conjunctival injection, and mood alteration are similar to those of cannabis. Most effects seem to fade 2–6 hours after use, with some reports stating that effects begin as soon as 10 minutes after inhalation.

Adverse Psychiatric Effects

When using SC products, adverse psychological effects are frequently experienced. These effects can include anxiety, difficulty thinking clearly, agitation, paranoia, and delusions. According to reports, SC can exacerbate pre-existing chronic psychotic disorders and cause acute psychosis, which is more common in users who have a family history of psychosis or underlying biological vulnerability. In documented cases, psychotic symptoms have been known to last anywhere from one week to five months. Some frequent cannabis users may use SC instead of THC to ease the symptoms of cannabis withdrawal; this is most likely a sign of cross-tolerance between the two compounds. SCs seem to be an adequate cannabis replacement, particularly in situations where cannabis is not accessible. Case studies have shown that using SC products can cause dependence syndrome and withdrawal symptoms that are comparable to those experienced with cannabis.

3.4.3 Adverse Physiologic Effects

Heaviness, dizziness, and dry mouth are among the most often reported side effects. Dystonia, dyspnea, tremors, and diaphoresis are additional undesirable physiological side effects. Similar to cannabis users, tachycardia is frequently experienced when using SC; this is probably not because of a direct sympathetic effect, but rather because of decreased peripheral vascular resistance and the ensuing need to sustain cardiac output by faster heartbeat. Along with hypertension and chest pain, the tachycardia could be quite severe. Also documented is a case of severe bradycardia accompanied by chest pain. Cannabinoid hyperemesis syndrome is a chronic disorder initially observed in chronic cannabis users who experienced cyclic episodes of vomiting and abdominal pain relieved by bathing or showering in hot water. These episodes have been linked to several SC compounds, specifically JWH-018, JWH-073, and AM-2201. Yet, hyperemesis syndrome associated with cannabis use is extremely uncommon. These symptoms could aid in distinguishing between the two types of intoxication to the extent that nausea and vomiting may be more common in SC.

Seizures, acute renal failure, and myocardial infarction are examples of severe SC-related toxicity that has required emergency care. Deaths from heart attacks and suicide brought on by severe anxiety have been linked to SC. The long-term effects of SC have not been studied. Several sources advise vaporization over smoking as a method of delivering cannabinoids because smoking SC products exposes smokers to burned plant material and SC, both of which may have negative effects on the respiratory system. Furthermore, anecdotal evidence suggests that prolonged use of JWH-018 can cause tolerance and withdrawal symptoms, raising the possibility that it is a carcinogen (Krueger et al., 2014).

3.4.4 Synthetic Hallucinogens

Pharmacology

Following the 1991 release of Alexander Shulgin's book PIHKAL, A Chemical Love Story, synthetic designer hallucinogens became increasingly popular. "Phenethylamines I Have Known and Loved," or PIHKAL, is an acronym that describes the synthesis of more than 200 hallucinogenic substances. The term "2C" refers to the two carbon molecules that are positioned between the amino group and the benzene ring in the series of hallucinogenic phenethylamines that Shulgin originally described. These substances stimulate serotonergic receptors to cause hallucinations; their structures are similar to those of MDMA. From the 2C series of phenethylamines, the substituted phenethylamine 4-iodo-2,5dimethoxy-N-(2-methoxybenzyl) phenethylamine (25I-NBOMe) is a relatively new derivative. One of the many N-benzyl phenethylamines that have gained popularity since October 2011 is 25I-NBOMe. S. Many of the chemicals sold as bath salts have been temporarily placed on Schedule I by the Drug Enforcement Administration. Originally created for serotonin receptor research, 25I-NBOMe is a highly effective, high-affinity agonist of the serotonin 2a (5HT2a) receptor. Additional NBOMe drugs that cause hallucinations are 25C-NBOMe and 25B-NBOMe.

Acute clinical effects

There have been reports of the use of 25I-NBOMe in both liquid and powder form. There are numerous possible ways to administer this medication, such as by inhaling vapors, insufflation of the nose, oral ingestion, sublingual/buccal administration, and intravenous injection. The most typical applications are buccal, sublingual, and oral; nasal insufflation is also not unheard of. When 25I-NBOMe is administered orally or through the oral mucosal route, it is absorbed as a powder or on blotter paper. The medication is usually taken once in a tiny dose of approximately 0.1 grams, or "cap." "After nasal use, clinical effects can happen quickly and usually peak in 20 minutes." Reports indicate a broad range of action duration, ranging from 3 to 13 hours. Agitation lasted for several days in cases of clinical toxicity that were reported. According to reports, 25I-NBOMe has effects akin to those of classic serotonergic hallucinogens like psilocybin or lysergic acid diethylamide. Consumers report experiencing varied degrees of stimulation during hallucinations. There have also been reports of depersonalization. Compared to traditional serotonergic hallucinogens, 25I-NBOMe was found to have more "negative effects while high" but better "value for money," according to 442 respondents to an online survey.

Adverse psychiatric effects

Many users experience psychiatric consequences in addition to the expected visual and auditory hallucinations, which lead them to seek medical attention. Delirium, agitation, aggression, violence, paranoia, dysphoria, extreme confusion, and self-harm are a few of these effects. A serotonergic or sympathetic toxidrome that includes an "excited delirium" and extreme agitation, aggression, and violence has been observed in certain patients. In one instance, a 19-year-old man who was supposedly naïve to hallucinogens perished in a multi-story fall after consuming 25I-NBOMe and exhibiting strange and paranoid behavior. In a different tragic instance, a male driver, age 21, who had consumed 25I-NBOMe, became extremely angry, drove his car off the road, and started destroying the interior of the car before passing away from an unidentified illness.

Adverse physiologic effects

The few clinical reports of 25I-NBOMe users often describe tachycardia, hypertension, and mydriasis. Numerous cases have also been reported involving hyperreflexia and clonus. Many of the cases involved seizures that eventually necessitated medical attention. Severe toxicity has resulted in pulmonary edema, trauma-related death, and hyperthermia. In one instance of a fatal exposure, a 15-year-old girl consumed 25I-NBOMe outside of a rave and went into unconsciousness. When she arrived at a nearby hospital, her rectal temperature was 39.9°C, indicating asystole. The physiological long-term effects are unknown.

3.4.5 Drug Testing Challenges

Clinicians face a significant diagnostic and monitoring challenge because not all designer drugs can be detected by urine or serum toxicology screens. The majority of clinical practice settings and laboratories do not currently offer widespread, standardized designer drug testing, despite the fact that laboratory testing is growing. Heterogeneity in the contents, concentration, and chemical constituents of designer drug products—all of which can differ between and within products—complicates the analytical task. In order to avoid regulation and detection, illicit manufacturers have shown an extraordinary degree of adaptability in manipulating the psychoactive ingredients of designer drugs. To get around legal restrictions, drug designers frequently modify functional groups, substitute substances, and change the moieties of substances in a quick and iterative process. Urine drug screening presents serious difficulties in detecting compounds or their metabolites as a result of this practice.

People often state that they use designer drug products because they are not detected by routine urine drug tests. For instance, people under the supervision of the criminal justice system might use designer drugs to avoid being discovered by probation officials. SCs are used by US military personnel who want the same mood-altering effects as cannabis but at a much lower risk of being caught. Most soldiers referred for addiction treatment are identified through urine drug testing. Urine collection is still useful clinically to test for unreported, co-occurring substance use, even though most emerging designer drugs will not be detected on a routine urine drug screening in a healthcare setting. To check for common drugs of abuse, a general laboratory screening battery of urine or serum should be sent. This aids in the clinician's awareness of possible toxicity resulting from drug interactions or the necessity of more frequent or intensive monitoring owing to the presence of non-designer substances. Understanding the most popular designer drugs and other substances of abuse in a particular area can help clinicians quickly identify intoxication and start managing serious complications when comprehensive designer drug testing is not available or is taking time.

3.4.6 Screening and Assessment

Detecting designer drug use can be challenging, as they are not typically picked up on routine drug screens. This is especially important to keep in mind when treating young adults seeking emergency medical care, as they are the most common demographic for designer drug-related incidents. Therefore, clinicians should directly inquire about designer drug use when treating young adults with symptoms of substance-related toxicity. Just because routine drug tests come back negative for illicit substances doesn't mean designer drugs weren't involved, as polysubstance use is common in this population. Clinicians should be aware of any inconsistencies in symptoms or behavior that could indicate recent designer drug use.

Based on differences in patient presentation, clinicians can be on the lookout for clinical clues that could indicate the use of designer drugs (see Table 3.2). Conjunctival injection and other cannabis products are markers of a state of intoxication in SC. It is possible that some patients who arrive for emergency care still have the package containing the designer medication. This can be checked to see if any common brand names for a particular class of designer drugs can be identified (refer to Table 3.1), and any leftover material may be sent to a lab for examination. Because substances can change their appearance quickly, websites can be useful for identifying the specific substances that have been consumed. However, a variety of websites that may or may not offer accurate information have emerged as a result of the lack of research-based information regarding the negative effects of designer drugs Kueppers and Cooke, 2015). The use of designer drugs or other smokable drugs may be indicated by the presence of smoking paraphernalia like a pipe, and a strong perfume or cologne scent may be an attempt to cover up the odor of recent smoking.

Table 3.2. Indicators of designer drug use

Body system	Finding	**Medical indication**	**Drug (s)**
General	Hyperthermia	Intoxication	Synthetic hallucinogens, bath salts
Head & neck	Conjunctival injection	Recent use	Synthetic cannabinoids
	Smoky chemical smell on breath	Recent smoking	Any smoked designer drug
	Epistaxis	Intranasal use	Bath salts, synthetic hallucinogens
	Nasal septal perforation	Intranasal use	Bath salts
	Poor dentition	Inadequate oral hygiene	Bath salts
	Jaw clenching, teeth grinding (bruxism)	Intoxication	Bath salts
Cardiac	Tachycardia	Recent use	Any designer drug
	Hypertension	Recent use	Any designer drug
	Chest pain	Cardiac ischemia, myocarditis	Bath salts, synthetic cannabinoids
Renal	Acute kidney injury	Recent use	Synthetic cannabinoids
Gastrointestinal	Nausea, vomiting	Recent use or withdrawal syndrome	Synthetic cannabinoids
	Enlarged and/or tender liver	Acute hepatitis	Any injected designer drug
Musculoskeletal	Muscle spasms	Intoxication	Bath salts
	Limb swelling and pain	Rhabdomyolysis	Bath salts, synthetic hallucinogens
Skin	Diaphoresis	Recent use	Bath salts
	Ecchymosis	Recent use or intoxication	Synthetic hallucinogens
	Fresh needle marks, track marks	Injection drug use	Any injected designer drug
Neurologic	Clonus	Recent use	Synthetic hallucinogens
	Seizures	Intoxication	Bath salts, synthetic hallucinogens, synthetic cannabinoids
Psychiatric	Agitation	Recent use	Any designer drug
	Hallucinations	Recent use	Any designer drug
	Psychosis	Intoxication	Any designer drug

Source: https://www.ncbi.nlm.nih.gov/pmc/articles/PMC4422150/

It is probably wise to routinely inquire about the use of designer drugs, especially in patients who have a history of SUD, those undergoing required urine testing (e.g., supervisors in criminal justice), or among individuals who have disclosed a past usage of designer drugs belonging to a distinct chemical class. Concurrent use of different classes of designer drugs may raise the risk of toxicity and unfavorable effects. Clinicians should ask patients about specific products by name or about "synthetics" in general, as patients might not be aware of the terms used by medical professionals or the various street names for identical products. Ask follow-up questions regarding frequency, usage patterns, and subjective effects for each affirmative response. A thorough investigation into the subjective effects may shed light on the designer drug class, especially in cases where the relationship between the brand and the compound is less clear-cut and has a broad range of contents. Table 3.1, while providing a list of designer drug compounds and classes, does not include all brand names; thousands of different trade-name brands are probably sold worldwide.

Additional clinical research should ask targeted questions concerning the variables linked to the use of designer drugs and the possible outcomes, such as health issues, interpersonal conflicts, financial difficulties, or legal issues. Chronic designer drug use can result in both a designer drug use disorder and physiologic dependence with tolerance and withdrawal associated with cessation. Thorough investigation of these aspects pertaining to the patient's designer drug use aids in the clinician's preliminary assessment of the condition and sheds light on the necessity of treatment. Routine laboratory testing should include a complete blood cell count and complete metabolic panel in addition to standardized urine drug testing for patients presenting with acute medical complications of designer drug use. If there are cardiac symptoms, cardiac enzymes should be ordered. If rhabdomyolysis is suspected due to severe muscle spasms, pain and swelling in the extremities, or severe seizures, creatine phosphokinase can be beneficial. Depending on the initial presentation, more diagnostic tests might be chosen.

3.4.7 Management of Acute Intoxication

The toxicity of designer drugs does not have a specific antidote. A significant oral ingestion is required before activated charcoal can be used. After receiving supportive treatment, the majority of nonpsychiatric symptoms seem to be self-limited and go away in a few days. Supportive therapy can help control unpleasant psychological consequences of acute intoxication, such as agitation, paranoia, or anxiety. Until the acute effects wear off, it's usually enough to place the distressed user in a quiet place and maintain gentle touch. Suspended observation has been used to treat intoxication with 25I-NBOMe and psychosis caused by SCBs. Anxiety, agitation, and seizures have been treated with benzodiazepines for psychopathological clinical features. Owing to the lowered seizure threshold caused by the use of designer drugs such as phenethylamine and cathinone, antipsychotics are considered second-line treatments for agitation. Should the patient be extremely agitated and a danger to themselves or medical personnel, sedation might be necessary. In particular, for those with persistent symptoms, psychiatric consultation is recommended, as some designer drug-associated psychoses may be severe and necessitate extended inpatient treatment.

Since abrupt cessation of stimulants or hallucinogens does not result in severe physiological side effects, during medically supervised withdrawal, they are not tapered off or substituted with a cross-tolerant medication. When abruptly stopping SC, withdrawal symptoms like nausea and irritability can occur, just like when quitting cannabis. On the other hand, there is no need for pharmaceutical replacement (e.g., dronabinol), as the withdrawal from SC poses no risk to life. In order to provide supportive care, patients may require intravenous fluids and, if necessary, antiemetics. In the event that the patient experiences significant psychological symptoms that last for more than a week after stopping the medication, a thorough evaluation is necessary to ascertain whether the patient has a primary mental illness that co-occurs and needs to be treated with specialized therapy (Kronstrand et al., 2014). Prolonged anxiety, depression, or psychosis are treated in the same way as if there has been no recent use of designer drugs.

A significant number of critically ill patients require admission to the intensive care unit. Intoxicated patients should undergo continuous cardiac monitoring, pulse oximetry, and frequent neurological assessments. It is important to administer intravenous fluids to maintain adequate urine output and prevent dehydration, especially in patients with rhabdomyolysis, to avoid acute renal failure. Intensive monitoring is crucial for early detection and intervention in cases of serious consequences, such as myocardial infarction. Patients may have ingested multiple drugs with varying pharmacological profiles, including stimulants and depressants. Clinicians should be vigilant for unexpected reactions to treatment or changes in patient condition as different designer drugs take effect. Flexibility in treatment strategies may be necessary to address changes in mental and cardiovascular status.

A Closer Look

Law for Designer Drugs

Since many designer drugs have emerged recently, there are currently no laws restricting or outlawing their use. In certain cases, new drugs have emerged in direct response to legislative action, taking the place of a similar substance that had recently been outlawed. Many of the chemicals are governed by different drug analog laws in different countries. However, the majority of countries lack general analog acts or comparable laws, so novel compounds may become illegal even with slight structural changes. The Controlled Substance Analogue Enforcement of 1986 amended the Controlled Substances Act in the United States in an attempt to outlaw designer drugs ahead of time by outlawing the production, distribution, or possession of chemicals that were strikingly similar in chemistry and pharmacology to Schedule I or Schedule II drugs.

Other nations have approached the problem in different ways. In certain countries, like Germany, Canada, the United Kingdom, and Sweden, new drugs are outlawed as soon as they cause problems. If the police believe that the purpose of the holding is connected to drug abuse, they have the authority to seize drugs that are not on the list of substances covered by the anti-drug laws in Sweden. Police have the option to destroy drugs they have seized, subject to a prosecutor's decision. The Criminal Justice (Psychoactive Substances) Act 2010 was enacted in Ireland as a catch-all to address the gap in time between the introduction of new substances and their individual prohibition. It prohibits substances based on their psychoactive effect. A similar strategy is used in the UK by the Psychoactive Substances Act of 2016. Certain nations, like Australia, have implemented generic drug prohibitions that are based more on chemical structure than psychoactive effect. A chemical is prohibited if it satisfies a set of requirements pertaining to changes and substitutions of previously banned drugs. In an ANVISA ruling issued recently, Brazil followed Australia's lead in defining what constitutes a drug.

Summary

- A designer drug is a structural or functional analog of a controlled substance that has been designed to mimic the pharmacological effects of the original drug while avoiding classification as illegal and/or detection in standard drug tests.
- The development of designer drugs may be considered a subfield of drug design. The exploration of modifications to known active drugs—such as their structural analogs, stereoisomers, and derivatives—yields drugs that may differ significantly in effects from their "parent" drug (e.g., showing increased potency or decreased side effects).
- Designer drugs are synthetic compounds developed to mimic the physiologic effects of other abused drugs. Many designer drugs are chemically similar to other abused drugs but are modified to avoid being classified as illegal.
- Designer doping agents have become increasingly popular outside of the professional athletic community and include anabolic steroids, peptide hormones, growth factor mimetics, and hormone and metabolic modulators.
- Hospitalization for the adverse effects of designer drugs affords an excellent opportunity (teachable moment) for advising patients to decrease their substance use and for engaging them in treatment. Healthcare provider awareness and patient education are cornerstones of public health initiatives to confront new challenges presented by designer drugs.
- Commonly used designer drugs, including synthetic cannabinoids, cathinones, and hallucinogens, exhibit diverse chemical structures and mechanisms of action that contribute to their psychoactive effects on the central nervous system.
- Legislation aimed at controlling the production, distribution, and usage of designer drugs faces significant challenges in keeping pace with rapidly evolving chemical formulations, thereby impacting its effectiveness.
- Designer drugs encompass a wide range of synthetic compounds designed to mimic the effects of traditional illicit substances, and their physiological and psychological effects on users can vary significantly depending on the specific compound, dosage, route of administration, and individual factors.
- Harm reduction approaches aimed at minimizing the risks associated with designer drug use encompass a range of strategies focused on reducing harm to individuals, communities, and society as a whole.
- Designer drug use is most prevalent among young adults, primarily males in their mid to late 20s, but ranging from teens to adults 40 years of age. Those who use designer drugs tend to be single and have lower levels of education and income.

References

1. King LA, Kicman AT. A brief history of 'new psychoactive substances' Drug Test Anal. 2011;3:401–3. doi: 10.1002/dta.319.
2. Johnson LA, Johnson RL, Portier RB. Current "legal highs" J Emerg Med. 2013;44:1108–15. doi: 10.1016/j.jemermed.2012.09.147.

3. Kelly JP. Cathinone derivatives: a review of their chemistry, pharmacology and toxicology. Drug Test Anal. 2011;3:439–53. doi: 10.1002/dta.313.

4. Brandt SD, Sumnall HR, Measham F, Cole J. Analyses of second-generation 'legal highs' in the UK: initial findings. Drug Test Anal. 2010;2:377–82. doi: 10.1002/dta.155.

5. Wiegand TJ, Wax PM, Schwartz T, Finkelstein Y, Gorodetsky R, Brent J. The toxicology investigators consortium case registry—the 2011 experience. J Med Toxicol. 2012;8:360–77. doi: 10.1007/s13181-012-0264-9.

6. Winstock A, Mitcheson L, Ramsey J, Davies S, Puchnarewicz M, Marsden J. Mephedrone: use, subjective effects and health risks. Addiction. 2011;106:1991–6. doi: 10.1111/j.1360-0443.2011.03502.x.

7. Winstock AR, Mitcheson LR, Deluca P, Davey Z, Corazza O, Schifano F. Mephedrone, new kid for the chop? Addiction. 2011;106:154–61. doi: 10.1111/j.1360-0443.2010.03130.x.

8. Spiller HA, Ryan ML, Weston RG, Jansen J. Clinical experience with and analytical confirmation of "bath salts" and "legal highs" (synthetic cathinones) in the United States. Clin Toxicol (Phila) 2011;49:499–505. doi: 10.3109/15563650.2011.590812.

9. Carhart-Harris RL, King LA, Nutt DJ. A web-based survey on mephedrone. Drug Alcohol Depend. 2011;118:19–22. doi: 10.1016/j.drugalcdep.2011.02.011.

10. Hu X, Primack BA, Barnett TE, Cook RL. College students and use of K2: an emerging drug of abuse in young persons. Subst Abuse Treat Prev Policy. 2011;6:16. doi: 10.1186/1747-597X-6-16.

11. Johnston L, O'Malley P, Miech R, Bachman J, Schulenberg J. Monitoring The Future National Survey Results on Drug Use: 1975-2013: Overview, Key Findings on Adolescent Drug Use. Ann Arbor: University of Michigan Institute for Social Research; 2014.

12. Kronstrand R, Thelander G, Lindstedt D, Roman M, Kugelberg FC. Fatal intoxications associated with the designer opioid AH-7921. *J Anal Toxicol.* 2014;38(8):599–604. doi: 10.1093/jat/bku057.

13. Krotulski AJ, Papsun DM, Friscia M, Swartz JL, Holsey BD, Logan BK. Fatality following ingestion of tetrahydrofuranylfentanyl, U-49900 and methoxy-phencyclidine. *J Anal Toxicol.* 2018;42(3):e27–e32. doi: 10.1093/jat/bkx092.

14. Krueger J, Sachs H, Musshoff F, Dame T, Schaeper J, Schwerer M, Graw M, Roider G. First detection of ethylphenidate in human fatalities after ethylphenidate intake. *Forensic Sci Int.* 2014;243:126–129. doi: 10.1016/j.forsciint.2014.07.017.

15. Kudo K, Usumoto Y, Kikura-Hanajiri R, Sameshima N, Tsuji A, Ikeda N. A fatal case of poisoning related to new cathinone designer drugs, 4-methoxy PV8, PV9, and 4-methoxy PV9, and a dissociative agent, diphenidine. *Leg Med (Tokyo)* 2015;17(5):421–426. doi: 10.1016/j.legalmed.2015.06.005.

16. Kueppers VB, Cooke CT. 25I-NBOMe related death in Australia: a case report. *Forensic Sci Int.* 2015;249:e15–e18. doi: 10.1016/j.forsciint.2015.02.010.

Chapter 4

STIMULANTS: AMPHETAMINES AND CATHINONES

Contents

Introduction

A wide range of psychoactive substances are referred to as stimulants because of their capacity to improve alertness, focus, and general cognitive function. Amphetamines and cathinones are two notable classes that have different, though occasionally overlapping, and effects on the central nervous system. A class of synthetic compounds known as amphetamines mainly works by releasing and blocking the reuptake of neurotransmitters like serotonin, norepinephrine, and dopamine. Through this process, these neurotransmitters are more concentrated at the synaptic cleft, which raises arousal, elevates mood, and improves cognitive function. Because of their stimulant qualities, amphetamines have historically been used extensively in the treatment of diseases like obesity, narcolepsy, and attention deficit ADHD. However, because of the possibility of abuse and addiction, their distribution is strictly regulated.

Conversely, catehinones are organically occurring alkaloids present in the native East African and Arabian Peninsula khat plant (*Catha edulis*). Synthetic cathinone derivatives, also known as "bath salts" in underground drug markets, are well-known for having stimulant properties similar to those of amphetamines (Aarde et al., 2015). Similar to amphetamines, but with different potencies and selectivities, catechinones mainly function by increasing the release of dopamine, norepinephrine, and serotonin. Increased energy, improved sociability, and increased feelings of euphoria are the outcomes of this spike in neurotransmitter activity. But with reports of severe adverse reactions and fatalities linked to their use, the relatively recent appearance of synthetic cathinones in black markets has sparked questions about their safety and long-term health effects. Although they have similar pharmacological properties, amphetamines and cathinones differ in terms of their molecular makeup and mode of action. The specific molecular interactions and affinities of the compounds in both classes target different monoamine neurotransmitter systems, which leads to variations in their overall effects and side effect profiles. Furthermore, there are notable differences in the legal and medical standing of these substances. Amphetamines are permitted for therapeutic use under stringent guidelines, while cathinones are primarily categorized as illegal drugs because of their high potential for abuse and lack of recognized medical benefits.

Cathinones and amphetamines are two different but related classes of stimulants that have important applications in medicine and recreational settings. Comprehending the pharmacological characteristics, modes of action, and possible hazards of these substances is imperative for making knowledgeable decisions about their administration and control in medical and social settings (Aarde et al., 2013). Amphetamines can be used therapeutically under medical supervision, but the introduction of synthetic cathinones has brought attention to the problems that new psychoactive substances (NPS) continue to present in today's drug markets and public health initiatives.

Orientation and Directional Terms:

Term	Definition	Illustration
Substances	A substance is a chemical element and its compounds in the natural state or the result of a manufacturing process.	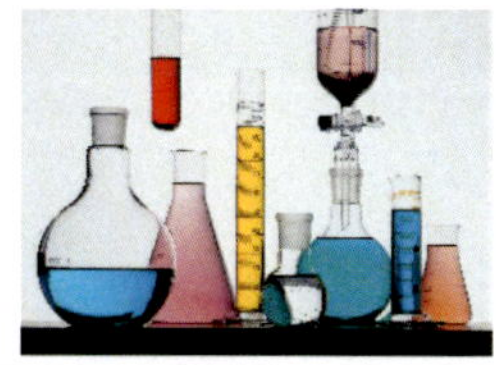
Phenethylamine	Phenethylamine is an organic compound, natural monoamine alkaloid, and trace amine, which acts as a central nervous system stimulant in humans.	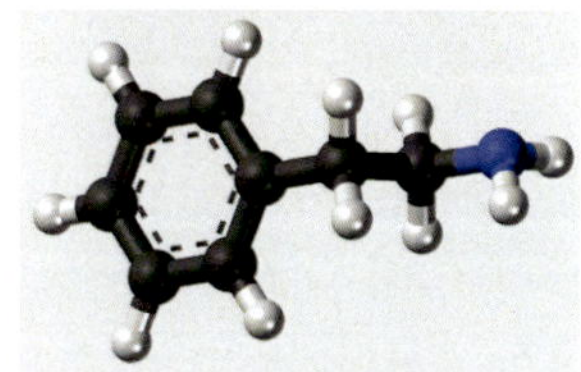
Norepinephrine transporter	The norepinephrine transporter (NET) is a protein that in humans is encoded by the solute carrier family 6 member 2 (SLC6A2) gene.	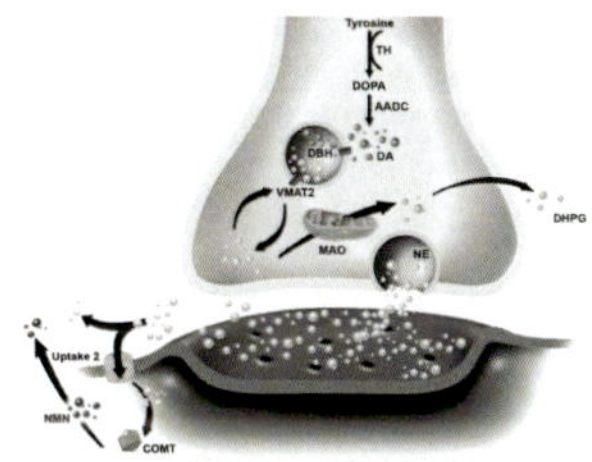
Cathinone	Cathinone is a monoamine alkaloid found in the shrub Catha edulis (khat) and is chemically similar to ephedrine, cathine, methcathinone and other amphetamines.	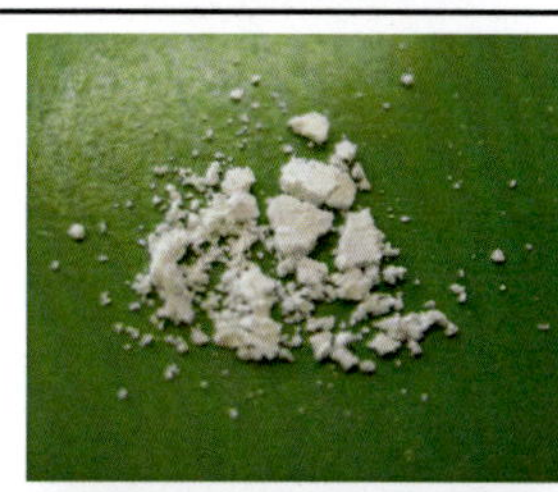
Amphetamine	It is a central nervous system stimulant that is used in the treatment of attention deficit hyperactivity disorder, narcolepsy, and obesity.	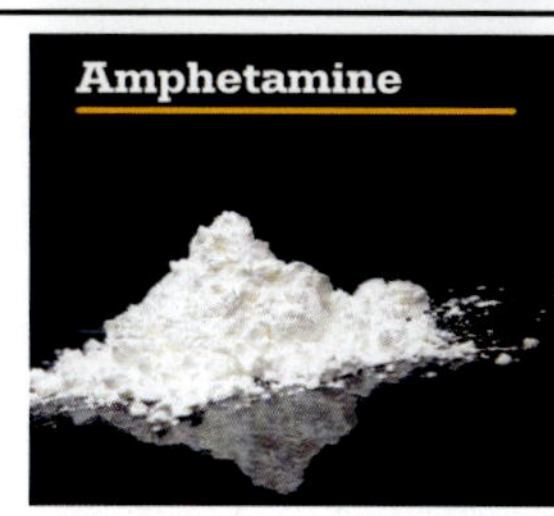

4.1 Chemistry, Pharmacology, and Effects of Amphetamine Derivatives

A wide range of substances with different chemical structures, pharmacological characteristics, and physiological effects are collectively referred to as amphetamine derivatives. Fundamentally, these derivatives are based on the same phenethylamine structure as amphetamine, a central nervous system stimulant that primarily functions by increasing the release and inhibiting the reuptake of monoamine neurotransmitters like serotonin, dopamine, and norepinephrine. Amphetamine derivatives affect mood, cognition, and physiological arousal in various ways by modifying the activity of these neurotransmitter systems.

Amphetamine derivatives are distinguished chemically by changes made to the amphetamine molecule, frequently by substituting it at various points along the phenethylamine scaffold. These changes may have an impact on the compound's potency, duration of action, and selectivity for particular monoamine transporters, among other pharmacokinetic and pharmacodynamic characteristics.

Amphetamine derivatives work pharmacologically by interfering with monoamine transporters, specifically the serotonin transporter (SERT), norepinephrine transporter (NET), and dopamine transporter (DAT). Amphetamine derivatives increase the synaptic concentrations of these neurotransmitters by blocking their reuptake into presynaptic neurons. This results in increased neurotransmission and postsynaptic receptor activation. Furthermore, certain derivatives might enhance synaptic transmission by encouraging the release of neurotransmitters from presynaptic vesicles (Baumann et al., 2013).

Amphetamine derivatives have a wide range of physiological effects, which can change based on dosage, mode of administration, and individual susceptibility. A common combination of side effects is decreased appetite and fatigue with elevated energy, alertness, and euphoria. Pleasure and motivation are the results of these effects, which are mediated by the brain's reward circuitry's dopaminergic and noradrenergic pathways being activated.

Chronic use of amphetamine derivatives, however, can result in tolerance, dependence, and a host of other unfavorable health outcomes. Extended stimulation of monoamine neurotransmitter systems can cause neuroadaptive alterations in the brain, interfere with regular neuronal activity, and exacerbate withdrawal symptoms when drug use is stopped. Long-term use may also lead to cognitive deficits, psychiatric disorders like anxiety and psychosis, and cardiovascular problems.

Clinical medicine has found several therapeutic uses for amphetamine derivatives despite their potential for abuse and negative effects. These include the management of obesity, narcolepsy, and attention deficit ADHD. For people with these conditions, amphetamine derivatives can effectively reduce symptoms and enhance quality of life when used under medical supervision and at the prescribed doses. The complex class of compounds known as amphetamine derivatives has a wide range of physiological, pharmacological, and chemical characteristics. Although they can be therapeutically useful in some medical situations, their widespread misuse and potential for harm make it crucial to comprehend their chemistry, pharmacology, and effects for regulatory and medical purposes (Bonano et al., 2013). Promoting safe and responsible use in clinical practice requires balancing the therapeutic benefits of amphetamine derivatives with the risks of abuse and dependence.

4.2 Synthesis and Structure-Activity Relationships of Cathinones (bath salts)

In the field of synthetic stimulants, the synthesis and structure-activity relationships (SAR) of cathinones, also referred to as bath salts, are a complicated and developing area. Analogs of beta-keto amphetamines and cathinones share structural similarities with the khat plant's naturally occurring alkaloid cathinone. The process of synthesizing cathinones generally entails modifying the amphetamine backbone by substituting different amino acids at different positions to change pharmacological characteristics like potency, duration of action, and selectivity for distinct neurotransmitter systems.

The term "beta-keto amphetamines" originates from the fact that cathinones are chemically defined by having a phenethylamine backbone with a ketone functional group at the beta position. By promoting interaction with monoamine neurotransmitter transporters, specifically the dopamine, norepinephrine, and SERTs, this structural motif confers stimulant properties. Since synthetic cathinones are easily synthesized from readily available precursor chemicals, they are attractive candidates for covert synthesis and distribution in black market drug markets.

Changes made to the cathinone structure can have a big effect on these compounds' pharmacological profile in terms of SAR. For monoamine transporters, substitutions at the aromatic ring, alkyl chains, or amino groups can affect the receptor's affinity, potency, and selectivity. For instance, adding electron-withdrawing groups to the phenyl ring, like fluorine or chlorine, frequently improves potency and metabolic stability, producing effects that are stronger and last longer (Bondarev et al., 2003). The pharmacokinetic properties of the compound can also be influenced by changes to the alkyl chain length or branching pattern, which can change lipophilicity and membrane permeability.

The stereochemistry of the chiral centers inside the molecule is another important component of SAR in cathinones. Numerous cathinones are found in enantiomeric pairs, with various stereoisomers displaying unique pharmacological characteristics. The pharmacological effects of synthetic cathinones are highly dependent on their enantiomeric purity, wherein one enantiomer frequently exhibits higher potency or selectivity in comparison to its mirror image.

The wide variety of synthetic cathinones that are sold in black markets emphasizes how crucial it is to comprehend these substances' synthetic aromatic residues (SAR) for forensic and legal reasons. Ongoing research into the synthesis, pharmacology, and toxicology of cathinones is crucial to inform public health initiatives aimed at mitigating the risks associated with their use as new analogs continue to emerge through covert synthesis and designer drug strategies. To effectively address the challenges posed by these synthetic stimulants, efforts to regulate and control the distribution of cathinones must also take into account their structural diversity and potential for rapid analog emergence.

4.2.1 Structure-Activity Relationships of Synthetic Cathinones

Studies on the SAR seek to characterize the qualitative impact of chemical structure on a particular biological action. They concentrate on determining which substituents and how much of them change activity (i.e., what kinds of substituents and how much of them change stereochemistry (i.e., potency, action). It is acknowledged—though not widely—that multiple SARs could be developed for a particular set of agents. Think about this: a group of agents' behavioral responses may be connected to their capacity to trigger a particular neurotransmitter receptor in the brain. A different SAR might be developed the capacity of these agents to function as agonists in an in vitro functional assay (e.g., an in vitro radioligand binding assay), while another SAR might be developed for these agents' ability to bind at the target receptor. Instead of acting as agonists at the receptor of interest, some of the agents that show affinity for the receptor may act as weak partial agonists or antagonists. Furthermore, substances that are unable to bind to the receptor may have allostery (Bondareva et al., 2002). Furthermore, because some of the agents may be quickly metabolized in vivo or may not be able to cross the blood-brain barrier to reach their intended target, the SARs for these actions may differ from the SARs derived from their behavioral actions. SAR is primarily associated with the assay that yielded the biological data, and it is not always easy to extrapolate the formulated SAR to other pharmacological actions/assays.

Studies on the quantitative SAR (QSAR) make an effort to elucidate the reasons behind/how specific structural characteristics affect a given set of agents' behaviors. Following the completion of SAR studies, a QSAR study can be carried out utilizing correlational analysis, also known as a "Hansch analysis," to determine whether action or potency within a group of agents may be connected to a particular physicochemical property of the substituent being changed. Among the metrics are electronic character (determined by the Hammett σ value or Taft steric parameter Es), steric size (e.g. volume), a general or particular shape (e.g., values), and lipophilicity (Verloop parameters). Additional parameters take the entire molecule into account.

SAR and QSAR studies are usually a means to an end rather than ends in and of themselves. Results from these studies can, for instance, be used in drug design to improve an agent's potency or selectivity, lessen side effects (or off-target effects), lower toxicity, change metabolism, or investigate mechanisms of action.

SAR and QSAR studies should, as a general rule, concentrate on data from a common assay; ideally, these data should be produced from the same laboratory and acquired under comparable circumstances. Other than maybe from a basic qualitative viewpoint, using biological data for one compound from one study with data from (an) other compound(s) from different laboratories or from unrelated studies does not produce reliable SAR results. When a new agent has been discovered, and efforts are being made to discover something of interest, the latter strategy is not unusual. Such data are undoubtedly unsuitable for QSAR research. Even better are data produced when a molecule's structure is changed one substituent at a time, allowing outcomes to be methodically connected to a common molecule (i.e., e. either where structures can be connected to one another by a single structural change (linear SAR; see Figure 4.1B) or non-linear SAR (see Figure 4.1A). Another approach to SAR is to "deconstruct" a molecule by removing one substituent at a time to identify its influence on a particular action (see Figure 4.1C); the latter is actually a combination of the above two approaches (Cameron et al., 2013a).

Every one of the aforementioned strategies is frequently used to formulate SAR; in fact, the majority of them have been utilized to look into the SAR of synthetic cathinones. It should be acknowledged, nevertheless, that the outcomes of these SAR investigations are not always clear-cut. For instance, substituents E and F (Figure 4.1C) may have an impact on one another when the "deconstruction" method is taken into consideration. That is, the adjacent substituent (i.e., F or E) may have an effect on the presence of substituent E, one of these substituents may change the other's orientation or function. For instance, E and F may hydrogen bond, but they cannot do so in the absence of F, or they may sterically repel one another, which would not occur if one of the two substituents were eliminated. Additionally, rotomeric binding is a possibility (Cameron et al., 2013a).

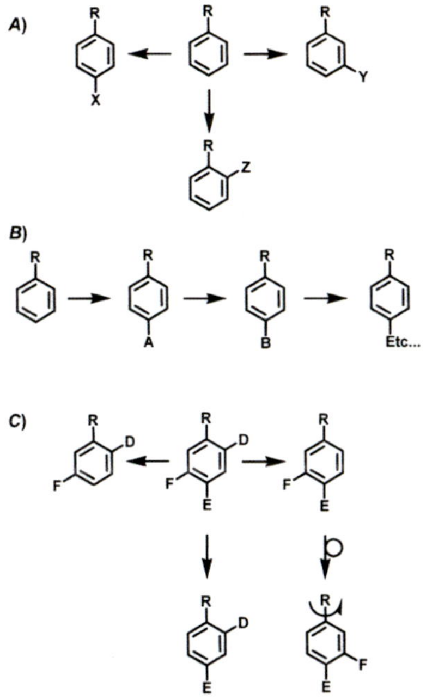

Figure 4.1. Examples of three types of structure-activity relationship (SAR) studies that can be pursued. Panel *A*) depicts a non-linear SAR study where the structure of a molecule is modified one substituent at a time; results can be related back to a common molecule in a systematic manner. Panel *B*) exemplifies how structures can be related to one another by a single and, usually, position-consistent, structural alteration. Panel C) is a combination of these two approaches and depicts the concept of "deconstruction".

Source: https://www.ncbi.nlm.nih.gov/pmc/articles/PMC5818155/bin/nihms942289f1.jpg

For instance, binding may take place in a way specified by the D substituent when the E and F substituents are present in addition to the D substituent. However, rotomeric binding could happen if the D substituent is missing. In other words, the compound substituted with E/F (only) may bind as indicated in the lower right corner Figure 4.1C. Consequently, SAR research, especially "deconstruction" research, needs to consider these possibilities and formulate SAR conservatively because different SAR interpretations might be possible.

4.2.2 Early Structure-Activity Relationship of Cathinone

These studies cover research done from the time that cathinone (1) was discovered until the mid- to late-1990s. Cathinone, more precisely S(−) cathinone or S(−)1 (the chemical structures of which are shown in Figure 4.2), was discovered in 1975 to be the primary stimulant found in the shrub Catha edulis. When S(−)cathinone (S(−)1) was first discovered, it was simply called "cathinone"; however, more recent studies have used the term "cathinone" to refer to racemic or (±)cathinone unless stereochemistry is specifically defined, while earlier studies used it to refer only to the S(−)-isomer. Prior to 1975, the predominant stimulant constituent of the plant was believed to be (+)cathine (Figure 4.2). Thus, it should come as no surprise that some of the initial studies concentrated on the stereochemical properties of cathinone as well as a pharmacological comparison of these two agents, cathinone and (+)cathine. In 1978, the United Nations Narcotics Laboratory created cathinone and its optical isomers, and soon after, it made samples of the compounds available (Cameron et al., 2013b). It was soon demonstrated that in rodents and other behavioral studies, cathinone (1) was a more potent locomotor stimulant than (+)cathine (2). Using rats trained to distinguish between S(+) amphetamine (AMPH; S(+)3, Figure 4.2), for instance, S(−)cathinone (S(−)1) was several times more potent than (+)cathine (2) and nearly as potent, usually more potent, than AMPH (S(+)3) in tests of stimulus generalization. S(−)cathinone was also more potent than (±)cathinone and R(+)cathinone in drug discrimination tests involving rats trained with AMPH and cathinone, as well as as a locomotor stimulant. Therefore, two of the first pertinent SAR discoveries were that the hydroxyl group of (+)cathine (2) was oxidized to its corresponding keto analog (i.e., S(-)cathinone was more potent than R(+) cathinone as a stimulant or amphetamine-like agent., cathinone, 1) led to a retention of stimulant action and an increase in behavioral potency (Carroll et al., 2009).

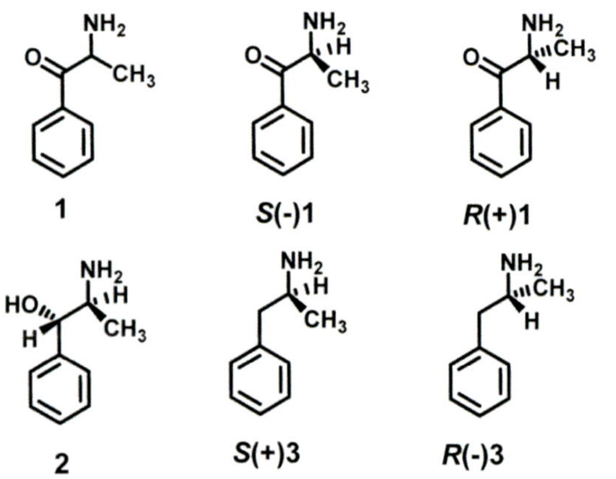

Figure 4.2. Structures of (±)cathinone (**1**), S(−) cathinone or **S(−)1**, *R*(+)cathinone or ***R*(+)1**, (+)cathine (**2**), *S*(+)amphetamine or ***S*(+)3**, and *R*(−)amphetamine or ***R*(−)3**.

Source: https://www.ncbi.nlm.nih.gov/pmc/articles/PMC5818155/bin/nihms942289f2.jpg

The lower lipophilicity of (+)cathine (2) (cLogP = 0.81 and 1.16, respectively) and its consequent decreased ability to penetrate the blood-brain barrier, as well as the fact that its target protein does not pharmacologically tolerate its hydroxyl group, could be the cause of its reduced in vivo potency in comparison to cathinone (1).

Amphetamine has two optical isomers, the (+)-isomer being the more potent of the two. The (−)-isomer symbolizes the cathinone eutomer; it is the eutomer. Nevertheless, the most accurate description of these isomers' structural relationship in three-dimensional space comes from their absolute configuration, the S-isomer in both cases (Figure 4.2), rather than from their optical rotation, denoted by + or −.

The following SAR questions were then addressed: i) Will N-alkylation change the potency of cathinone? ii) What is the effect of aryl substitution? iii) Does the α-methyl group of cathinone contribute to its stimulant/stimulus actions? Initially, since cathinone was a central stimulant, these questions were addressed by looking at their locomotor actions in rodents and discriminative stimulus effects in rats (such studies are still being employed). As time went on, it was shown that cathinone was a dopamine (DA) releasing agent, just like amphetamine, and subsequent research focused on this to look into SAR (Fantegrossi et al., 2013).

α-*Demethylation*

α-desmethylcathinone (Figure 4.3), which is a locomotor stimulant in mice but lacks the α-methyl group, was inactive at multiple times the cathinone's effective dose. Four drug discrimination studies did not succeed in substituting (i.e., produced vehicle-appropriate responding) in rats trained to discriminate or (±) cathinone from saline vehicle at doses up to 10 times the ED50 dose of S(−)cathinone (S(−)1). S(−)cathinone was about four times more potent as tritiated dopamine ([3H]DA) release agent than α-desmethyl cathinone from the rat caudate nucleus. Much more recently, it was demonstrated that in a rat brain synaptosome preparation, 4 is roughly one-third as potent as cathinone (EC_{50} = 208 nM and 83 nM, respectively) as a DA-releasing agent. It seems that α-desmethylcathinone (4) either does not readily enter the brain or is rapidly metabolized in vivo if the behavioral effects of cathinone are related to the release of dopamine via the DAT, as are those of amphetamine. Therefore, some effects might have been expected for the doses examined. It should be mentioned that even though β-phenylethylamine (PEA), the α-desmethyl analog of amphetamine, is only roughly one-third as effective as AMPH as a depolarizing agent (i.e., the indication of a release agent) at the dopamine transporter in humans. showed that PEA's dopamine-releasing agent potency is roughly 1/4 that of AMPH. Additionally, a 4-chain extension produced only weakly active compounds (Glennon, 2014).

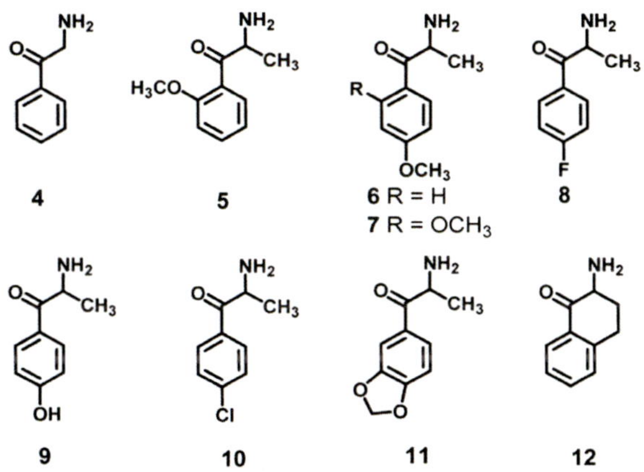

Figure 4.3. Structures of some cathinone analogs involved in early structure-activity relationship investigations.

Source: https://www.ncbi.nlm.nih.gov/pmc/articles/PMC5818155/bin/nihms942289f3.jpg

Aryl-substitution

The analysis of ring-substituted cathinone analogs is rather limited. Even at multiple times the active dose of S(−)cathinone, 2-methoxycathinone, 4-methoxycathinone, 2,4-dimethoxycathinone, and 4-fluorocathinone (5–8), respectively, failed to stimulate locomotor activity in mice. 4-methoxycathinone (6), 4-hydroxycathinone (9) and 4-chlorocathinone (10) produced saline-like effects and only partial generalization in rats trained to distinguish (±)cathinone from vehicle. 3,4-methylenedioxycathinone (MDC; 11) caused partial (50 %) substitution in rats trained to respond to AMPH; at slightly higher doses, the animals' behavior was disrupted. This suggested that MDC (11) likely has central effects in addition to or separate from its AMPH-like action. In fact, MDC (11) completely replaced rats that had been taught to distinguish between the empathogen MDMA (i.e., from vehicle, such as 1-(3,4-methylenedioxyphenyl)-2-aminopropane; ecstasy. MDMA's β-keto or β-carbonyl counterpart, MDC (11), has been suggested to have behavioral characteristics similar to MDMA in drug discrimination studies.

Conformational constraint

One example of a conformationally-constrained analog of cathinone is 2-amino-1-tetralone (12; Figure 4.3). 12 produced saline-like responses in rats trained to distinguish AMPH from the saline vehicle at ten times the ED_{50} dose of S(−)cathinone; however, it was only roughly five times less effective than S(−)cathinone as a releasing agent of [^{3}H]DA from the rat caudate nucleus (Gregg et al., 2015).

N-Alkylation

Cathinone is a central stimulant and DA releaser, just like amphetamine. N-(mono) methylcathinone was prepared and called "methcathinone" (MCAT, 13; Figure 4.4), analogous to amphetamine/methamphetamine terminology, because N-monomethylation of amphetamine, to afford methamphetamine, enhances its stimulant potency. Even though this substance was first created in the early 20th century and its ability to stimulate locomotion in rodents was observed, it wasn't until the term "methcathinone" was introduced that compound 13 attracted significant research attention. Not long after, it was discovered that methcathinone (13) posed a significant risk for drug abuse in the former Soviet Union, where it was referred to as ephedrone. Nevertheless, there were no reports of its use in the scientific literature at the time.

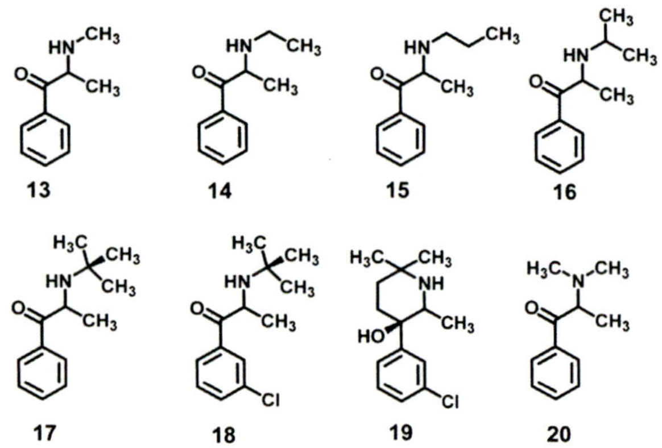

Figure 4.4. Some amine-modified methcathinone (**13**) analogs.

Source: https://www.ncbi.nlm.nih.gov/pmc/articles/PMC5818155/bin/nihms942289f4.jpg

Methcathinone (13) was found to be a strong DA releaser, a locomotor stimulant in rodents, and an agent more potent than methamphetamine in stimulus generalization tests conducted on AMPH-trained rats for drug discrimination studies (see Table 4.1). S(−)Methcathinone also replaced S(+) methamphetamine in rats that were trained with (−)ephedrine. Comparing enantiomeric comparisons, behavioral research on drug discrimination (Table 4.1) and mouse locomotor studies revealed that S(−)methcathinone was more potent than its R(+)-enantiomer (Kolanos et al., 2011).

Table 4.1. Comparison of stimulus generalization potencies of several amphetamine and cathinone analogs to substitute for training drug using rats trained to discriminate *S*(+)amphetamine from saline vehicle.

Agent	**ED_{50} (mg/kg)**
(±)Amphetamine (3)	0.71
(±)Methamphetamine	0.49
(±)Methcathinone (**13**)	0.37
S(−)**13**	0.25
R(+)**13**	0.66
(±)Ethcathinone (**14**)	0.77
(±)*N*-*n*-Propylcathinone (**15**)	2.02
(±)*N*,*N*-Dimethylcathinone (**20**)	0.61
S(−)**20**	0.44

Source: https://www.ncbi.nlm.nih.gov/pmc/articles/PMC5818155/

The N-methyl group of methcathinone (13) is homologous to an ethyl (i.e., Drug discrimination studies using rats trained to distinguish AMPH from vehicle showed slight declines in potency in response to ethcathinone) or n-propyl group (14 and 15, respectively; Figure 4.4).

More recently, ethcathinone (**14**) was shown to behave both as a weak DA reuptake inhibitor (IC_{50} = 1,014 nM) as well as a weak DA releasing agent (EC_{50} = 2,118 nM), whereas its propyl homolog **15** was found inactive as a DA reuptake inhibitor.

N-Isopropylcathinone (**16**) and N-*tert*-butylcathinone (**17**) produced stimulant-characteristic hyperlocomotion in rats at a doses of 7.5 mg/kg and 10 mg/kg, respectively, that were approximately half that seen following administration of methcathinone at 5 mg/kg. Compound **17** is the des-chloro analog of the antidepressant bupropion (**18**; Figure 4.4), and bupropion was also found to be a locomotor stimulant in the same study mentioned above at doses of 10 and 15 mg/kg. In rats trained to discriminate AMPH from saline vehicle, bupropion (**18**) (ED_{50} = 5.4 mg/kg) fully generalized to (+)amphetamine, but was 18 times lower in potency; of six bupropion metabolites, only one substituted for the AMPH stimulus: *S,S*-hydroxybupropion (**19**; Figure 4.4) (ED_{50} = 4.4 mg/kg).

Many years later, an extensive surface pharmacological retrieval (SAR) study was carried out on thirty bupropion analogs. The study included an analysis of the compounds' binding to the DAT, NET, and serotonin (5-HT) transporter (SERT), as well as their actions as reuptake inhibitors at all three major transporters, their effects as locomotor stimulants in mice, and the ways in which the rats were trained to distinguish cocaine from vehicle (Kolanos et al., 2015a). The majority of the analogs had the bupropion-shared tert-butyl amine substituent (18). Bupropion's des-chloro analog, or (i. e., 17) was about half as potent as bupropion (18) as a locomotor stimulant, showed about one-sixth the affinity of bupropion (18) at DAT, was equipotent at NET and inactive at SERT, and replaced in rats trained on cocaine. Another interesting observation was that extension of the α-methyl side chain had a pronounced influence on affinity at DAT with the following rank-order of potency: -methyl < -ethyl < -n-propyl > n-butyl >n-pentyl > n-hexyl, with the n-hexyl analog still binding with an affinity comparable to bupropion (**18**). A conformationally-constrained bupropion analog (i.e., the N-tert-butyl 5-chloro counterpart of **12**) displayed little affinity for DAT (or NET or SERT) but was twice as potent as **18** as a locomotor stimulant.

All of these results pointed to the accommodation of fairly large substituents on the terminal amine of cathinone, and to the tendency of those substituents to lessen the effectiveness of the resulting agents as stimulants similar to amphetamines. The mechanism or mechanisms of action of these agents were not well understood at the time ((Kolanos et al., 2015b).

N,N-Dimethylation of cathinone (i.e., *N,N*-dimethylcathinone or *N*-methylmethcathinone, **20**; Figure 4.4) resulted in retention of AMPH-like stimulus action, but with about half the potency of methcathinone (**13**); the *S*(−)-isomer of **20** was more potent than racemic **20** (Table 4.1). It might be mentioned that **20**, also termed dimethylpropion, metamfepramone, and DMCN, was once examined as an anorectic agent; investigation of its metabolism in human subjects revealed that nearly half of an orally administered dose of **20** was metabolically demethylated to what is now termed methcathinone (**13**) (Foley et al., 2004). Hence, some of the behavioral actions ascribed to **20** might be the result of its metabolism to **13**.

4.2.3 The Methcathinone Years

Research on cathinone's structural modification predominated until the mid-1990s. Then, with the discovery of methcathinone as a powerful central stimulant, the focus shifted to analogs of the latter. The possibility that methcathinone and some of its analogs function as DA-releasing agents was also better understood. Studies that concentrated more on the SAR for their releasing action at the DAT started to modestly outweigh SAR derived from behavioral studies. Methcathinone eventually turned into a U. S. substance listed in Schedule I.

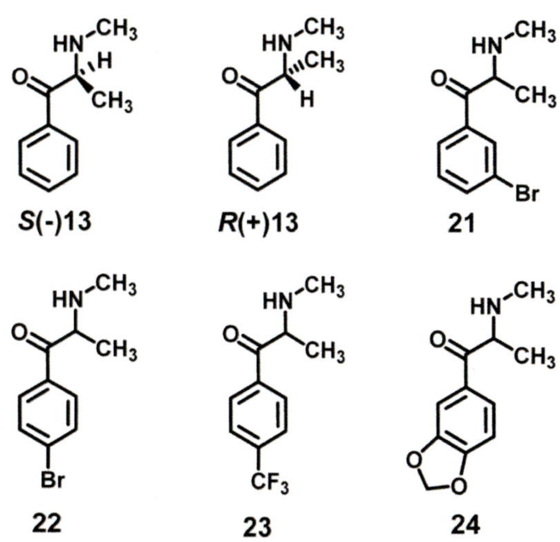

Figure 4.5. Some early methcathinone analogs.

Source: https://www.ncbi.nlm.nih.gov/pmc/articles/PMC5818155/bin/nihms942289f5.jpg

In a locomotor assay in rats, 3-bromomethcathinone (**21**; Figure 4.5) produced hyperlocomotion at doses of 7.5

and 10 mg/kg comparable to that produced by methcathinone at 5 mg/kg, whereas 4-bromomethcathinone (**22**), now termed brephedrone or 4-BMC, was inactive at these doses. Subsequently, in a related assay in rats, 4-trifluoromethyl-methcathinone (4-CF_3 MCAT; **23**) was inactive as a locomotor stimulant.

In cocaine-trained rats, stimulus generalization occurred with the following order of potency (ED_{50} values given in parenthesis): *S*(−)MCAT (0.18 mg/kg) > (±)MCAT (0.39 mg/kg) > *R*(+)MCAT (0.51 mg/kg) > cocaine (2.6 mg/kg).

Unlike MDC (**11**), methylenedioxymethcathinone (MDMC, methylone, **24**), the N-methyl analog of MDC, was substituted in AMPH-trained rats; however, it was six times less potent than methcathinone. MDMC (**24**) also substituted in MDMA-trained rats (Gatch et al., 2015).

S(−)Methcathinone was demonstrated to serve as a training drug in rats, and stimulus generalization occurred upon administration of other central stimulants with the following order of potency (ED_{50} values given in parentheses): *S*(−)MCAT (0.11 mg/kg; 0.5 µM/kg) > *S*(+) methamphetamine (0.17 mg/kg; 0.9 µM/kg) > (±)MCAT (0.25 mg/kg; 1.2 µM/kg) > *R*(+) MCAT (0.43 mg/kg; 2.1 µM/kg) ~ (±)cathinone (0.41 mg/kg; 2.2 µM/kg). As an aside, it might be noted that the *S*(−)methcathinone stimulus is also generalized to cocaine (ED_{50} = 1.47 mg/kg; 4.3 µM/kg)) (Majchrzak et al., 2016).

Because methcathinone (**13**) had been shown to act as releasing agents at the DAT, an SAR study was conducted and several agents were compared for their ability to release DA, norepinephrine, and 5-HT from rat brain synaptosomes. Some of the data are shown in Table 4.2.

Table 4.2. Biogenic amine releasing potency of several agents of interest.

Agent	**EC_{50} (nM)**		
	DAT	**NET**	**SERT**
S(+)Amphetamine **S(+)3**	24.8	7.1	1765
S(+) Methamphetamine	24.5	12.3	736
S(−)Cathinone ***S*(−)1**	18.5	12.4	2386
S(−)Methcathinone ***S*(−)**13	14.8	13.1	1772
(+)Cathine **2**	88.3	15.0	Inactive
(−)Cathine **25**	1371.0	137.0	Inactive

The S-isomers of cathinone (1), methcathinone (13), amphetamine (3), and methamphetamine, which are behaviorally more potent, showed similar potencies at DAT and NET, as well as similar potencies as releasing agents (Table 4.2). Each of them had a lesser potency when it came to 5-HT release. As a norepinephrine-releasing agent, (+)cathine (2) had potency similar to the other agents mentioned above; however, at DAT, it was several times less potent than the others and inactive at SERT (Table 4.2). Table 4.2 displays the data for (−)cathine (25) for comparative purposes. What's interesting is that an AMPH-stimulus, which supported a potential role for dopamine and/or DA in their actions, generalized to all of the agents in Table 2, with the exception of (−)cathine (25). When the -CF3 group was introduced, it had a negative impact on DAT and NET release and increased selectivity for SERT (Marusich et al., 2014). Additionally, 23 was found to be inactive as a locomotor stimulant in rats, and its actions were compared to those of its 2- and 3-substituted positional isomers (the other two positional isomers were not examined).

These investigations confirmed that S(−) methcathinone is a more potent central stimulant than R(+)methcathinone. It was also shown that S(−)methcathinone is a potent dopamine and norepinephrine-releasing agent. Additionally, the studies demonstrated that the introduction of aryl substituents decreases the stimulant and dopamine-releasing effects of methcathinone. Furthermore, S(−)methcathinone can be used as a training drug to examine the stimulus effects of other cathinone and non-cathinone central stimulants.

4.2.4 Current Structure-activity Relationship Studies

One early drug combination that gained popularity in 2010 was called "bath salts," though it went by several other names as well. Mephedrone (26), methylone (MDMC; 24), methylenedioxypyrovalerone (MDPV; 27), or a combination of one, two, or more of these and/or other agents were present in bath salts.

Methylone (24) was already well-documented (see supra), but the other two agents were largely unknown. Mephedrone (26) was predicted to be a DA-releasing agent with less potency and selectivity than methcathinone (13), based on SAR already developed for cathinone and amphetamine analogs. MDPV (27) was something "new," as previous research on the therapeutic potential of several related pyrovalerones—but not MDPV—as DA reuptake inhibitors had been done (Kolanos et al., 2013).

Using methamphetamine-trained and cocaine-trained rats, as well as MDPV-trained mice, a number of investigators showed that these three synthetic cathinones (methylone, mephedrone, and MDPV), among others (see below), behaved as locomotor stimulants in rodents, were self-administered by rats, and produced discriminative stimulus effects similar to other central stimulants (Glennon and Young, 2011). Because the studies were not SAR-focused, there is significant difficulty in developing a trustworthy SAR for these agents (which was not the goal of the original investigations and is extremely challenging in retrospect).

This is due to the lack of structural diversity and scarcity of agents examined in the individual studies, the various animal species used, the various routes (e.g., i.v. versus i.p. or i.m.) of medication administration, as well as the different time intervals used. the finding that while locomotor activity was a reliable indicator for the dose ranges that would be looked at in their later drug discrimination studies, the degree of locomotor stimulation may not be a reliable indicator of the propensity of the agent for abuse. Additionally, they hypothesized that minor variations might not matter and that behavioral effects might be produced by reaching a threshold level of neurotransmitter release or reuptake (Negus et al., 2007).

The capacity of synthetic cathinones to act at neurotransmitter transporters of biogenic amines (i.e., DAT, NET, SERT) may be responsible for their impacts on behavior. It was demonstrated that mephedrone (26) acted as a DA releaser. It was demonstrated that MDPV (27) exhibited traits of a DA reuptake inhibitor. Mephedrone (26) and MDPV (27) were found to produce dopamine-like depolarization and cocaine-like hyperpolarization, respectively, using a frog oocyte preparation transfected with hDAT.

These are the telltale signs of a reuptake inhibitor and a releasing agent, respectively. After looking into a number of synthetic cathinones, it was discovered that mephedrone (26) had a significantly higher potency as an inhibitor of NET than it did as an inhibitor and releaser of DA and 5-HT. On the other hand, MDPV (27) did not release DA or 5-HT but was a strong reuptake inhibitor at DAT and NET and a very weak inhibitor of SERT (Negus et al., 2007).

Table 4.3. Effect of several synthetic cathinones on synaptosomal release and reuptake inhibition at biogenic transporters; data for amphetamine and cocaine included for comparison.

	Release EC_{50} (nM)			Reuptake Inhibition IC_{50} (nM)		
	DAT	NET	SERT	DAT	NET	SERT
Methylone (**24**)	117	140	234	1,232	1,031	1,017
Mephedrone (**26**)	51	58	122	762	487	422
MDPV (**27**)	2.3*	13*	Inactive	4.1	26	3,349
S(+)Amphetamine	5.8	6.6	698	93	67	3,418
Cocaine	151*	2,190	Inactive	211	292	313

*Extent of release was <35%.

Expanding the methylenedioxy ring of methylone (24) to an ethylenedioxy ring (EDMC; 30) resulted in a 2- to 3-fold decrease in potency as a releasing agent at all three transporters. Changing the α-methyl group of methylone (24) to an α-ethyl group (butylone; 31) and replacing the methylenedioxy group of MDPV (27) with a fused phenyl ring (naphyrone; 32) transformed them into reuptake inhibitors at the three transporters. Naphyrone (32) exhibited 5- to 10-fold greater potency than butylone (31) at DAT, NET, and SERT and was weaker than MDPV (27) at DAT and NET but stronger at SERT. These studies, as well as others, highlighted the significant impact of substituents on the terminal amine and/or at the α-position of cathinone analogs on their actions as releasing agents or reuptake inhibitors, as well as on their selectivity for the major biogenic amine transporters.

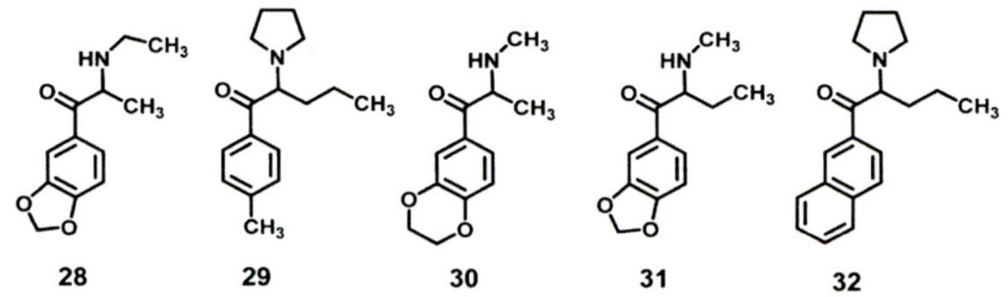

Figure 4.6. Structures of ethylone (**28**), pyrovalerone (**29**), ethylenedioxymethcathinone (EDMC) (**30**), butylone (**31**), and naphyrone (**32**).

Synthetic Cathinones as Reuptake Inhibitors

Source: https://www.ncbi.nlm.nih.gov/pmc/articles/PMC5818155/bin/nihms942289f7.jpg

Among the synthetic cathinones that were making an appearance on the black market, MDPV (27) stood out since it was the first to be recognized as a DA reuptake inhibitor. A methodical SAR deconstruction of MDPV (27) is depicted in Figure 4.7 in order to ascertain which of its numerous structural characteristics, and to what degree, contribute to its activities as a DA reuptake inhibitor. The compounds depicted in Figure 4.7 exhibited reuptake inhibitory behavior, albeit with notable variations in potency. When the carbonyl group was removed from MDPV, it became its amphetamine analog (33) and lost approximately 8 times its potency. On the other hand, when the methylenedioxy substituent (i.e., α-PVP; 34) had very little impact. It seems that the α side chain's length is crucial; if the side chain is shorter (i.e., MDPPP; 35) leads to >25 times drop in potency. The amine was the next most crucial component, provided the side chain remained intact. The amine's transformation from the most basic tertiary amine (i.e., 36; dimethylone) to either a primary or secondary amine (i.e., pentylone, 37, and 38, respectively) eventually caused a 200-fold reduction in potency (Rothman et al., 2003).

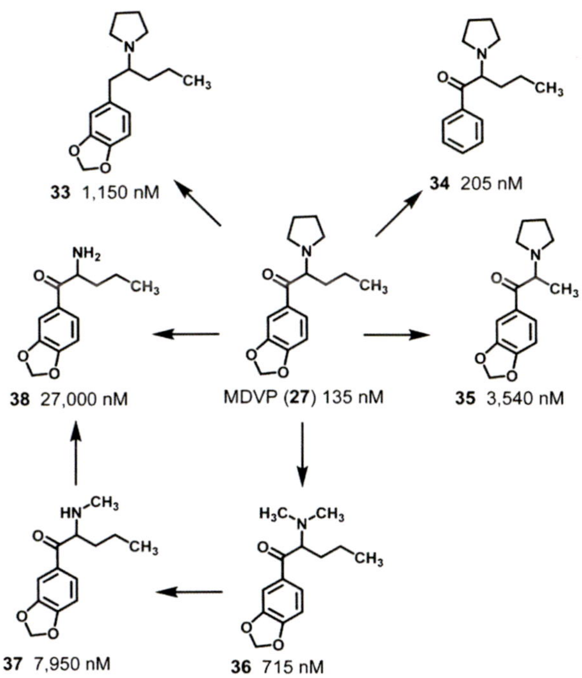

Figure 4.7. Deconstruction of methylenedioxypyrovalerone (MDPV) (**27**). Values represent the potency of the analogs to block the reuptake of DA.

Source: https://www.ncbi.nlm.nih.gov/pmc/articles/PMC5818155/bin/nihms942289f8.jpg

Because the methylenedioxy group played a minimal role in the ability of MDPV (**27**) to act as a DAT inhibitor, a series of analogs lacking this functionality was examined with a focus on SAR. These analogs might be viewed as being derived from α-PVP (*"flakka"*; **34**) (Figure 4.8 and Table 4.4) – currently, a very popular drug of abuse. Using the deconstruction process, the α-*n*-propyl group of **34** was shortened in a stepwise manner (Sakloth, 2015). Truncation of the α-propyl substituent to an α-ethyl group (i.e., α-PBP; **41**; Table 4.4) reduced potency by about 3-fold, and further contraction to an α-methyl group (i.e., α-PPP; **40**) resulted in an overall >10-fold decrease in potency. Elimination of the α-*n*-propyl group altogether – that is, replacement by -H (i.e., **39**; Table 4.4), resulted in a nearly 200-fold decrease in potency. Nevertheless, all of the analogs behaved as DA reuptake inhibitors.

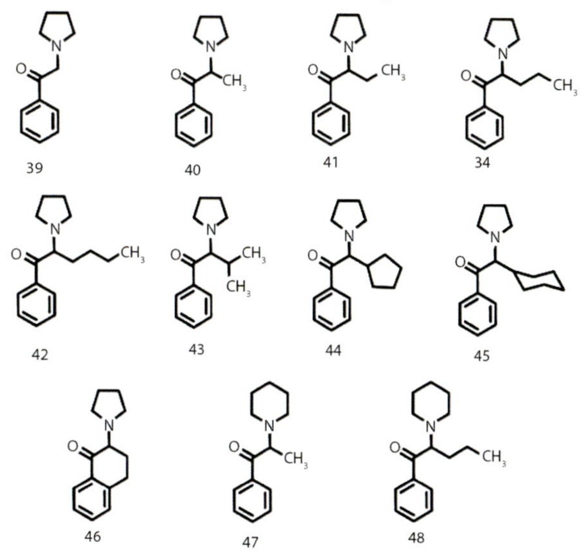

Figure 4.8. Deconstructed (**39–41**) and **e**laborated (**42–48**) analogs of α-pyrrolidinovalerophenone (α-PVP) (**34**).

Source: https://www.ncbi.nlm.nih.gov/pmc/articles/PMC5818155/bin/nihms942289f9.jpg

The findings support those shown in Figure 4.7 in that the α-substituent of the synthetic cathinones plays a major role in their actions as reuptake inhibitors at DAT when the amine substituent is held constant as a pyrrolidine moiety. In addition, none of the analogs was effective as a reuptake inhibitor at SERT (IC_{50} >10,000 nM). From these data, it can be surmised that the length of the α-substituent is influential for DAT action, but that action at SERT might not readily accommodate a pyrrolidine moiety regardless of the length of the α-substituent (Tang et al., 2015).

Table 4.4. Potency of deconstructed and elaborated α-pyrrolidinovalerophenone (α-PVP) (**34**) analogs to inhibit synaptosomal reuptake at DAT.

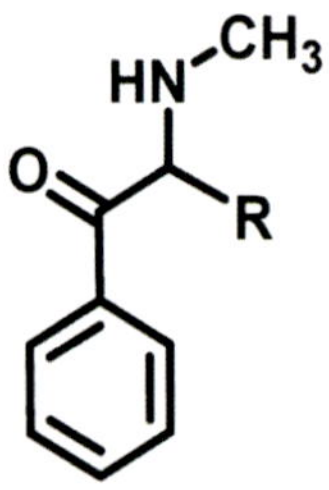

Agent	R	IC_{50} (nM)
39	-H	3,250
40	$-CH_3$	196.7
41	$-CH_2CH_3$	63.3
34	$-CH_2CH_2CH_3$	17.5
42	$-CH_2CH_2CH_2CH_3$	11.6
43	$-CH(CH_3)_2$	92.3
44	$-C_5H_9$	17.1
45	$-C_6H_{11}$	8.3

Because the length/bulk of the α-substituent seemed important for these agents to act as reuptake inhibitors at DAT, additional compounds were examined. Increasing the length of the α-substituent from *n*-propyl (i.e., **34**) to *n*-butyl (i.e., α-PHP; **42**) resulted in a slight increase in potency (Table 4.5). Branching of the α-ethyl side chain of **41** to its isopropyl counterpart **43** reduced potency by about 50% (Table 4.4). But, as might now be expected based on the information provided in Table 4.4, increasing the bulk of this branched analog should result in increased potency. Elaborated analogs **44** and **45** (IC_{50} = 17.1 and 8.3 nM; Table 4.5) were at least as potent as α-PVP (**34**).

Compound **46** is a conformationally-constrained analog of **41**; its potency (IC_{50} = 12,900 nM) is >200-fold less than that of **41**. Ring expansion of the pyrrolidine ring of α-PVP (**34**) to a piperidine ring (i.e., **48** IC_{50} = 128 nM) resulted in a 7-fold decrease in potency; likewise, the piperidine analog of **40** (i.e., **47** IC_{50} = 2,490 nM) also displayed reduced potency.

Pyrovalerone (29) has a chiral center and can have two optical isomers; as a reuptake inhibitor at DAT, the S-isomer was 100 times more effective than the R-enantiomer. At NET and SERT, the potency of both isomers was lower (Watterson et al., 2014).

There are two optical isomers of MDPV (27) as well (Figure 4.9). Both were prepared and investigated for their neurochemical effects on neurotransmitter reuptake as well as their behavioral effects in an intracranial self-stimulation (ICSS) assay in rats, a behavioral technique used to assess abuse potential. In assays of DAT uptake inhibition, *S*(+)MDPV (IC_{50} = 2.13 nM) was twice as potent as (±)MDPV (IC_{50} = 4.85 nM) and 180-fold more potent than *R*(−)MDPV (IC_{50} = 382.80 nM); as such, the *S*-isomer was 100-fold more potent than cocaine (IC_{50} = 198.80 nM).

The three were less potent at NET uptake inhibition but with the same rank order of potency: IC_{50} = 9.86 nM, 16.84 nM, and 726 nM, respectively, relative to cocaine IC_{50} = 395.9 nM (Saha et al., 2015). Neither (±)MDPV nor either of its optical isomers inhibited the reuptake at SERT. *S*(+)MDPV produced abuse-related and dose-dependent facilitation of ICSS in rats, and the potency of *S*(+)MDPV (significant facilitation at doses ≥0.1 mg/kg) was greater than that of (±)MDPV whereas *R*(−)-MDPV failed to alter ICSS at doses up to 100 times greater than the lowest effective dose of *S*(+)MDPV.

Table 4.5. Potency of selected 4-substituted methcathinone analogs as releasing agents at DAT and SERT, and in a rat intracranial self-stimulation (ICSS) assay.

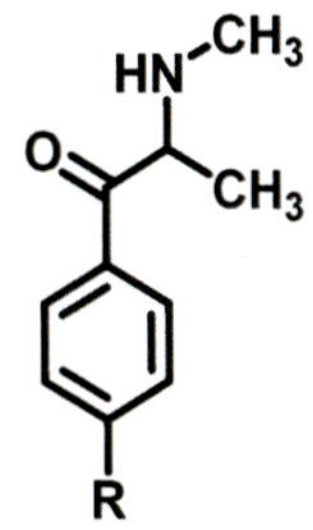

Agent	R	DAT EC_{50} (nM)[a]	SERT EC_{50} (nM)[a]	DAT Selectivity[b]	ICSS Maximum % Baseline Facilitation[c]
Methcathinone (**13**)	-H	12.5	3,860	309	191.9
Flephedrone (**50**)	-F	83.4	1,290	15.4	156.3
Methedrone (**51**)	$-OCH_3$	506	120	0.24	110.9
4-Chloromethcathinone (**52**)	-Cl	42.2	144	3.40	114.9
4-Bromomethcathinone (**22**)	-Br	59.4	60	1.01	118.0
Mephedrone (**26**)	$-CH_3$	49.1	118	2.41	102.5
4-Trifluoromethylmethcathinone (**23**)	$-CF_3$	2,700	190	0.07	90.9

[a]EC_{50} values and ICSS.

[b]DAT selectivity calculated as $(\text{DAT } EC_{50})^{-1} \div (\text{SERT } EC_{50})^{-1}$; higher values indicate greater DAT selectivity.

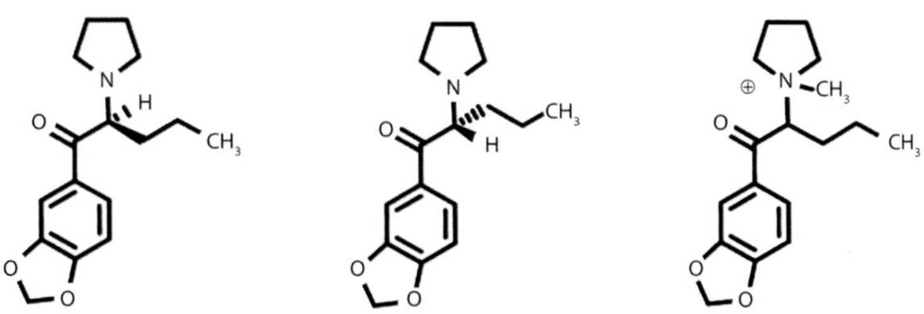

S(+) 27 R(-) 27 49

Figure 4.9. Newer methylenedioxypyrovalerone (MDPV) (**27**) analogs: *S*(+)MDPV, *R*(−)MDPV, and Q-MDPV (**49**).

Source: https://www.ncbi.nlm.nih.gov/pmc/articles/PMC5818155/bin/nihms942289f10.jpg

Further research is necessary, but preliminary results also indicate that the N-methyl quaternary amine counterpart of MDPV (i.e., frog oocytes transfected with hDAT experienced hyperpolarization due to Q-MDPV; 49, Figure 4.9. These findings imply that 49 may have DAT reuptake inhibitory effects. Potency of synthetic cathinones to inhibit reuptake at DAT is related to the "size" of the α side chain, according to one of the first QSAR studies on the topic published. That is, potency was significantly correlated with both the volume (r = 0.909) and the lipophilicity (π value; r = 0.917) of their α-substituents, based on the data displayed for the eight agents in Table 4.4. On the other hand, volume and π showed a strong high correlation (r = 0.997) for the substituents in this set. It is obvious that further research will be needed to ascertain which of these two parameters is more crucial for activity as well as the ideal volume and/or lipophilicity for this action (UNODC, 2013; Tang et al., 2015).

4.2.5 Synthetic Cathinones as Releasing Agents

It has previously been noted that mephedrone (26), while not as strong or specific as MCAT (13), was discovered to function as a releasing agent at DAT. Numerous related methcathinone analogs share this property. Numerous studies on these agents have been described in the literature. The majority of these investigations did not specifically address SAR and QSAR endpoints; only those that did will be mentioned here.

The ability of seven methcathinone analogs to act as substrates at DAT and SERT and to modulate in vivo ICSS in rats was investigated. These analogs differed only in their 4-position substituents. Table 4.5 shows a wide range of potencies and selectivities for these agents. In the ICSS assay, 4-trifluoromethymethcathinone (23), which was the least potent analog, was the least potent analog, and MCAT (13) was the most potent analog. The potencies of the other agents were in the middle. The in vivo efficacy to produce ICSS facilitation was correlated (r=0.92) with the selectivity of DAT versus SERT in vitro.

Additionally, the Taft steric parameter (i.e., the magnitude of ICSS facilitation (r=0.81) and DAT versus SERT selectivity (r=0.78) were correlated with the ES value of the 4-position substituents. The electronic (σ) or lipophilic (π) nature of the substituents did not correlate with ICSS facilitation, DAT potency, or SERT potency (Reith et al., 2015). Further research looked at more precise steric parameters, such as substituent volume and Verloop size (i.e., minimum or maximum substituent width, B1 and B5, and substituent length, L, respectively). The four steric parameters, minimum width (B1) (r=−0.778), maximum width (B5) (r=−0.814), length (L) (r=−0.773), and volume (Å3) (r=−0.915), all showed negative correlations with maximal ICSS facilitation. Internal correlations were found between a few parameters: volume and maximal width (r=0.935), substituent length (r=0.814), and length (r=0.798). While potency at SERT was positively correlated with increasing volume (r=0.825) and length (r=0.903) of the 4-position substituent, it was negatively correlated with increasing volume (r=−0.803) and maximal substituent width (r=−0.807) in the ability of the agents to promote in vitro monoamine release via DAT. Selectivity between DAT and. Volume (r= -0.972) and maximal width (r= -0.917) showed a correlation with SERT (Watterson et al., 2014).

While the interactions of MCAT analogs at DAT and SERT may be expected to be influenced by a variety of structural elements, such as the aromatic ring and terminal amine, these structural elements are shared by all of the analogs listed in Table 4.5. In other words, the only variable that differs between these analogs is the substituent at the 4-position; hence, they constitute a matched set with only one variable substituent. It was discovered that potency at DAT decreased while potency at SERT increased as the size of the 4-position substituent increased.

This reciprocal relationship was also evident with DAT versus SERT selectivity. Therefore, it would appear that the steric characteristics of the 4-position substituent are crucial to the way the studied MCAT analogs function. However, it was impossible to single out one steric parameter as being the most significant due to internal correlations among some of the steric parameters. However, it was conjectured that due to the reliable identification and greater correlation coefficients linked to steric volume (i.e., ˝3), indicating that the most significant characteristic for these interactions is probably the total volume of the 4-position substituent.

New hDAT and hSERT models were produced by homology modeling studies using the dDAT crystal structure as a template. Docking studies using the agents in Table 4.5 demonstrated that hSERT was more effective than hDAT at accommodating large substituents at the MCAT (13) 4-position. The outcomes matched those of the previously mentioned QSAR research. Moreover, hydrophobic interactions provided by the 4-position substituent are required for potency at hSERT, whereas unfavorable polar interactions at the 4-position might influence potency at hDAT, according to a hydropathic interaction (HINT) analysis that took into account potential interactions of the 4-position substituents with particular nearby transporter amino acid residues (Watterson et al., 2014). Overall, the results showed that bulky substituents are not easily accommodated in the MCAT binding pocket linked to the 4-position substituent in hDAT, but they are more easily accommodated in the larger and less polar binding pocket in hSERT. These QSAR and modeling/docking studies have led to the general conclusions that: i) MCAT analogs with small 4-position substituents prefer binding at DAT rather than SERT; ii) larger substituents prefer binding at SERT; and iii) these substituents' hydrophobic nature modulates potency at SERT.

New hDAT and hSERT models were produced by homology modeling studies using the dDAT crystal structure as a template. Docking studies using the agents in Table 4.5 demonstrated that hSERT was more effective than hDAT at accommodating large substituents at the MCAT (13) 4-position. The outcomes matched those of the previously mentioned QSAR research. Moreover, hydrophobic interactions provided by the 4-position substituent are required for potency at hSERT, whereas unfavorable polar interactions at the 4-position might influence potency at hDAT, according to a hydropathic interaction (HINT) analysis that took into account potential interactions of the 4-position substituents with particular nearby transporter amino acid residues (Suyama et al., 2016). Overall, the results showed that bulky substituents are not easily accommodated in the MCAT binding pocket linked to the 4-position substituent in hDAT, but they are more easily accommodated in the larger and less polar binding pocket in hSERT. These QSAR and modeling/docking studies have led to the general conclusions that: i) MCAT analogs with small 4-position substituents prefer binding at DAT rather than SERT; ii) larger substituents prefer binding at SERT; and iii) these substituents' hydrophobic nature modulates potency at SERT (Iversen, 2010).

Rats were implanted with bilateral guide cannulae targeting the nucleus accumbens (NAc) in a QSAR study that used in vivo microdialysis to investigate the relationship between the volume of the 4-position substituent and the in vivo neurochemical selectivity of cathinone analogs to alter nucleus accumbens (DA) DA and 5-HT levels. MCAT (13) and five of the 4-substituted MCAT analogs listed in Table 4.6 (i.e., 22–26, 50–52). The levels of 5-HT and/or NAc DA increased in a dose-dependent manner for each of the six compounds. A correlation was found between in vitro selectivity to promote monoamine release via DAT and SERT (r = 0.95) and the molecular volume (i.e., the dose required to increase peak 5-HT levels by 250 % divided by the dose required to increase peak DA levels by 250 %) and in vivo selectivity. (ie., Å3) of the substituent at position four (r = −0.85). The outcomes provide more evidence for the connection between the above-discussed molecular, neurochemical, and behavioral measures.

Table 4.6. Potencies of stereoisomers of several simple cathinone analogs for the synaptosomal release of neurotransmitters from DAT, NET, and SERT.

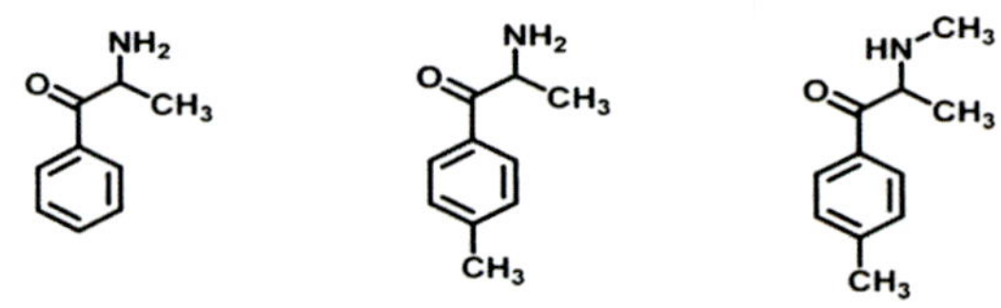

Cathinone 4-Methylcathinone Mephedrone

	EC_{50} (nM)*			DAT vs SERT Selectivity
	DAT	NET	SERT	
S(−)Cathinone ***S*(−)1**	25	14	9,267	370
R(+)Cathinone ***R*(+)1**	184	72	>10,000	>50
S(−)4-Methylcathinone ***S*(−)53**	150	89	179	1.2
R(+)4-Methylcathinone ***R*(+)53**	391	115	1,592	4.1
S(−)Mephedrone ***S*(−)26**	74	-	61	0.8
R(+)Mephedrone **R(+)26**	31	-	1,470	47

*Some values have been rounded off to the nearest whole number

Racemates are defined as an equal mixture of an agent's two optical isomers or antipodes. The "active" isomer is frequently one isomer (i.e., the eutomer) in contrast to the other, which is "inactive" or less active. (i.e. the distomer). The action is known as stereospecific (or enantiospecific) when the distomer is dormant, and the eutomer has twice the potency of the racemate. The maximum theoretical potency of the eutomer is twice that of the racemate, and the "inactive" isomer merely dilutes the potency of the "active" isomer by 50%. In other situations, the optical isomers are said to have a stereoselective (or enantioselective) effect when both isomers—the eutomer and the distomer—are "active," but one is more potent than the other (Marusich et al., 2012).

Methcathinone (13) is stereoselective in terms of its behavioral actions and potency as a DA-releasing agent, as previously mentioned; S(−)methcathinone stands for the eutomer. A less selective release agent is mephedrone (26) (Table 4.5). Mephedrone (26), which is 4-methylmethcathinone, can be broken down into 4-methylcathinone (53) and cathinone (1) by taking out the N-methyl group. Understanding the difference between the stereoselective and stereospecific aspects of the actions of these agents can be gained by looking at their optical isomers. When it comes to release at DAT as opposed to NET, S(−)Cathinone (Table 4.6) is stereoselective but not selective. In other words, both isomers are "active," but the S(−)-isomer has several times the potency of its R(+)enantiomer (Table 4.6). But at SERT, both cathinone isomers are essentially dormant. The 4-methyl group is introduced, i.e., 4-methylcathinone; 53) led to a reduction in DAT/NET release selectivity compared to release at SERT, as well as a decrease in stereoselectivity for DAT/NET release (<3-fold). (Table 4.6). Adding an N-methyl group (i.e., mephedrone; 26) caused the two optical isomers to be almost equipotent, further reducing stereoselectivity at DAT. (i.e. the potency of S(−)- and R(+)mephedrone differs by only about twofold. Furthermore, S(−)mephedrone no longer exhibits DAT versus SERT selectivity.

Biogenic amine-releasing agents have the potential to be abused because they can facilitate a higher release through DAT than through SERT, making DAT-selective agents more prone to abuse. This idea is supported by the fact that rats treated with R(+)mephedrone, which had a 50-fold selectivity for DAT over SERT, exhibited more rewarding qualities and locomotor stimulation than rats treated with its S(-)enantiomer, which showed no rewarding qualities and only mild locomotor stimulation as determined by conditioned place preference and facilitation of ICSS. R(+)53 for 4-methylcathinone (53), however, showed somewhat higher DAT versus SERT selectivity and produced abuse-related effects in ICSS despite being less potent than its S-enantiomer in terms of promoting release at DAT (Meltzer et al., 2006). As previously mentioned, the actions of synthetic cathinones can be modified by the type of terminal amine, α-substituents, aryl substituents, and stereochemistry. In other words, methcathinone (13) functions mainly as a releasing agent at DAT, but the addition of a 4-methyl group (i.e., methcathinone exhibits >300-fold selectivity for DAT, while mephedrone only shows slightly more than 2-fold selectivity (Table 4.5), mephedrone; 26) increases its potency as a releasing agent at SERT. Cathinone analogs' ability to inhibit DAT reuptake is generally enhanced by increasing the bulk of their terminal amine (see Figure 4.7). Furthermore, ethcathinone (14), the N-ethyl homolog of methcathinone, is a weak DA releaser and reuptake inhibitor (Hutsell et al., 2016). Hence, some cathinone analogs may have "mixed" or "hybrid" actions by "mixing and matching" the right substituents. Investigated this by comparing the effects of three agents—mephedrone (26), its N-ethyl homolog 4-methyl-N-ethylcathinone (54; 4-MEC), and its pyrrolidine counterpart 4-′-methyl-α-pyrrolidinopropiophenone (55; 4-MePPP)—with progressively increasing steric bulk on the terminal amine (Figure 4.10).

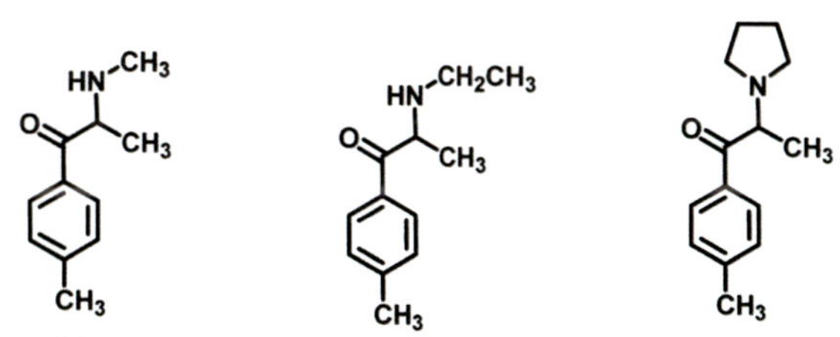

26 *54* 55

Figure 4.10. A structural comparison of mephedrone (**26**), 4-MEC (**54**), and 4-MePPP (**55**).

Source: https://www.ncbi.nlm.nih.gov/pmc/articles/PMC5818155/bin/nihms942289f11.jpg

Mephedrone (**26**) and 4-MEC (**54**) were nearly equipotent at inhibiting reuptake at DAT (IC_{50} *ca.* 800 nM) and SERT (IC_{50} *ca.* 500 nM), whereas 4-MePPP (**55**) was more potent as an inhibitor at the former (IC_{50} = 215 nM) as opposed to the latter (IC_{50} >10,000 nM). However, in a synaptosomal release assay, mephedrone (**26**) and 4-MEC (**54**) were similar in potency to evoke release from SERT (EC_{50} *ca.* 100 nM), whereas 4-MePPP (**55**) was inactive. In contrast, mephedrone was an effective releaser at DAT (EC_{50} = 39 nM), whereas 4-MEC (**54**) and 4-MePPP (**55**) were inactive (Reith et al., 2015). The overall conclusion was that changing the nature of the N-alkyl substituent of cathinone analogs has a profound influence on their actions; 4-MEC (**54**) is a SERT-releasing agent/DAT blocker, whereas 4-MePPP (**55**) is a selective DAT blocker.

4.3 Risks and Consequences of Stimulant Abuse

Abuse of stimulants has serious negative effects on social and societal well-being, as well as risks to one's physical and mental health. Stimulant abuse can have serious, sometimes irreversible consequences. It can involve the misuse of prescription drugs like amphetamines or the use of illegal substances like cocaine or methamphetamine. Overdosing on stimulants is one of the immediate risks involved in their abuse. Stimulants have the potential to severely tax the cardiovascular system, resulting in dangerously high heart rates, spikes in blood pressure, and arrhythmias in the heart. In extreme situations, this can put the person's life in danger by causing heart attacks, strokes, or sudden cardiac arrest (Gatch et al., 2013).

Abuse of stimulants on a regular or chronic basis may also result in tolerance, requiring higher doses to produce the desired results. This pattern of increasing use raises the risk of addiction and dependence, which are characterized by obsessive drug-seeking behavior despite drawbacks. An individual's life can be severely disrupted by stimulant addiction, which can result in monetary troubles, strained relationships, and legal issues.

The effects of stimulant abuse on the nervous system are concerning. Extended exposure to elevated dopamine levels, a neurotransmitter linked to pleasure and reward, can desensitize the brain's reward circuitry, compromising dopamine signaling naturally and resulting in anhedonia, which is the incapacity to derive pleasure from previously pleasurable activities. Chronic stimulant abuse can also alter the structure and function of the brain, which may lead to mental illnesses like psychosis, depression, and anxiety, as well as cognitive deficits and memory problems (Foley et al., 2013).

Abuse of stimulants also has serious social and financial repercussions. Abuse of substances can cause impairments in judgment and decision-making, which raises the possibility of mishaps, injuries, and dangerous behaviors like illicit or unsafe sexual activity. Stimulant abuse imposes a burden on individuals, families, and communities through increased healthcare costs, criminal justice expenditures, and lost productivity.

Preventing, intervening, and treating stimulant abuse calls for a multimodal strategy that addresses its risks and effects (Sakloth et al., 2015). Campaigns for education and awareness can help raise public awareness of the risks associated with stimulant abuse and encourage the use of healthy coping mechanisms. To recover and take back control of their lives, people with stimulant addiction must have access to evidence-based treatment programs, such as behavioral therapies and medication-assisted treatments.

The social effects of stimulant abuse can also be lessened by initiatives to restrict the availability of illegal stimulants through law enforcement and regulatory actions. We can endeavor to lessen the frequency of stimulant abuse and lessen its severe effects on both individuals and communities by addressing the systemic and individual factors that contribute to it.

4.3.1 Risks of Stimulant Abuse

Stimulant abuse poses a range of risks to both physical and mental health, as well as to social and societal well-being (Del Bello et al., 2015). Here are some of the key risks associated with the misuse of stimulant drugs:

- **Cardiovascular Effects:** Stimulants can significantly increase heart rate, blood pressure, and vasoconstriction, placing excessive strain on the cardiovascular system. This can lead to adverse events such as heart palpitations, arrhythmias, hypertension, and even heart attacks or strokes, particularly in individuals with pre-existing cardiovascular conditions.
- **Neurological Effects:** Prolonged stimulant abuse can lead to alterations in brain structure and function. Chronic use may result in neurotoxicity, affecting neurotransmitter systems such as dopamine, serotonin, and norepinephrine. These changes can lead to cognitive impairments, memory deficits, and increased risk of psychiatric disorders such as anxiety, depression, and psychosis.
- **Addiction and Dependence:** Stimulant drugs have a high potential for addiction and dependence. Continued use can lead to tolerance, requiring higher doses to achieve the desired effects and withdrawal symptoms upon cessation. Addiction to stimulants is characterized by compulsive drug-seeking behavior despite negative consequences, which can severely disrupt an individual's life and lead to a cycle of substance abuse.
- **Psychological Effects:** Stimulant abuse can induce intense euphoria, increased energy, and heightened arousal. However, these effects are often followed by dysphoria, irritability, and mood swings as the drug's effects wear off. Long-term stimulant use can exacerbate underlying mental health conditions or precipitate the onset of new psychiatric disorders.
- **Physical Health Complications:** In addition to cardiovascular issues, stimulant abuse can lead to a range of physical health complications. These may include gastrointestinal problems, appetite suppression leading to malnutrition, dental issues (such as "meth mouth" associated with methamphetamine use), and compromised immune function, increasing susceptibility to infections.
- **Behavioral Risks:** Stimulant abuse can impair judgment, decision-making, and impulse control, leading to risky behaviors such as reckless driving, unsafe sexual practices, and involvement in criminal activities. These behaviors not only endanger the individual but also pose risks to others in their environment.
- **Social and Economic Consequences:** Stimulant abuse can have far-reaching social and economic consequences. It can strain relationships with family, friends, and colleagues, disrupt employment or educational opportunities, and lead to financial instability. The societal burden of stimulant abuse includes healthcare costs, criminal justice expenses, and lost productivity.

An all-encompassing strategy that incorporates harm reduction techniques, education, prevention, and access to evidence-based treatment and support services is needed to address the risks associated with stimulant abuse. We can endeavor to lessen the prevalence and effects of stimulant abuse on people and communities by increasing awareness of the risks connected with its misuse and putting into place efficient interventions (Simmler et al., 2013).

4.3.2 Synthetic Cathinones

A class of medications known as synthetic cathinones is connected to the khat plant that grows naturally. They are stimulants, which means that they work similarly to amphetamines by accelerating the transmission of messages between the brain and the body. NPS are a class of drugs that includes synthetic cathinones as well. NPSs are a class of drugs that first came onto the recreational drug scene in the middle of the 2000s. They are made to look and act like popular illegal substances like cocaine, ecstasy, cannabis, and lysergic acid diethylamide (LSD).

With 130 detected in total, including 12 detected for the first time in 2017, synthetic cathinones are the second largest group of new substances monitored by the European Monitoring Centre for Drugs and Drug Addiction (EMCDDA) (EMCDDA, 2015).

Synthetic cathinones are mostly white or brown powders but can also be in the form of small, chunky crystals. They are sometimes found as capsules and less commonly as tablets.

Other types of cathinones:

- Mephedrone (4-MMC), M-CAT)
- Methylone
- Methcathinone
- Buphedrone
- Bupropion
- Pyrovalerone
- Alpha-pyrrolidinovalerophenone (alpha-PVP) MDPV.

How are they used?

Typically, synthetic cathinones are injected, swallowed, or snorted. The desired effects usually manifest within 15 to 45 minutes of oral administration. The desired effect is anecdotally reported to happen within a few minutes of snorting. Usually, the effects linger for two to four hours (Uchiyama et al., 2014).

4.3.3 Effects of Synthetic Cathinones

There is no safe level of drug use. The use of any drug always carries some risk. It's important to be careful when taking any type of drug.

Synthetic cathinones affect everyone differently based on:

- the amount taken
- a person's size, weight and health
- whether the person is used to taking it
- whether other drugs are taken around the same time
- the strength of the drug (which can vary from batch to batch).

The individual effects and toxicity of each cathinone are distinct and can vary greatly between each person using them.

Generally speaking, in small doses, the following effects may be experienced and may last for approximately 2-4 hours:

- rush of intense pleasure
- feeling happy, energetic and wanting to talk more
- intense connection with music
- restless sleep
- muscle tension (face and jaw)
- blurred vision
- light-headedness, dizziness
- distorted sense of time
- enlarged (dilated) pupils, blurred vision
- dry mouth, thirst
- sweating
- memory loss
- Reduced appetite.

Higher doses may result in the following adverse effects:

- anxiety
- paranoia
- nose bleeds from snorting the drug
- stomach pains, nausea, vomiting
- skin rashes
- fast or irregular heartbeat
- high blood pressure and hot flushes
- strong urge to re-dose
- chest pain
- tremors, convulsions, death.

4.3.4 Mixing Synthetic Cathinones with Other Drugs

Mixing synthetic cathinones with other drugs can have unpredictable effects and increase the risk of harm.

- Synthetic cathinones and opioids can increase the risk of heart strain and respiratory arrest.
- Synthetic cathinones and MDMA: can cause anxiety, heart strain, and increased neurotoxic effects.
- Synthetic cathinone and cocaine can cause anxiety and heart strain, which can lead to stroke.
- Synthetic cathinones and benzodiazepines: can decrease/mask the effects of both. Risk of overdose if one wears off before the other – depending on the amount taken.
- Synthetic cathinone and alcohol: may feel less intoxicated due to the stimulant effects of amphetamine and lead to drinking more.

Reducing harm

To ensure you know what to expect and what a typical dose is, try to find out which particular cathinone you are using. Advice on harm reduction with synthetic cathinones is based in part on what is known about related drugs, such as MDMA and amphetamines since there is a lack of research on individual synthetic cathinones (Cozzi et al., 2013).

There are ways in which you can reduce the risks associated with using synthetic cathinones:

- Always test a small amount first and wait to feel the effects before taking more
- try to eat regularly even if you are not hungry. Eat fresh healthy food such as fruit and vegetables that are high in vitamins and nutrients.
- try to rest and get sleep.
- stay hydrated. People can become dehydrated when using synthetic cathinones, take small sips of water regularly.
- Avoid if you have a history of mental health issues.
- Regular use of synthetic cathinones can increase the risk of heart attack or other heart problems. Using less frequently and smaller amounts of amphetamines may reduce this risk.

In Australia, poisons information centres and clinical toxicology units around Australia are often contacted for advice on poisonings from synthetic cathinones. Features of these poisonings include:

- agitation
- tachycardia (increased heart rate)
- hypertension (high blood pressure)
- delirium

- aggressive behavior
- hallucinations
- hyperthermia
- cardiac dysrhythmia (irregular heartbeat)
- Seizures. Deaths have also occurred due to alpha-PVP toxicity. Injecting synthetic cathinones can cause soft tissue and vascular damage. Sharing needles may also transmit:
- tetanus
- hepatitis B
- hepatitis C
- HIV/AIDS.

Dependence and tolerance

Although there is little information on those seeking treatment for synthetic cathinone dependence, users have noted a strong urge to redose in addition to their dependence (Eshleman et al., 2013).

Coming down

In the days after synthetic cathinone use, the following may be experienced:

- restless sleep
- tiredness
- dizziness
- low mood wounds, sores taking longer to heal
- memory loss
- depression
- anxiety
- tremors
- problems sleeping
- Paranoia.

A Closer Look

Cathinones

Synthetic stimulant medications known as "cathinones" are structurally similar to the naturally occurring psychoactive alkaloid called "cathinone," which is produced by the khat plant (Catha edulis). These artificial substances, also known as bath salts or designer drugs, have become more well-known in recent years because of their extensive availability and strong stimulant properties.

The main way that catechinones work in the brain is by raising the concentrations of neurotransmitters like serotonin, norepinephrine, and dopamine. Like other stimulant drugs like amphetamines and cocaine, this action increases arousal, euphoria, and energy levels. However, because of their different chemical structures, cathinones may also have special pharmacological qualities and adverse effects. Methcathinone, which was first created in the 1920s and has been used recreationally for its stimulant effects, is one of the most well-known cathinones. Since then, a large number of synthetic cathinones have been created and sold as substitutes for illegal drugs or as legal highs. Methylone, alpha-pyrrolidinopentiophenone (alpha-PVP), and mephedrone are a few examples.

There are several serious risks associated with using cathinones, such as addiction, heart problems, mental health issues, and even death. Cathinones have a history of overdose and adverse reactions because of their strong stimulant qualities and erratic effects. Furthermore, it is challenging to regulate and control these drugs due to their covert production and distribution, which often results in their sale online or in black markets. Many nations have enacted laws restricting or outlawing the manufacture, distribution, and ownership of these drugs in response to the growing threat of abuse of cathinones. Nonetheless, law enforcement and public health authorities continue to face difficulties due to the covert nature of the illicit drug market. In order to address this expanding public health issue, it is still imperative that initiatives be made to increase awareness, offer education, and provide support to those who are battling with cathinone abuse.

Summary

- Amphetamine derivatives encompass a diverse class of compounds with varying chemical structures, pharmacological properties, and physiological effects.
- The synthesis and structure-activity relationships (SAR) of cathinones, commonly known as "bath salts," represent a complex and evolving field within the realm of synthetic stimulants.
- Structure-activity relationship studies aim to define the qualitative influence of chemical structure on a given biological action and are focused on identifying what, and to what extent, substituents and – where applicable – the stereochemistry, of substituents alter activity (i.e., action, potency).
- All of the above approaches are commonly used to formulate SAR, and most have been employed to investigate the SAR of synthetic cathinones.
- The abuse-related potential of biogenic amine-releasing agents appears to be related to their ability to promote greater release via DAT than via SERT, such that DAT-selective agents possess higher abuse liability.
- Stimulant abuse poses significant risks and consequences to both physical and mental health, as well as to social and societal well-being.
- Synthetic cathinones is the name of a category of drugs related to the naturally occurring khat plant. They are stimulants, meaning that they speed up the messages between the brain and the body and have similar effects to amphetamines.

References

1. Aarde SM, Creehan KM, Vandewater SA, et al. In vivo potency and efficacy of the novel cathinone α-pyrrolidinopentiophenone and 3,4-methylenedioxypyrovalerone: self-administration and locomotor stimulation in male rats. Psychopharmacology (Berl) 2015;232:3045–3055.
2. Aarde SM, Huang PK, Creehan KM, et al. The novel recreational drug 3,4-methylenedioxypyrovalerone (MDPV) is a potent psychomotor stimulant: self-administration and locomotor activity in rats. Neuropharmacology. 2013;71:130–140.
3. Baumann MH, Partilla JS, Lehner KR, et al. Powerful cocaine-like actions of 3,4-methylenedioxypyrovalerone (MDPV), a principal constituent of psychoactive 'bath salts' products. Neuropsychopharmacology. 2013;38:552–562.
4. Bonano JS, Banks ML, Kolanos R, et al. Quantitative structure-activity relationship analysis of the pharmacology of para-substituted methcathinone analogues. Br J Pharmacol. 2015;172:2433–2444.
5. Bondarev ML, Bondareva TS, Young R, et al. Behavioral and biochemical investigations of bupropion metabolites. Eur J Pharmacol. 2003;474:85–93.
6. Bondareva TS, Young R, Glennon RA. Central stimulants as discriminative stimuli: asymmetric generalization between (−)ephedrine and S(+)methamphetamine. Pharmacol Biochem Behav. 2002;74:157–162.
7. Cameron K, Kolanos R, Solis E, et al. Bath salts components mephedrone and

methylenedioxypyrovalerone (MDPV) act synergistically at the human dopamine transporter. Br J Pharmacol. 2013a;168:1750–1757.

8. Cameron K, Kolanos R, Vekariya R, et al. Mephedrone and methylenedioxypyro- valerone (MDPV), major constituents of "bath salts," produce opposite effects at the human dopamine transporter. Psychopharmacology (Berl) 2013b;227:493–499.

9. Carroll FI, Blough BE, Abraham P, et al. Synthesis and biological evaluation of bupropion analogues as potential pharmacotherapies for cocaine addiction. J Med Chem. 2009;52:6768–6781.

10. Cozzi NV, Brandt SD, Daley PF, et al. Pharmacological examination of trifluoromethyl ring-substituted methcathinone analogs. Eur J Pharmacol. 2013;699:180–187.

11. Del Bello F, Sakloth F, Partilla JS, et al. Ethylenedioxy homologs of N-methyl-(3,4-methylenedioxyphenyl)-2-aminopropane (MDMA) and its corresponding cathinone analog methylenedioxymethcathinone: Interactions with transporters for serotonin, dopamine, and norepinephrine. Bioorg Med Chem. 2015;23:5574–5579.

12. EMCDDA. Trends and Developments. European Monitoring Centre for Drugs and Drug Addiction; Luxembourg: 2015. European Drug Report.

13. Eshleman AJ, Wolfrum KM, Hatfield MG, et al. Substituted methcathinones differ in transporter and receptor interactions. Biochem Pharmacol. 2013;85:1803–1815.

14. Fantegrossi WE, Gannon BM, Zimmerman SM, et al. In vivo effects of abused 'bath salt' constituent 3,4-methylenedioxypyrovalerone (MDPV) in mice: drug discrimination, thermoregulation, and locomotor activity. Neuropsychopharmacology. 2013;38:563–573.

15. Foley KF, Cozzi NV. Novel aminopropiophenones as potential antidepressants. Drug Dev Res. 2003;60:252–260.

16. Gatch MB, Dolan SB, Forster MJ. Comparative behavioral pharmacology of three pyrrolidine-containing synthetic cathinone derivatives. J Pharmacol Exp Ther. 2015;354:103–110.

17. Gatch MB, Taylor CM, Forster MJ. Locomotor stimulant and discriminative stimulus effects of 'bath salt' cathinones. Behav Pharmacol. 2013;24:437–447.

18. Glennon RA. Bath salts, mephedrone, and methylenedioxypyrovalerone as emerging illicit drugs that will need targeted therapeutic intervention. Adv Pharmacol. 2014;69:581–620.

19. Glennon RA, Young R. Drug Discrimination: Applications to Medicinal Chemistry and Drug Studies. Wiley; Hoboken: 2011.

20. Gregg RA, Baumann MH, Partilla JS, et al. Stereochemistry of mephedrone neuropharmacology: enantiomer-specific behavioural and neurochemical effects in rats. Br J Pharmacol. 2015;172(3):883–894.

21. Hutsell BA, Baumann MH, Partilla JS, et al. Abuse-related neurochemical and behavioral effects of cathinone and 4-methylcathinone stereoisomers in rats. Eur Neuropsychopharmacol. 2016;26:288–297.

22. Iversen LE. Consideration of the cathinones. Advisory Council on the Misuse of Drugs. 2010 A report submitted to the Home Secretary of the UK (March 31, 2010)

23. Kolanos R, Cameron KN, Vekariya RH, et al. "Bath salts": an imitation of methamphetamine plus cocaine? Abstract #249. Southeast Regional American Chemical Society Meeting; Richmond, Virginia. 2011.

24. Kolanos R, Sakloth F, Jain AD, et al. Structural modification of the designer stimulant α-pyrrolidinovalerophenone (α-PVP) influences potency at dopamine transporters. ACS Chem Neurosci. 2015a;6:1726–1731.
25. Kolanos R, Partilla JS, Baumann MH, et al. Stereoselective actions of methylenedioxypyrovalerone (MDPV) to inhibit dopamine and norepinephrine transporters and facilitate intracranial self-stimulation in rats. ACS Chem Neurosci. 2015b;20:771–777.
26. Kolanos R, Solis E, Jr, Sakloth F, et al. "Deconstruction" of the abused synthetic cathinone methylenedioxypyrovalerone (MDPV) and an examination of effects at the human dopamine transporter. ACS Chem Neurosci. 2013;4:1524–1529.
27. Majchrzak M, Rojkiewicz M, Celiński R, et al. Identification and characterization of new designer drug 4-fluoro-PV9 and α-PHP in the seized materials. Forensic Toxicol. 2016;34:115–124.
28. Marusich JA, Antonazzo KR, Wiley JL, et al. Pharmacology of novel synthetic stimulants structurally related to the "bath salts" constituent 3,4-methylenedioxypyrovalerone (MDPV) Neuropharmacology. 2014;87:206–213.
29. Marusich JA, Grant KR, Blough BE, et al. Effects of synthetic cathinones contained in "bath salts" on motor behavior and a functional observational battery in mice. Neurotoxicology. 2012;33:1305–1313.
30. Meltzer PC, Butler D, Deschamps JR, et al. 1-(4-Methylphenyl)-2-pyrrolidin-1-yl-pentan-1-one (pyrovalerone) analogues: a promising class of monoamine uptake inhibitors. J Med Chem. 2006;49:1420–1432.
31. Negus SS, Mello NK, Blough BE, et al. Monoamine releasers with varying selectivity for dopamine/norepinephrine versus serotonin release as candidate "agonist" medications for cocaine dependence: studies in assays of cocaine discrimination and cocaine self-administration in rhesus monkeys. J Pharmacol Exp Ther 2007. 2007;320:627–636.
32. Reith MEA, Blough BE, Hong WC, et al. Behavioral, biological, and chemical perspectives on atypical agents targeting the dopamine transporter. Drug Alcohol Depend. 2015;147:1–19.
33. Rothman RB, Vu N, Partilla JS, et al. In vitro characterization of ephedrine-related stereoisomers at biogenic amine transporters and the receptorome reveals selective action as norepinephrine transporter substrates. J Pharmacol Exp Ther. 2003;307:138–145.
34. Saha K, Partilla JS, Lehner KR, et al. 'Second-generation' mephedrone analogs, 4-MEC and 4-MePPP, differentially affect monoamine transporter function. Neuropsychopharmacology. 2015;40:1321–1331.
35. Sakloth F. PhD Dissertation. Virginia Commonwealth University; Richmond, VA: 2015. Psychoactive synthetic cathinones (or 'bath salts'): Investigation of mechanisms of action.
36. Sakloth F, Kolanos R, Mosier PD, et al. Steric parameters, molecular modeling and hydropathic interaction analysis of the pharmacology of para-substituted methcathinone analogues. Br J Pharmacol. 2015;172:2210–2218.
37. Simmler LD, Buser TA, Donzelli M, et al. Pharmacological characterization of designer cathinones in vitro. Br J Pharmacol. 2013;168:458–470.
38. Suyama JA, Sakloth F, Kolanos R, et al. Abuse-related neurochemical effects of para-substituted methcathinone analogs in rats: microdialysis studies of nucleus accumbens dopamine and serotonin. J Pharmacol Exp Ther. 2016;356:182–190.

39. Tang QY, Kolanos R, De Felice LJ, et al. Structural analysis of dopamine- and amphetamine-induced depolarization currents in the human dopamine transporter. ACS Chem Neurosci. 2015;6:551–558.

40. Uchiyama N, Matsuda S, Kawamura M, et al. Characterization of four new designer drugs, 5-chloro-NNEI, NNEI indazole analog, α-PHPP and α-POP, with 11 newly distributed designer drugs in illegal products. Forensic Sci Int. 2014;243:1–13.

41. UNODC. The challenge of new psychoactive substances. United Nations Office of Drugs and Crime; Vienna, Austria: 2013.

42. Watterson LR, Olive MF. Synthetic cathinones and their rewarding and reinforcing effects in rodents. Adv Neurosci (Hindawi) 2014;2014:209875.

43. Watterson LR, Kufahl PR, Nemirovsky NE, et al. Potent rewarding and reinforcing effects of the synthetic cathinone 3,4-methylenedioxypyrovalerone (MDPV) Addict Biol. 2014;19:165–174.

Chapter 5

HALLUCINOGENS: PSYCHEDELIC AND DISSOCIATIVE DRUGS

Contents

Introduction

Hallucinogens encompass a fascinating array of psychoactive substances that have been used by humans for centuries if not millennia. These drugs alter perception, mood, and cognition, often leading to profound sensory experiences and alterations in consciousness. Two major categories within the realm of hallucinogens are psychedelic and dissociative drugs.

Psychedelic drugs induce profound alterations in perception, mood, and thought, often leading to a heightened sense of awareness and sensory experiences. Substances like LSD, psilocybin, and mescaline fall into this category. Users may experience vivid visual hallucinations, alterations in time perception, and profound spiritual or mystical experiences. These drugs have been used for spiritual, therapeutic, and recreational purposes, with some cultures incorporating them into religious ceremonies for centuries (Domino et al., 1965).

On the other hand, dissociative drugs produce a sense of detachment or disconnection from reality, often accompanied by feelings of depersonalization and derealization. Substances like ketamine, phencyclidine (PCP), and dextromethorphan (DXM) belong to this category. Dissociative drugs can induce hallucinations, sedation, and alterations in perception, similar to psychedelic drugs, but they typically create a sense of detachment from the environment and the self, leading to experiences of "floating," detachment, or out-of-body sensations.

Despite their classification into distinct categories, psychedelic and dissociative drugs share some overlapping effects, including alterations in sensory perception, hallucinations, and changes in mood and cognition. Both types of drugs have a complex pharmacology, acting on various neurotransmitter systems in the brain, including serotonin, glutamate, and dopamine (Johnstone et al., 1959).

In recent years, there has been a resurgence of interest in the therapeutic potential of both psychedelic and dissociative drugs for treating various mental health conditions, including depression, anxiety, post-traumatic stress disorder (PTSD), and substance use disorders (SUDs). Research into their mechanisms of action and therapeutic applications has expanded, offering new insights into how these drugs may be used to improve mental health and well-being.

However, the recreational use of hallucinogens also carries risks, including the potential for adverse psychological reactions, impaired judgment, and, in some cases, life-threatening medical complications. Understanding the effects, risks, and potential benefits of psychedelic and dissociative drugs is essential for promoting safe and responsible use, whether for therapeutic or recreational purposes.

Orientation and Directional Terms

Term	Definition	Illustration
Psilocybin	Psilocybin is a naturally occurring psychedelic prodrug compound produced by more than 200 species of fungi. The most potent are members of genus *Psilocybe*, such as *Psilocybe azurescens*, *P. semilanceata*, and *P. cyanescens*, but psilocybin has also been isolated from about a dozen other genera.	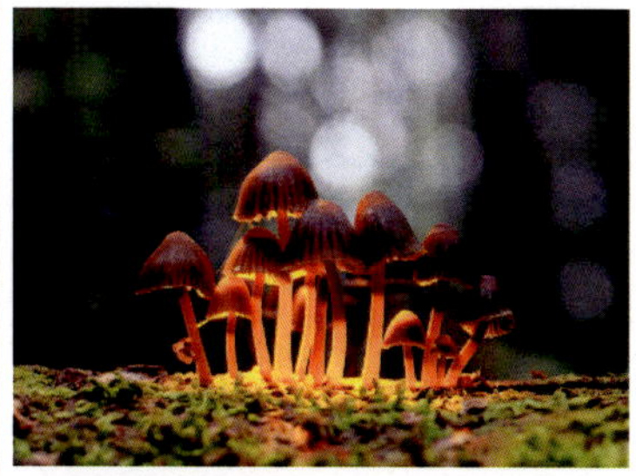
Dextromethorphan (DXM)	Dextromethorphan (DXM) is a cough suppressor found in more than 120 over-the counter (OTC) cold medications, either alone or in combination with other drugs such as analgesics (e.g., acetaminophen), antihistamines (e.g., chlorpheniramine), decongestants (e.g., pseudoephedrine), and/ or expectorants (e.g., guaifenesin).	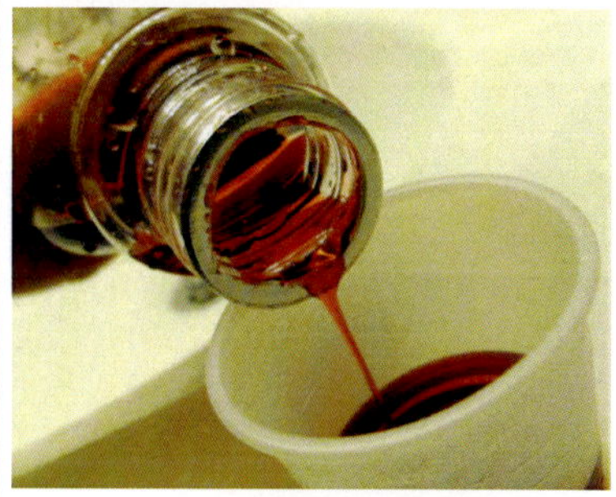
Therapeutics	Therapeutics, treatment, and care of a patient for the purpose of both preventing and combating disease or alleviating pain or injury. The term comes from the Greek therapeutikos, which means "inclined to serve."	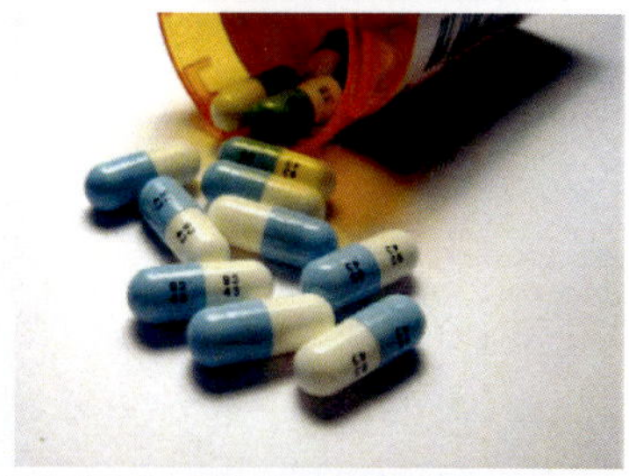
Lysergic acid diethylamide (LSD)	LSD is a potent hallucinogen that has a high potential for abuse and currently has no accepted medical use in treatment in the United States.	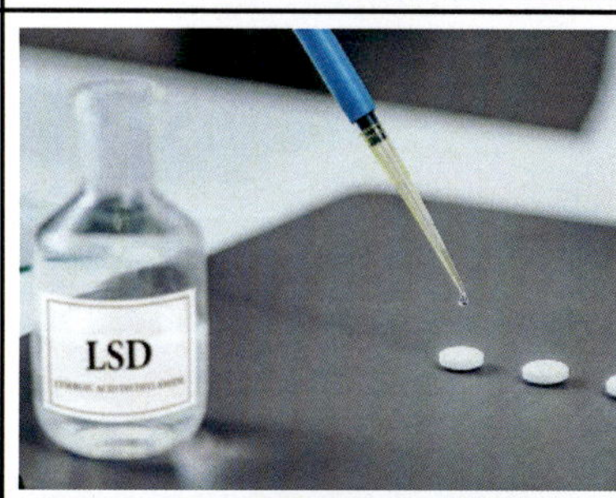
N, N-Dimethyltryptamine	N, N-Dimethyltryptamine is a substituted tryptamine that occurs in many plants and animals, including humans, and is both a derivative and a structural analog of tryptamine.	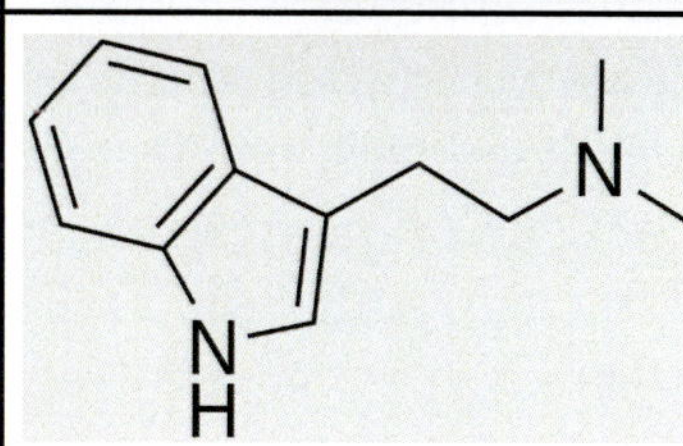

5.1 Classification and Effects Of Psychedelic Substances

Psychedelic substances encompass a diverse group of compounds that share the ability to alter perception, cognition, and mood. They can be classified based on various criteria, including their chemical structure, primary effects, and cultural or traditional use. Here's an overview of the classification and effects of psychedelic substances:

5.1.1 Lysergic Acid Diethylamide (LSD)

The highly potent hallucinogen LSD was first synthesized in 1938. When something appears real but is not, you experience hallucinations when you see, hear, feel, taste, or smell it. We call it Acid most of the time.

The fungus ergot, which grows on rye and other grains, contains lysergic acid, which is used to make LSD synthetically. Due to its extreme potency, its doses are typically in the microgram (mcg) range. It has stimulating, enjoyable, and mind-altering effects that are frequently referred to as a "trip.". It may result in an unpleasant, occasionally terrifying experience known as a "bad trip" in certain circumstances (Edwards et al., 2001).

Within the U.S.A Since LSD has no recognized medical use, is illegal, and is listed as a Schedule 1 drug by the Drug Enforcement Agency (DEA), it carries a high risk of abuse and lacks accepted safety when used under medical supervision. Notwithstanding its Schedule 1 status, there has been a renewed focus on the possible therapeutic applications of LSD, including the management of depression and alcoholism. There are currently studies being conducted that adhere to contemporary research standards and could contribute to our understanding of the use of LSD.

LSD is produced in crystalline form and then mixed with other inactive ingredients or diluted as a liquid for production in ingestible forms. It is odorless, colorless, and has a slightly bitter taste.

Active doses for LSD are between 0.5 and 2 mcg/kg (100–150 mcg per dose). Its half-life is about 3 hours but ranges between 2 hours and 5 hours, and the psychoactive effects can last up to 12 hours.

LSD is usually found on the streets in various forms, for example:

- blotter paper (LSD soaked onto sheets of absorbent paper with colorful designs; cut into small, individual dosage units) - the most common form
- thin squares of gelatin (commonly referred to as window panes)
- tablet form (usually small tablets known as Microdots) or capsules
- liquid on sugar cubes
- pure liquid form (may be extremely potent)

Some people may inhale LSD through the nose (snort) or inject it into a vein (shoot it up). There is no way to predict the amount of LSD that is contained in any form consumed (Persson et al., 2002).

Effects of Lysergic Acid Diethylamide Use

The effects of LSD use are complex and multifaceted, encompassing a wide range of psychological, perceptual, and emotional changes. As one of the most potent hallucinogenic substances known to humanity, LSD has captured the fascination of scientists, psychologists, and artists alike. Its effects are highly subjective and can vary greatly depending on factors such as dosage, set (mindset), and setting (environment). In this exploration, we delve into the intricate tapestry of LSD's effects, from the profound alterations in perception to the potential risks and therapeutic possibilities.

Altered Perception and Sensory Experience

At the core of the effects LSD lies a profound distortion of perception and sensory experience. Users often report vivid visual hallucinations characterized by intricate patterns, geometric shapes, and vibrant colors. Everyday objects may appear to morph and transform before one's eyes, leading to a heightened sense of wonder and awe. Auditory hallucinations are also common, with sounds taking on new meanings and textures. Music, in particular, can evoke intense emotional responses and synesthetic experiences, where sounds are perceived as visual or tactile sensations (Geisslinger et al., 1995).

Changes in Consciousness and Thought Patterns

LSD induces a state of altered consciousness marked by a profound shift in thought patterns and cognitive processes. Users often describe a loosening of the ego or sense of self, leading to a feeling of interconnectedness with the universe or a sense of unity with others. This dissolution of boundaries can result in a heightened sense of empathy and compassion, as well as a deepening of existential insights and philosophical contemplation. Time and space may lose their usual constraints, leading to a sense of timelessness or infinity.

Emotional Intensity and Spiritual Experiences

The effects of LSD on mood and emotions are complex and unpredictable. While some users report feelings of euphoria, bliss, and awe, others may experience anxiety, fear, or existential dread, commonly referred to as a "bad trip." Emotional experiences on LSD can be deeply cathartic, leading to profound personal insights and spiritual revelations. Many users describe a sense of transcendence or mystical union with the cosmos, often accompanied by feelings of reverence, gratitude, and interconnectedness with all life (Ihmsen et al., 2001).

Potential Risks and Adverse Effects

Despite its profound effects, LSD use carries inherent risks and potential adverse effects. Bad trips, characterized by extreme anxiety, paranoia, or delusions, can occur, leading to acute psychological distress and trauma. Flashbacks, or recurrences of LSD-like experiences, may occur days, weeks, or even months after the drug was last taken, contributing to a condition known as Hallucinogen Persisting Perception Disorder. Additionally, LSD use can impair judgment and perception, leading to accidents, risky behavior, or self-harm. Individuals with underlying mental health conditions, such as anxiety, depression, or psychosis, may be particularly vulnerable to the negative effects of LSD.

Therapeutic Potential and Research Findings

Despite its recreational use, LSD has also attracted interest from researchers for its potential therapeutic applications. Early studies from the mid-20th century suggested that LSD could be effective in treating various psychiatric disorders, including depression, anxiety, post-traumatic stress disorder (PTSD), and SUDs. More recent research has revived interest in LSD-assisted psychotherapy as a promising approach for addressing treatment-resistant mental health conditions. Studies have shown that LSD can facilitate introspection, emotional processing, and neuroplasticity, leading to lasting improvements in mood, cognition, and well-being. However, further research is needed to fully understand the therapeutic benefits and risks of LSD.

Health Hazards and Flashbacks with Lysergic Acid Diethylamide

When under the influence of LSD, a person's capacity to make reasonable decisions and recognize everyday threats is compromised, increasing the risk of harm or even death. Following an LSD trip, the user may experience acute anxiety, depression, and flashbacks (also known as hallucinogen persisting perception disorder), which are the effects of LSD, reoccurring days or even months after the last dose was taken.

- A flashback occurs suddenly, often without warning, usually in people who use hallucinogens chronically or have an underlying personality problem.
- Healthy people who only use LSD occasionally may also have flashbacks.
- Bad trips and flashbacks are only part of the risks of LSD use. LSD users may also manifest relatively long-lasting psychoses, such as schizophrenia or severe depression.

Tolerance to LSD is a side effect of the drug, requiring higher doses for the same effect. Some drug users who use the substance frequently need to take increasingly larger doses in order to reach the same level of intoxication as before. Considering how unpredictable the drug is, this is a very risky practice (Henthorn et al., 1999).

Extent of Lysergic Acid Diethylamide Use

Rates of LSD and hallucinogens in general use remain low among youth in the U.S.A

- The *National Survey on Drug Use and Health* (NSDUH) in 2020 estimated that 7.1 million people aged 12 or older were past-year users of hallucinogens, corresponding to 2.6% of the population.
- Hallucinogens include LSD, PCP, peyote, mescaline, psilocybin mushrooms, Ecstasy, ketamine, DMT/AMT/"Foxy," (DMT is the main active ingredient in Ayahuasca), and *Salvia divinorum.*

The percentage of use among adults aged 18 to 25 (7.3% or 2.4 million people) was higher than that among adolescents aged 12 to 17 (1.5% or 370,000 people) or adults aged 26 or older (2% or 4.3 million people).

In 2021, based on data from NIDA's *Monitoring the Future 2021 Survey Results: Overall Findings*, past year illicit drug use for LSD among surveyed 12th graders was 2.5%, a drop of 1.4%. As a comparison, this was far below illicit drug use for marijuana, which stood at 30.5% (compared to 35.2% in 2020) for 12th graders.

Past MTF surveys found that "generational forgetting" -- students stating that they are not familiar with the drug -- has resulted in a decline in perceived risk of LSD among younger groups, which may put them at higher risk of use in future years. This points to the need for continued education overtime on all illicit drugs (including hallucinogens) that may be a risk for youth.

5.1.2 Psilocybin

Magic mushrooms, also known as psilocybin, are ingested for their hallucinogenic properties and are found naturally. Since they are psychedelic substances, their effects can be felt through all senses, changing a person's perception of time, thought processes, and emotions. A person using psychedelics may experience hallucinations, seeing or hearing distorted or nonexistent objects. Psilocybin is the main component of magic mushrooms. The chemical with the psychoactive qualities, psilocin, is created in the body when psilocybin is consumed (Malinovsky et al., 1996).

Effects of Magic Mushrooms

There is no safe level of drug use. The use of any drug always carries some risk. It's important to be careful when taking any type of drug.

Magic mushrooms can affect everyone differently, based on:

- size, weight, and health
- whether the person is used to taking it
- whether other drugs are taken around the same time
- the amount taken
- the strength of the mushroom (varies depending on the type of mushroom)
- the environment (where the drug is taken)

The effects of magic mushrooms usually begin in 30 minutes when eaten, or within 5–10 minutes when taken as a soup or tea and can last approximately four to six hours.[3]

During this time, the person may experience:

- euphoria and wellbeing
- change in consciousness, mood, thought, and perception (commonly called a trip)
- dilation of pupils
- perceptual changes, such as visual and auditory hallucinations (seeing or hearing things that aren't there or are distorted)
- stomach discomfort and nausea
- headaches
- fast or irregular heartbeat
- increased body temperature
- breathing quickly
- vomiting
- facial flushes, sweating, and chills.

Overdose

The use of magic mushrooms rarely results in any life-threatening symptoms (Geisslinger et al., 1991). If a large amount or a strong batch of mushrooms is consumed, the person may experience:

- agitation
- vomiting
- diarrhoea
- muscle weakness
- panic or paranoia
- psychosis
- seizures
- coma.

Bad trips

Sometimes, a person may experience the negative effects of magic mushrooms and have a 'bad trip.'

A bad trip might include:

- unpleasant or intense hallucinations
- anxiety
- paranoia
- panic or fear.

Coming down

After taking magic mushrooms, delayed

headaches can happen. These usually don't last longer than a day.[5]

A person who has taken mushrooms may experience feelings of:

- exhaustion
- depression
- anxiety.

Some people who use magic mushrooms frequently might get flashbacks to experiences they had with the mushrooms in the past. Usually, they are perceptual or emotional distortions combined with visual distortions. Weeks, months, or even years after the drug was last taken can cause flashbacks. This may be unsettling, particularly if it brings back memories of a terrifying incident or hallucination. Flashbacks typically last a minute or two and can be triggered by using other drugs, stress, fatigue, or exercise.

Impact of Mood and Environment

Psychoactive drugs, or drugs that alter mental states, can also have distinct effects based on an individual's mood (sometimes referred to as their "set") or the environment they are in (also known as their "setting"). Set refers to an individual's mental state, prior experiences with psychedelic drugs, and anticipated outcomes. For instance, if you're stressed or anxious before taking magic mushrooms, it could ruin your trip (Noppers et al., 2010).

Setting refers to the conditions in which a person uses a psychedelic drug, including the type of music and light, the location, the people they are with, and whether the place is known or unfamiliar.

For instance, taking magic mushrooms in a peaceful, quiet, and relaxed setting can result in or contribute to a positive experience, but taking them in a busy, noisy area can have the opposite effect. Being in a good state of mind, with trusted friends and a safe environment before taking magic mushrooms reduces the risk of having a bad trip.

Using Magic Mushrooms with Other Drugs

The effects of taking magic mushrooms with other drugs – including over-the-counter or prescribed medications – can be unpredictable and dangerous.

Magic mushrooms + ice, speed , or ecstasy: This can increase the chances of a bad trip and lead to panic.

Magic mushrooms + some psychiatric medications: Mushrooms should not be taken by people on psychiatric medications as a relapse or worsening of the condition could occur.

5.1.3 Dimethyltryptamine (DMT)

Dimethyltryptamine, or DMT, is a powerful hallucinogenic compound that has captivated the interest of scientists, spiritual seekers, and psychonauts alike. Often referred to as the "spirit molecule," DMT is renowned for its ability to induce profound alterations in consciousness, perception, and reality. In this exploration, we delve into the multifaceted world of DMT, examining its chemistry, effects, cultural significance, therapeutic potential, and mysteries that continue to intrigue researchers and explorers of the human mind.

Chemistry and Pharmacology

DMT, chemically known as N, N-dimethyltryptamine, is a naturally occurring compound found in various plants, animals, and even the human brain. Structurally, it belongs to the tryptamine family, sharing similarities with neurotransmitters like serotonin and melatonin. DMT's psychoactive effects stem from its ability to bind to serotonin receptors in the brain, particularly the 5-HT2A receptor, leading to alterations in neural activity and neurotransmitter release (Sprenger et al., 2006).

Effects and Experiences: The effects of DMT are notoriously intense and immersive, often described as transcending ordinary reality and opening the doors of perception to otherworldly dimensions. While experiences can vary widely among individuals, common themes and phenomena emerge:

- **Rapid Onset and Intensity**: DMT is known for its rapid onset of action, with effects typically manifesting within seconds to minutes after administration. Users often describe an abrupt transition from baseline consciousness to a profoundly altered state characterized by a rapid escalation of sensory and perceptual phenomena.
- **Visual Hallucinations**: DMT induces vivid and intricate visual hallucinations that unfold in a rapid, kaleidoscopic fashion. Users may encounter a vast array of geometric patterns, fractal shapes, and vibrant colors, often described as more vivid and intense than anything experienced in ordinary waking consciousness.
- **Encounters with Entities**: Many users report encounters with seemingly autonomous entities or beings during DMT experiences. These entities can take on a wide range of forms, from benevolent guides and teachers to enigmatic aliens or spirits. These encounters are often described as deeply meaningful and profound, leaving a lasting impression on the user's psyche.
- **Time and Space Distortion**: DMT can induce a profound distortion of time and space, leading to a sense of timelessness or infinity. Users may feel as though they have entered a timeless dimension or alternate reality where conventional notions of space and time no longer apply.
- **Ego Dissolution and Mystical Experiences**: DMT often induces a state of ego dissolution, where the boundaries of self and other dissolve, leading to a sense of unity with the universe or a higher power. Many users describe DMT experiences as profoundly mystical or spiritual, characterized by feelings of awe, reverence, and interconnectedness with all life.
- **Physical Sensations**: Alongside the profound alterations in consciousness, users may also experience physical sensations such as tingling, vibrations, or a sense of weightlessness. These sensations are often described as integral to the overall DMT experience, contributing to a sense of immersion and embodiment within the psychedelic realm.

Cultural and Spiritual Significance

DMT has a long history of use in indigenous cultures around the world, where it is often revered as a sacred medicine or sacrament. In the Amazon basin, for example, DMT-containing plants like ayahuasca have been used for centuries in shamanic rituals for healing, divination, and spiritual growth. Similarly, in the Andes region, DMT-containing snuffs like yopo and vilca have been used by indigenous peoples for ceremonial purposes. These traditions highlight the deep cultural and spiritual significance of DMT as a tool for accessing higher states of consciousness and communing with the divine (Rogers et al., 2004).

Therapeutic Potential and Research Findings

In recent years, there has been a resurgence of interest in the therapeutic potential of DMT and related psychedelics for treating various mental health conditions. Preliminary research suggests that DMT may hold promise for addressing conditions such as depression, anxiety, PTSD, and SUDs. Studies have shown that DMT can facilitate profound emotional processing, insight generation, and neuroplasticity, leading to lasting improvements in mood and well-being. However, further research is needed to fully understand the therapeutic benefits and risks of DMT, as well as the optimal dosing and treatment protocols.

Mysteries and Unanswered Questions

Despite decades of research, DMT continues to mystify scientists and researchers with its enigmatic properties and profound effects on consciousness. Key questions remain unanswered, such as the role of endogenous DMT in the human brain, the mechanisms underlying DMT-induced hallucinations and mystical experiences, and the nature of the entities encountered during DMT experiences. These mysteries underscore the need for continued scientific inquiry and exploration into the nature of consciousness and the human mind.

5.1.4 Mescaline

Mescaline is a hallucinogenic drug that is obtained from various cacti that contain mescaline, such as the Peruvian torch cactus, San Pedro cactus, and the small, spineless cactus Peyote (*Lophophora williamsi*). It can be synthesized and is also present in some members of the bean family, Fabaceae.

Hallucinogens have been used by humans for hundreds of years, primarily in religious ceremonies and rituals. Rich, vivid visual hallucinations are caused by mescaline. Native Americans in the southwest region of the United States and northern Mexico have been using peyote for religious purposes since the beginning of recorded history (Wieber etal., 1975). It functions similarly to other hallucinogenic drugs, such as LSD and psilocybin (magic mushrooms).

How is Mescaline Used or Abused?

The top of the cactus above ground, or the crown, consists of disc-shaped buttons cut from the roots and dried. These buttons are generally chewed or soaked in water to produce an intoxicating tea. It can be consumed raw or dried but is extremely bitter. The hallucinogen may also be ground into powder for oral capsules, or smoked with marijuana and tobacco.

The hallucinogenic experience typically begins 60 minutes after consumption and lasts about 8 to 12 hours. However, different doses can affect people in various ways, and doses extracted from plants can vary widely.

Mescaline is used primarily as a recreational drug and is also used to supplement various types of meditation and psychedelic therapy.

- It is classified as a Schedule I drug in the U.S., making it illegal in all forms (including peyote); however, it remains legal in certain religious ceremonies registered by the Native American Church
- Schedule I drugs have a high potential for abuse, no currently accepted medical use in treatment in the United States, and a lack of accepted safety for use under medical supervision.

What are the effects from mescaline?

"Trips", the intense psychedelic experience for the user, may be pleasurable and enlightening or anxiety-producing and unpleasant (known as a "bad trip"). There is no way to know how a user's mescaline experience may ultimately play out.

Common effects during mescaline use may include:

- visual hallucinations and radically altered states of consciousness (psychedelic experience)
- open and closed-eye visualizations
- euphoria
- dream-like state
- altered body image
- slowed passage of time
- altered perception of space
- laughter
- a mixing of senses (synesthesia, such as "seeing a sound" or "hearing colors")
- pupil dilation

Side effects or risks

Intense nausea, vomiting, dilation of the pupils, increased heart rate, increased blood pressure, a rise in body temperature that causes heavy perspiration, headaches, muscle weakness, and impaired motor coordination

Side effects or risks of mescaline use may include:

- anxiety, fear
- racing heartbeat (tachycardia)
- increased blood pressure
- dizziness
- weakness
- diarrhea
- elevated body temperature
- excessive sweating
- tremors
- intense nausea, vomiting
- headache
- accidental injury
- psychosis, panic or paranoia
- seizures
- amnesia (loss of memory)
- post-hallucinogen perceptual disorder (flashbacks)
- rarely, suicidal thoughts or actions

Like most psychedelic hallucinogens, mescaline is not physically addictive; however, it can cause tolerance, meaning higher doses are needed to achieve the same hallucinogenic effect. Mescaline-containing cacti can induce severe vomiting and nausea, which is an important part of traditional Native American or Shaman ceremonies and is considered a cleansing ritual and a spiritual aid (Kharasch et al., 1992).

If you take prescription medications, there are no well-controlled studies to determine the overall effect of drug interactions.

- Medications that have an effect on the brain and may affect serotonin levels (for example, antidepressants, antipsychotic agents, and medications for bipolar disorder) may have the potential for dangerous drug interactions when combined with mescaline.
- Drugs that affect the circulatory system and heart or have stimulant effects may lead to rapid pulse and dangerous cardiovascular outcomes.
- Other drug interactions are also possible, although scientific data are limited.

5.2 Dissociative Drugs

Dissociative drugs are a class of psychoactive substances that induce a state of dissociation, characterized by feelings of detachment from one's surroundings, body, or sense of identity.

5.2.1 Phencyclidine

A notorious hallucinogen known for producing delusions of euphoria, omnipotence, superhuman strength, and social and sexual prowess is PCP (sometimes known as "angel dust"). The name 1-(1-phenylcyclohexyl) piperidine, which refers to its relatively easy synthesis from arylcyclohexylamine piperidine, is the source of the acronym PCP.

Before piperidine and its derivatives were outlawed in the US in 1978, there were over 60 designer analogs that were more toxic than PCP but could evade clinical detection. Because of its effects similar to PCP, ketamine—the only drug approved for medical use—was frequently stolen from veterinary clinics. PCP has street names like "horse tranquilizer," "hog," and "elephant" because, like ketamine, it was once used as an animal tranquilizer and pre-induction anesthetic. It was highly regarded for its capacity to induce anesthesia and analgesia without inducing cardiorespiratory depression, but it was quickly withdrawn when patients developed post-operative psychosis, agitation, and dysphoria (Sigtermans et al., 2009).

Following a decline after the 1980s, PCP has become more of a drug of abuse in this decade. Only 3.9% of twelfth graders used PCP in 1997, compared to 12.8% in 1979. PCP, however, is still present in PCP-laced marijuana cigarettes, also known as "whacko tobacco," and it has been found in as many as 24% of marijuana samples taken from the street. Unfortunately, numerous cases of occult pediatric PCP intoxication have been linked to exposure to the smoke and butts of these cigarettes.

Pharmacology

PCP can be taken in many different forms, including liquid ("whack"), tablets ("PeaCe Pill"), crystals, and white crystalline powder ("angel dust"). It can also be smoked, snorted, swallowed, or injected intravenously or subcutaneously. A standard marijuana cigarette laced with PCP has 1–10 mg of the drug. The weight of an average tablet ranges from 1 to 6 mg. Compared to 10 mg needed by ingestion or inhalation, only 0–25 mg of IV solution is needed to cause sedation.

However, due to the rapid onset of action (usually within 2-4 minutes) and lack of injection complications, 70% of usage occurs through inhalation. When taken orally, effects could appear 15–60 minutes later. Because PCP is a weak base that dissolves in lipids, water, and alcohol, it has an unusually large volume of distribution—6.22 L/kg. As a result, body habitus, nutritional status, and alcohol consumption all affect the relationship between dose, serum level, and effects.

Walberg et al. did not find any direct relationship between the serum concentration of PCP and the clinical pattern of intoxication in a case series of 216 patients with "pure" PCP intoxication. This lack of correlation between plasma concentration and the clinical effects of PCP is poorly understood. Additionally, no relevant data or literature could be found to correlate PCP concentrations in the cerebrospinal fluid with the clinical effects of the drug (Clements et al., 1981).

PCP-binding antibodies were found to increase serum concentrations of PCP in animal experiments, suggesting that they only modify its distribution. The half-life of PCP is thought to be three days due to its uneven and slow release from lipid stores, with the highest levels found in adipose tissue. The brain's high lipid content and ion trapping can cause cerebral PCP levels to be nine times higher than serum levels, which can prolong the drug's central nervous system effects in chronic users from seven hours to seven days.

The weakly basic PCP is actively secreted into the stomach's acid environment in significant amounts, regardless of the mode of administration. It can accumulate to levels 50 times higher than serum levels in the stomach before being reabsorbed in the small intestine. Thankfully, the liver uses oxidative hydroxylation to metabolize 90% of the medication during its initial pass. The 9 % of the active drug that is excreted directly is then combined with these metabolites to form glucuronidated salts for renal excretion.

Anesthesia and analgesia are thought to be produced by PCP's multiple sites of action in the central nervous system, which work in concert with one another. It is most receptive to NMDA (N-methyl-D-aspartate) receptor complexes found in the limbic system, neocortex, hippocampal regions, and basal ganglia. PCP has three main effects on neurons, and its serum concentrations up to 1 μM/mL are safe for human health. PCP's affinity for NMDA receptors, neuronal dopamine (DA), serotonin (5-HT) reuptake system, norepinephrine (NE), and σ opioid receptors decreases with time. PCP causes dopaminergic and sympathomimetic effects when taken orally in moderate doses of 1 to 5 mg. It also inhibits serotonin reuptake and increases the production of dopamine and norepinephrine by stimulating tyrosine hydroxylase. A calcium channel activated by excitatory neurotransmitters like glutamate, glycine, and aspartate but inhibited by phencyclidine at a binding site specific to PCP is part of the NMDA-Phencyclidine complex. Ironically, PCP also activates the central nervous system by releasing glutamate at presynaptic metabotropic receptors. Rather than being ion-gated channels, metabolotropic receptors are G-proteins (Table 5.1).

Table 5.1. Pharmacology of phencyclidine (PCP) in the central nervous system

• PCP has contrary actions on glutamate transmission, explaining its different effects
  • Inhibits the ion flux at the NMDA glutamate receptor
  • Increases glutamate transmission at non-NMDA receptors (G-protein mediated response)
• Inhibits the GABAergic output
• Decreases DA and NE uptake
• Increases the DA and NE levels by stimulating the enzyme tyrosine hydroxylase

GABA: γ - aminobutyric acid
NMDA: N-methyl D-aspartate
DA: dopamine
NA: norepinephrine

Source: https://www.ncbi.nlm.nih.gov/pmc/articles/PMC2859735/

Clinical Manifestations

The classic toxidrome of PCP intoxication—violent behavior, nystagmus, tachycardia, hypertension, anesthesia, and analgesia—presents in more than 50% of adult patients.

Due to PCP's ability to cause both central nervous system (CNS) stimulation and depression through various CNS effects, the clinical picture may fluctuate between extreme agitation and sedation. The drug stimulates σ-opioid receptors, nicotinic, muscarinic, and γ-aminobutyrique acid (GABA) receptors, binds to NMDA receptors, and functions as a monoamine reuptake inhibitor at increasing concentrations (Domino et al., 1984). Ataxia, hyperthermia, seizures, slurred speech, violent behavior, blank staring, horizontal, vertical, or rotatory nystagmus, and seizures are among the CNS findings associated with dosages of 1 to 5 mg that typically result in sedation and loss of inhibition (Table 5.2).

Table 5.2. Neuropsychiatric and clinical effects of phencyclidine (at different doses

Estimated ingested amount	Clinical effects
2–5 mg (Stage I)	Unpredictable, drunk, euphoric, disoriented, combativeness, rage obscenity.
	Alternating periods of lethargy and fearful agitation: waxing and waning.
	Decreased but intact pain perception, midpoint pupils, nystagmus, and ataxia differentiate PCP from stimulants.
5–25 mg (Stage II)	Stupor, mild coma, intact response to deep pain, muscle contractions, bizarre postures.
More than 25 mg (Stage III)	Comatose with no response to deep pain, hyperthermia, convulsions, death.

Source: https://www.ncbi.nlm.nih.gov/pmc/articles/PMC2859735/

The most peculiar aspect of PCP is that oral dosages of 5 to 10 mg can cause acute schizophrenia, which manifests as agitation, psychosis, catatonia, and audiovisual hallucinations. Coma is typically the result of doses higher than 10 mg. PCP is used in animal experiments to study the neurochemical underpinnings of schizophrenia. Rodent brains treated with low doses of PCP have shown neurochemical and metabolic alterations that are similar to those seen in schizophrenic patients' brains. The classic sign of a PCP-induced coma is an unresponsive patient with open eyes.

At higher recreational doses, PCP can be dangerous due to the same qualities that make it ideal for anesthesia at moderate doses: lack of muscle hypotonia or cardiorespiratory depression. It causes cholinergic symptoms like bronchospasm, salivation, urine retention, flushing, and miosis, similar to opiates, and sympathomimetic signs like hypertension, tachycardia, and diaphoresis, similar to cocaine. The two most prevalent ones are hypertension and tachycardia (Noppers et al., 2011).

PCP has also been demonstrated to directly irritate the heart, possibly causing arrhythmias and vasospasm. Furthermore, patients experience an increase in muscle tone, hyperreflexia, and myoclonic, dystonic, or choreoathetoid movements, including torticollis and opisthotonos. Hyperthermia and rhabdomyolysis are two side effects of this hypertonic muscle activity. Patients may experience episodes of both tachypnea and apnea, but respiratory depression necessitating intubation is rare in PCP intoxication. In addition, the patient's already obtunded state increases the risk of airway obstruction due to bronchorrhea caused by sympathomimetic effects and hyperactive pharyngeal and laryngeal reflexes. In patients with PCP intoxication, respiratory depression necessitating intubation is rare; however, patients may present with dyspnea and tachypnea episodes. Additionally, the patient experiences bronchorrhea due to sympathomimetic effects and hyperactive pharyngeal and laryngeal reflexes, which increase the risk of airway obstruction in an already obtunded patient (Idwall et al., 1979).

Cardiopulmonary arrest, intracranial hemorrhage in hypertension, and hyperkalemia due to rhabdomyolysis are examples of non-traumatic causes of death. However, rather than the drug's direct effects, aggressive behavior by the patients causes the majority of deaths in PCP-intoxicated patients. In addition to its analgesic effects, PCP can cause violent and strange behavior that can lead to significant self-inflicted trauma. Patients have even managed to enucleate their own eyes and walk into oncoming traffic.

As the drug is removed from the body, patients recovering from PCP exposure may experience a reaction that can last for days to weeks and manifest as psychosis, odd behavior, or depression. Extended psychosis is associated with a poor prognosis, as the patient may progress to full-blown schizophrenia. It is more common in chronic abusers. As little as one day of abstinence has been reported to cause depression, anxiety, irritability, restlessness, anergia, and disruptions in thought and sleep in chronic abusers. In monkeys given PCP on a chronic basis, oculomotor hyperactivity, tremor, diarrhea, and piloerection were noted within 8 hours of cessation.

Effects of Phencyclidine in Children

Ikonomidou et al. point out that during the period of rapid growth of the mammalian brain, neuronal apoptosis can be triggered by the transient blockade of glutamate. Olney's animal experimental findings support the induction of neuronal cell death by NMDA antagonists like PCP. Different brain regions display different age-dependent vulnerabilities to NMDA receptor-blocking drugs, leading to different patterns of neuronal loss depending on the time of exposure. In humans, the brain growth spurt period starts in the sixth month of gestation and extends to the third year of life.

Thus, young children are very sensitive to PCP and develop serious neurologic signs with minimal exposure. They can become intoxicated from passive inhalation of secondhand smoke or by ingesting the butts of PCP-impregnated cigarettes. These signs may present as listlessness, irritability, and poor feeding in newborns, and should immediately raise suspicion for intoxication. Different forms of choreoathetosis were seen in half of the cases. Hypertension and seizures are the next most common signs in infants, observed 30 and 20% of the time, respectively. Blood pressure elevations are common during the first 6 hours of intoxication but usually resolve spontaneously (Pedraz et al., 1987).

Seizures, apnea, and respiratory depression are documented more frequently in children than adults; however, they rarely require intubation. Violent behavior is less common in children, which may explain the lack of mortality reported in children. Mild intoxication in children may present as lethargy alternating with agitation, a dull trance-like stare, horizontal or vertical nystagmus, miosis, truncal ataxia, choreoathetosis, hypersalivation, and mild hypertension, and may last from 12 hours to over three days. Severe intoxication, including unresponsiveness with an open-eyed stare and short intermittent generalized seizures, may last up to six days.

Diagnosis

It is necessary to establish a clinical suspicion of PCP intoxication before ordering the necessary tests for confirmation. Other intoxications, schizophrenia, intracranial pathology, hypoxia, hypoglycemia, hyponatremia, sepsis, meningitis and encephalitis, thyroid storm, and neuroleptic malignant syndrome are among the differential diagnoses of the clinical picture produced by PCP. A lot of the characteristics of PCP intoxication are similar to those of cocaine overdoses, amphetamine overdoses, anticholinergic drugs, hallucinogens, and benzodiazepine withdrawal. As such, the standard of care for any patient, infant or adult, with an altered mental status of unknown etiology is now a qualitative urine toxicologic screen. Despite the fact that previous research has identified three dose-related phases of PCP intoxication, clinical management should not be guided by quantitative PCP levels because they do not exhibit a strong correlation with clinical findings (Thomson et al., 1988).

Since the kidneys excrete 9 % of the active drug directly, a qualitative chromatographic or immunologic urine drug screen is the most straightforward method of verifying a suspicion of PCP intoxication. After using PCP, the urine typically tests positive for 2-4 days; however, in cases of chronic exposure, the results may remain positive for more than a week. Several medications, such as diphenhydramine, DXM, and venlafaxine and its derivatives, can result in a positive PCP test result from a urine specimen when tested using techniques other than gas chromatography/mass spectrophotometry, like high-pressure liquid chromatography or fluorescence polarization immunoassay.

Bond et al. report a case of a 13-year-old girl who presented with a massive venlafaxine overdose and a false positive fluorescent-polarized immunoassay for PCP in the urine. The GS/MS, however, identified venlafaxine as the only substance present in the serum. Conversely, urine drug screens may be negative in the face of alkaline urine since PCP is a weak base. In this situation, saliva or gastric contents can be analyzed for PCP.

Serum potassium, blood urea nitrogen, creatinine, and creatine phosphokinase should be ordered whenever rhabdomyolysis is suspected due to the potential for PCP-induced seizures, myoclonic activity, and trauma to result in this condition. The best way to screen for rhabdomyolysis is with serum creatine phosphokinase because urine myoglobin can be temporary. It is also advised to check serum and capillary blood glucose levels, as PCP has been linked to hypoglycemia in 20% of patients.

Management

PCP intoxication is managed in the same way as any other intoxication. Priorities should be given to stabilizing the patient's breathing, circulation, airway, thermoregulation, and neurologic status. The most common cause of morbidity and death in these patients is self-inflicted injury, which should be prevented by restraining and sedating the patient if needed.

Physical restraints increase the risk of rhabdomyolysis; chemical restraints are preferred. Since antipsychotics can exacerbate PCP-induced hyperthermia, dystonic and anticholinergic reactions, and lower the seizure threshold, benzodiazepines are advised for patients who do not exhibit psychosis. If the patient is not overheating, haloperidol has been suggested as a helpful treatment for PCP-induced psychosis. Haloperidol use in patients with PCP intoxication is restricted due to the risks of torsade de pointes, prolongation of the QT interval, and adverse neurologic effects. When treating PCP-induced agitation and psychosis, atypical antipsychotics such as olanzapine or ziprasidone would be a better option than haloperidol due to their more favorable side effect profile. Diphenhydramine, which may cause the specimen to test falsely positive for PCP, can be used to treat dystonic symptoms caused by PCP (or haloperidol). However, it is best to administer diphenhydramine after obtaining a urine sample for toxicologic screening. Diphenhydramine has anticholinergic properties that can also result in tachycardia and issues with thermoregulation, so the advantages of using it should be balanced against these possible drawbacks. In order to prevent violent outbursts, patients should then be closely monitored in a quiet, dark environment with little auditory or tactile stimulation (White et al., 1982).

A blood glucose reading should be taken, as with all intoxications, and if the blood sugar is abnormally low, 100 mg of thiamine and 50% dextrose should be given. In patients with adequate breathing, naloxone is not required to treat potentially co-ingested opiates.

Because gastric lavage is debatable, it should only be applied after speaking with a toxicologist. In cases of suspected PCP ingestion, serial doses of activated charcoal may be required to stop the drug's later redistribution from lipid stores. A standard dose of 1 g/kg of activated charcoal is strongly advised to prevent further drug absorption during entero-hepatic recirculation. Before giving charcoal to a drunk patient, it is important to evaluate them for mental decline, aspiration risk, and potential airway complications.

Patients must undergo continuous cardiac monitoring because of the frequency and severity of cardiac symptoms. Diastolic hypertension >115 mmHg may be transient, or fall after sedation, eliminating the need for further treatment.

There are case reports of intracerebral hemorrhage secondary to hypertension. Additionally, Welch et al. describe several cases of intracerebral hemorrhage in infants that were not visualized on CT and have been diagnosed by lumbar puncture, suggesting that physicians should have a low threshold for performing this procedure in the face of hypertension and neurologic abnormalities, especially in children.

Urinary acidification with ammonium chloride or ascorbic acid was previously thought to improve PCP elimination; however, this is no longer advised as acidic urine raises the risk of acute tubular necrosis secondary to myoglobinuria in rhabdomyolysis. Moreover, the amount of PCP excreted in urine is only 9%. The 91 % that is metabolized by the liver will not be impacted by urinary acidification, and as a result, the total amount of drug removed will not increase. The fact that hemodialysis only eliminates the medication from the serum, allowing it to be redistributed from lipid stores, makes it ineffectual as well. However, hemodialysis is an option for treating rhabdomyolysis-related renal failure. Sodium bicarbonate, mannitol, furosemide, and fluids should be administered to patients with rhabdomyolysis aggressively because renal failure is thought to be far more dangerous than PCP intoxication (Wong et al., 1996).

Treatment for status epilepticus should involve IV benzodiazepines or phenobarbital as well as airway protection. After rapid sequence intubation, it is best not to paralyze the patient because, absent continuous electroencephalogram (EEG) monitoring, it is nearly impossible to determine whether the seizures are still occurring. If the temperature rises above 40°C, it could be the result of seizures, rhabdomyolysis, and PCP-induced myotonic activity. In this case, mechanical cooling techniques should be used aggressively to treat the patient. Benzodiazepines work well as a sedative and prevent shivering adjuncts.

Disposition

Hospitalization is necessary for patients who have rhabdomyolysis, hyperthermia, seizures, altered mental status, severe injuries or are younger than 18 years old. Children need to be closely observed in order to record changes in their level of consciousness, cardiorespiratory stability, and the suction of extra oral secretions. Patients with mild intoxication should be able to resume normal activities four to eight hours after consumption, while more severe intoxications might take weeks. It has been noted that infants may require anywhere from 48 hours to 4 days to recuperate. Patients who experience delayed recovery in the ICU should be closely monitored as they may go through severe psychiatric disturbances, depression, and anxiety during the post-high period.

Finally, it is important to investigate the source of intoxication, whether it be in an adult who is unknowingly inhaling PCP-laced marijuana cigarettes or, more tragically, a child who is unwillingly exposed to secondhand smoke.

5.2.2 Ketamine

Ketamine is a dissociative anesthetic with mildly psychedelic properties. It warps visual and auditory perceptions, leaving the user with a disoriented and powerless feeling. This injectable, fast-acting anesthetic can be used on both people and animals. Because it causes patients to feel cut off from their surroundings and pain, it is known as a "dissociative anesthetic.". Ketamine can cause amnesia (having no memory of events while under the influence of the drug), immobility, sedation (feeling calm and relaxed), and relief from pain. Because it can cause dissociative experiences and hallucinations, it is abused (Park et al., 1987). Sexual assault has also been made easier with the use of ketamine.

Physicochemical Characteristics

With a molecular mass of 238 g/mol and a pKa of 7.5, ketamine is a hydrosoluble aryl-cyclo-alkylamine (Figure 5.1). Benzethonium chloride or chlorobutanol are occasionally added to ketamine as preservatives when it is used as a chlorhydrate in a slightly acidic (pH 3.5–5.5) aqueous solution. The radical cyclohexanone has an asymmetric second carbon. The racemic mixture (optically inactive) of two equal enantiomers—isomers that diverge light in opposite directions—is known as ketalar. Two times stronger than the racemic form and four times stronger than the R(−)-ketamine isomer, the active enantiomer is S(+)-ketamine ("S" spatial structure, light diverged to the right). S(+) ketamine is accessible in Germany, Austria, Italy, and the Netherlands, among other European nations.

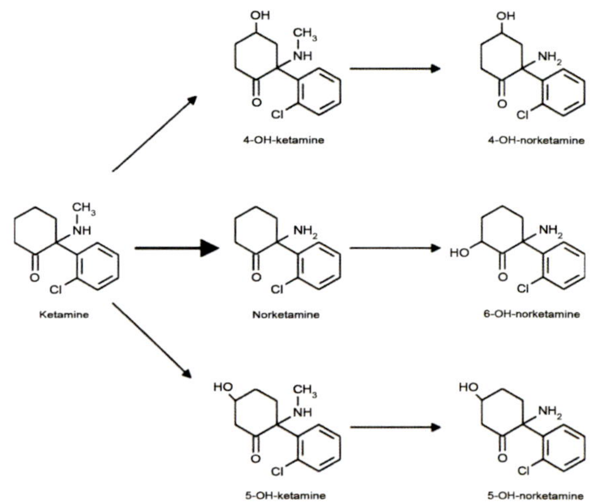

Figure 5.1. Metabolism. Ketamine is metabolized mainly to norketamine (80%), itself secondarily transformed into hydroxy-norketamine (15%), mainly 6-hydroxy-norketamine. Accessory pathway passes directly through the transformation of ketamine in hydroxy-ketamine (5%).

Source: https://www.ncbi.nlm.nih.gov/pmc/articles/PMC6493357/figure/cns12099-fig-0001/

Pharmacokinetics

Ketamine Metabolism

The metabolism of ketamine is typified by a low binding percentage (10–30%) to plasma proteins. Ketamine has a wide distribution due to its liposolubility, which is five times greater than that of thiopental. About 70 l is the volume of the central compartment, and 200 l, or 2.3 l/kg, is the distribution volume at steady state. Ketamine is mostly metabolized into norketamine (80%), an active metabolite that is primarily a hydroxylated into 6-hydroxy norketamine (15%) and ultimately excreted in bile and urine after glucuronoconjugation due to oxidation by a microsomal enzyme system (N-demethylation). Additionally, three other, less significant metabolites are produced (Figure 5.1). Ketamine can also be directly converted to hydroxy-ketamine (5 %) in another method. Particularly in animals, the liver is not the only organ involved in this metabolism; the kidneys, the intestine, and the lungs all play important roles. Although R(−)-ketamine can be converted into S(+)-norketamine, it appears that the enantiomers are unrelated in vivo. The rate at which ketamine is eliminated is high (1000–1600 ml/min or 12–20 ml/min/kg), equal to the blood flow in the liver, and subsequently dependent on it. Ketamine has a 2-3 hour half-life of elimination. One way to conceptualize its pharmacokinetics is as a tree compartment model. Women may have a 20% higher clearance rate than men (Grant et al., 1983).

Although the cytochromes that are part of the cytochromes P450 system and are in charge of ketamine metabolism are not fully understood, norketamine demethylation in humans is caused by a number of microsomal enzymes. Some P450 complex cytochromes are inhibited by ketamine, which may help to explain the tachyphylaxis that is seen when the drug is used repeatedly.

S(+) isomer demethylation is superior to that of R(−) isomer, which explains a 22% higher clearance compared to R(−)ketamine. S(+) isomer distribution volume is also higher. Racemic mixture pharmacokinetics is less favorable than that of S(+)-ketamine, because R(−) isomer otherwise inhibits S(+) isomer demethylation to a proportion of 30%. This interaction seems to exist in both ways; S(+) isomer also inhibits R(−) metabolism, probably by the same enzyme competition. However, differences in enantiomers are essentially pharmacodynamic because their cerebral and blood concentrations are similar. For an i.v. perfusion (50 mg/min), racemic, and S(+)-ketamine induce narcosis in 3 ± 1 min for a duration of 6 ± 2 min, but S(+)-ketamine has a better pharmacokinetics than the racemic mixture, with a shorter emergence phase.

Norketamine Pharmacokinetics

Norketamine appears in blood 2–3 min after a ketamine i.v. bolus administration and reaches a peak about 30 minute later. Norketamine is an analgesic molecule whose power is about 20–30% that of ketamine. Its pharmacokinetics is not well known, but time plasma concentration analysis after a unique ketamine administration demonstrates a slow elimination: norketamine persists more than 5 h after administration. Ketamine elimination half-time is inferior to that of norketamine, which strongly participates in the pharmacological effects observed in the elimination phase, particularly the analgesic effect. Because of norketamine accumulation, the need for ketamine, when administered in continuous perfusion, decreases over time.

Kinetics and Metabolism's Modification Due to Other Drugs

Enzyme inducers like rifampicin boost the metabolism and clearance of norketamine

(200%) and ketamine (13%). The opposite is true of enzyme inhibitors like clarithromycin. Ketamine N-demethylation appears to be inhibited by benzodiazepines.

Administration Routes

By i.v. route, the study of the transfer to the action site demonstrates that ketamine reaches its receptors very quickly with a transfer half-life of less than 1 minute. Ketamine can also be administered through intramuscular (i.m), intrarectal, oral, or intranasal routes. Ketamine i.m. administration has a high bioavailability (93%), with a plasma peak obtained in 5 minute. Per os, its bioavailability is limited (20%) because of the hepatic metabolism. The concentration peak occurs in 20–30 min. Intrarectal and intranasal ketamine bioavailabilities are, respectively, about 25 and 50%. After a unique epidural dose, ketamine rapidly goes to the systemic circulation: this can explain the high frequency of psychodysleptic effects observed after intrathecal or epidural injection (Schuttler et al., 1987).

Relationship with Renal and Liver Functions

Kidney function has little effect on the pharmacokinetics of ketamine or its active metabolite. Ketamine concentrations (obtained after the same dose) are 20% higher in patients with kidney dysfunction than in patients with normal kidney function; at a steady state, this translates to a moderate decrease in clearance. Patients with renal dysfunction only have statistically higher concentrations of dehydronorketamine. Ketamine has very little effect on the liver's portal or arterial blood flow in experiments.

Pharmacokinetics in Children

Intramuscular absorption is faster in children than in adults. This phenomenon could be linked to muscle weakness in children and to differences in regional flows. Distribution volume is slightly lower (1.9 l/kg) but plasma clearance is more important (16.8 ml/kg/min) than in adults. Elimination half-life is also shorter in children: 100 min. After an identical dose expressed in mg/kg, norketamine plasma concentrations are higher in children. However, in children from 4 to 10 years old and after an i.v. 2 mg/kg or i.m. 6 mg/kg injection, ketamine plasma concentrations are similar to those observed in adults. On the other hand, in the first 3 months of life, ketamine plasma clearance is shorter, probably due to a diminution of liver transformation and of kidney excretion. In this case, there is an increase in the elimination half-life in newborns and infants. Distribution volume seems to be comparable to older children.

Pharmacodynamics

Neurophysiological Effects

Clinical Aspects, Site of Action, and Modification of EEG:

When compared to other anesthetic medications (barbiturates, propofol, benzodiazepines, halogenated volatile anesthetics, etc.), ketamine produces an entirely different state of anesthesia.), also referred to as "dissociative anesthesia.". In this cataleptic state, the laryngeal, corneal, and papillary reflexes are conserved, and the eyes remain open along with the usual nystagmus. There are also some noticeable muscle contractions and hypertonia. The depth of anesthesia is appropriate for carrying out surgery because there won't be any motor responses directed toward the nociceptive stimulus (Park et al., 1987).

The thalamo-neocortical and limbic systems are functionally and electrophysiologically dissociated; sensory inputs can reach cortical receiving areas but not always register in some association areas.

Thanks to modern functional magnetic resonance imaging, it has been shown in humans that ketamine plasma concentrations of 200 ng/mL, which reduce pain scores, concomitantly decrease insular cortex and thalamus activities, usually activated by a nociceptive stimulation. Sprenger et al. investigated the effects of subanesthetic IV S(+)-ketamine doses (0.05–0.15 mg/kg/h) on the perception of painful heat stimuli in healthy volunteers. During placebo administration, a typical pain activation network (thalamus, insula, cingulate, and prefrontal cortex) was found, whereas decreased pain perception with ketamine was associated with a dose-dependent reduction of pain-induced cerebral activation. Analysis of the dose-dependent ketamine effects on pain processing showed a decreasing activation of the secondary somatosensory cortex (S2), insula, and anterior cingulate cortex, which has been linked to the affective pain component that underlines the potency of ketamine in modulating affective pain processing. Honey et al. showed that, even when overt behavior is unimpaired, ketamine has an impact on episodic memory task performance.

Spinal action is significant, even though supraspinal action predominates. Without altering the spinothalamic pathway's conduction, ketamine suppresses afferent signals from the spinoreticular pathways. Both the medial thalamic nuclei and the medial reticular formation, which relay the emotional side of pain perception, are selectively depressed. Ketamine has been shown to block the reticularis formation signal in cats, which is thought to be a crucial relay in the nociceptive transmission from the spine to the supraspinal level. Ketamine increases the descending inhibiting serotoninergic pathway, in contrast to other anesthetics (Dayton et al., 1983).

Compared to other anesthetics, ketamine alters the EEG in a different way. The most common EEG feature is the decrease in alpha rhythm amplitude (or even elimination of it) without changing its frequency and the emergence of theta waves, which do not exhibit any discernible correlation with the depth of narcosis. Furthermore, neither the amplitude of somatosensory evoked potentials nor mid-latency auditory evoked potentials is reduced by ketamine. Lastly, R(−)-ketamine has no effect on the EEG, but S(+)-ketamine likewise reduces the amplitude of the alpha rhythm. The bispectral index (BIS) is not decreased by ketamine; in fact, it may even rise. This effect is dose-dependent: in a randomized controlled trial, patients receiving propofol and fentanyl during general anesthesia showed a significant increase in BIS (from 40 to 63) at a dose of 0.05 mg/kg, whereas 0.0 2 mg/kg had no effect.

Doses and Concentration-Effect Relationship:

Ketamine alters memorization for a concentration of 70 ng/ml and provokes a lateral nystagmus for about 200 ng/mL. ED_{50} for narcosis (absence of verbal response) is 0.4–0.7 mg/kg. ED_{50} and ED_{95} for anesthesia (absence of response to the nociceptive stimulus) are, respectively, 0.6 and 1.3 mg/kg. These ED correspond to an efficient concentration of about 10 µm. The ketamine analgesic effect persists for steady-state plasma concentrations superior to 100–160 ng/ml (about 0.5 µm). After a peripheric neurological lesion, ketamine-efficient analgesic concentrations to reduce hyperalgesia and allodynia are at least superior to 100 ng/mL. After oral administration, ketamine-efficient analgesic concentrations are lower (40 ng/mL), because of the more important action of norketamine.

Psychodysleptic Effects:

Psychodysleptic effects, sometimes referred to as psychedelic effects, are phenomena that manifest during the "emergence phase" or "awakening phase" and involve disruptions of time, mood, body image, and auditory and visual perceptions. A sense of unreality, floating, or depersonalization, as well as conscious dreams or hallucinations, maybe the outcome of these disruptions. Following anesthesia, concentrations range from 600 to 1100 ng/ml during the awakening phase. These effects start to show up at 50 ng/mL. A linear dose-effect relationship was observed in healthy volunteers (concentrations between 50 and 200 ng/mL), with progressive effects corresponding to ketamine concentration. Around 500 ng/mL, more severe effects such as anxiety and paranoid feelings start to manifest. "Emergence phenomena" isn't really the right term because using a subanesthetic dose to induce sedation can also have psychodysleptic effects and hallucinations. Excessive dosages or a rushed i.v. Acute delirium may occur when low doses (between 5 and 10 mg) are administered. When using the dextrogyre isomer, these effects are not as noticeable (Corssen et al., 1966).

Psychosis, Ketamine, and Antidepressive Effect:

A continuous subanesthetic S-ketamine infusion was given in a double-blind study involving fifteen healthy participants, and cortical activation was assessed using functional magnetic resonance imaging. Subjects completed an overt word generation task while they were being scanned. Administration of ketamine resulted in formal thought disorder, difficulties with abstract thinking, and a lack of spontaneity and flow in conversation. Formal thought disorder scores were positively correlated with activation measures that included the precuneus, the left superior temporal gyrus, and the right middle and inferior frontal gyrus. Prominent activations in the prefrontal and anterior cingulate regions were linked to difficulty with abstract thought, while hyperactivations in the left superior temporal gyrus were linked to a lack of spontaneity and flow in conversation. NMDAR blockade elicited psychopathological symptoms and cortical activations in regions previously reported in patients with schizophrenia, without causing behavioral impairments during verbal fluency.

Ketamine-induced psychic disorders in healthy volunteers and in schizophrenia have shown some similarities and have led to pharmacological research.

Ketamine may make it possible to pinpoint a biochemical or biophysical mechanism linked to psychosis or assess the effectiveness of a substance as an antipsychotic in preventing ketamine's effects in volunteers in good health. It has been shown that the activation of prefrontal cortex and locus ceruleus are based on neurophysiological principles. From a pharmacological perspective, NMDA receptors are altered and may exhibit hypofunction in a hyperglutamatergic state.

Depression is linked to the NMDA receptor and is closely related to the glutamatergic system, as recent research has shown. Research unequivocally demonstrated that ketamine had antidepressant effects, quickly ending suicidal thoughts even in cases of bipolar disorder. Tiny ketamine dosages also help depressed patients feel better after surgery, and it's possible that this antidepressant effect contributes to the antalgic effect in chronic pain (White et al., 1985).

Mechanisms of Action

The neuropharmacology of ketamine is intricate. Ketamine primarily affects non-NMDA (N-Methyl-D-Aspartate) and glutamate binding sites. The unique effects of ketamine (such as amnesic and psychosensory effects, analgesia, and neuroprotection) are caused by the antagonistic interaction with the NMDA receptor. Other glutamate-independent mechanisms exist as well.

Glutamate-Independent Mechanisms

Numerous binding sites, including opioid, monoaminergic, cholinergic, nicotinic, and muscarinic receptors, are impacted by ketamine. Chlorine conductance increases due to the most common inhibiting neurotransmitter, GABA. Ketamine potentializes the GABA inhibition (GABA-A complex), just like other anesthetics do, but the analgesic effects are not primarily explained by this interaction. It has been established that ketamine agonism on spinal GABA receptors contributes to spinal analgesia, but only at high concentrations (greater than 500 μM), far higher than those achieved in human practice.

Mu, delta, and kappa opioid receptors are binding sites for ketamine. Although S(+)-ketamine has a two to three times higher affinity for opioid receptors than the R(−) isomer, its analgesic effect is not really caused by this interaction because naloxone does not counteract this effect in humans. Nonetheless, kappa opioid receptors may be involved in certain psychic effects.

It is obvious that the action of monoaminergic system is crucial. Ketamine induces a hyperadrenergic state (release of norepinephrine, dopamine, and serotonin) by stimulating noradrenergic neurons and inhibiting catecholamine uptake. Norepinephrine uptake inhibition is stereospecific; the R(−) isomer only blocks neuronal uptake, whereas the S(+) isomer also blocks extra-neuronal uptake. Extended synaptic activity results in a greater norepinephrine transfer in the bloodstream. Not only can alpha-2 agonists reduce this hyperadrenergic state, but they can also lessen ketamine-induced psychic phenomena. Ketamine also prevents the uptake of serotonin and dopamine due to its interaction with the serotonin transporter. Furthermore, ondansetron inhibits the emetic effects of ketamine, indicating a possible serotoninergic mechanism (Honey et al., 1985). The hypnotic, psychedelic, and analgesic effects of the molecule are partially explained by these interactions involving noradrenergic neurons.

Acetylcholine release is regulated by cholinergic neurons in the striatum and hippocampal regions. These cholinergic neurons in the prefrontal cortex may be triggered by muscarinic and nicotinic receptors. These receptors are directly inhibited by ketamine, which is a significant factor in the manifestation of psychic phenomena. As a result, physostigmine, an anticholinesterasic, can counteract the hypnotic effects of ketamine and reverse the central anticholinergic effects. Balmer and Wyte showed that physostigmine (0.05 mg) counteracted the analgesic effects of ketamine but preserved its sedative and hypnotic effects when they injected a ketamine perfusion (50 μg/kg/min) afterward. Ketamine may also promote the release of acetylcholine in the hippocampal regions by raising dopamine levels. Nevertheless, in certain models, ketamine may block acetylcholine liberation triggered by NMDA receptors at clinically relevant doses. At clinically effective concentrations of 2.8 ± 0.6 mm, ketamine inhibits nicotinic receptors. It exhibits antagonistic activity on muscarinic receptors, with a two-fold increase in affinity for S(+)ketamine over the R(−) enantiomer.

Some ketamine effects involve the purinergic system, like toxic effects on the urinary tract.

Ketamine interacts with potassium, L-type calcium, and sodium channels, which have the ability to act as local anesthetics, among other channels. L-type calcium channels may be the source of some of the psychodystrophic effects that nimodipine can counteract. The tachycardia brought on by ketamine could also be explained by the inhibition of sodium currents in the cardiac parasympathetic neurons in the nucleus ambiguous. Local anesthetic effects are related to antagonism on sodium channels. In terms of molecular weight and pKa, ketamine is comparable to lidocaïne. It is effective when applied topically as a local analgesic and may bind to the same site within the sodium channels as local anesthetics. A portion of the neuroprotective properties of (S)+isomer may be explained by the inhibition of neuron potassium channels that ketamine causes.

Glutamate-Dependant Mechanisms

NMDA Receptor:

Ketamine's most significant pharmacological effects are caused by blocking the NMDA receptor at concentrations between 2 and 50 µm. In the central nervous system (CNS), glutaminergic synapses are involved, and glutamate is the most common amino acid. Upon release, it triggers multiple postsynaptic and presynaptic receptors on ion channels. N-methyl-D-aspartate (NMDA) and non-NMDA (like AMPA [alpha-amino-3-hydroxy-5-methyl-4-isoxazole-propionic acid] and KA [kainate]) receptors are the two main categories of isotropic glutamate receptors. NMDA receptors are found on almost all CNS cells, especially in those parts of the brain associated with nociception, like the spinal dorsal horn and primary afferents. The release of glutamate in the synaptic cleft triggers the activation of postsynaptic ionotropic receptors, resulting in the opening of ion channels and subsequent membrane depolarization. The NMDA receptor is notable for its calcic conductance and is permeable to sodium-potassium exchanges. Presynaptic location is present in some. A heteromeric multimer, the NMDA receptor is similar to the AMPA receptor. The most likely structure is tetrameric, with two subunits making up the basic structure (dimers of dimers). Two NR1 and two NR2 subunits make up the majority of NMDA receptors in the central nervous system. PSD-95 (postsynaptic density 95) protein serves as their anchor in the plasmic membrane (Figure 5.3A) (Schuttler et al., 1987). The three subunit types—NR1, NR2, and NR3, also known as GluN1, GluN2, and GluN3—share sequences with the AMPA and kainate receptors. These subunits are arranged in three transmembrane domains (M1, M3, and M4) and contain four hydrophobic segments (M1 to M4) in their central region. Figure 5.2 shows the receptor's ionic channel, which is represented by the M2 segment facing the cytoplasm. There are two broad extracellular domains: the NTD N-terminal extremity (N-terminal domain) and the agonist-binding domain (ABD), which permit glutamate binding on NR2 and glycine binding on NR1. Figure 5.2 depicts the spatial clam structure of these two domains, NTD and ABD (Park et al., 1987).

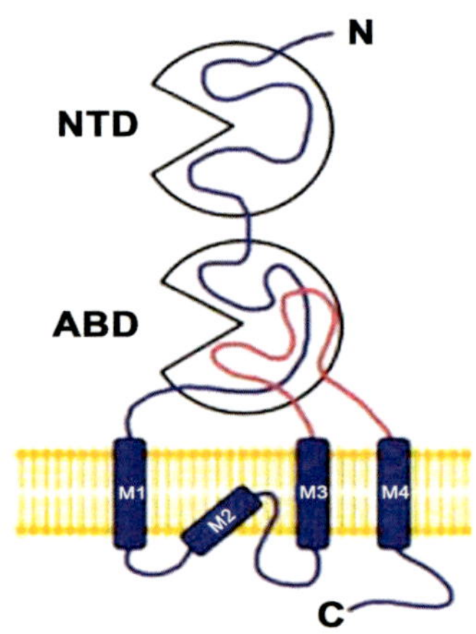

Figure 5.2. Structure of the four subunits of the N-methyl D-aspartate (NMDA) receptor. NTD, N-terminal domain, ABD, agonist-binding domain. The M2 segment faces the cytoplasm and would be the receptor ion channel.

Source: https://www.ncbi.nlm.nih.gov/pmc/articles/PMC6493357/figure/cns12099-fig-0002/

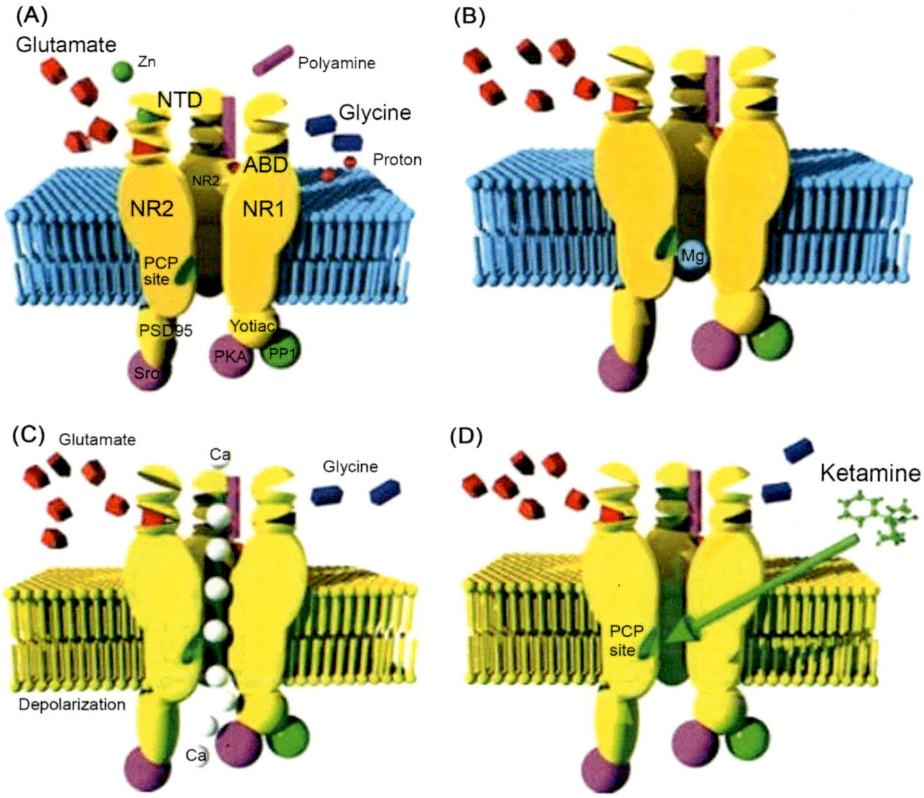

Figure 5.3. The N-methyl D-aspartate (NMDA) receptor is anchored in the membrane (sky blue) by the PSD-95 protein, linked to the Src tyrosine kinase. The four sub-units (2 NR1 and 2 NR2) form an NMDA receptor channel selective for the cathions.

Source: https://www.ncbi.nlm.nih.gov/pmc/articles/PMC6493357/figure/cns12099-fig-0003/

In this structure's slot, antagonists and competitive antagonists bind. There are seven NR1 subunit subcategories (h–g). The NR2/NR2 heteromeric complex, which contains NR2 subunits, appears to be involved in pathological processes, such as schizophrenia, that are linked to aberrant NMDA channel function. The type of receptor is based on four subtypes, denoted by the letters A through D. The two most prevalent types are A and B. The NR2A subtype is widespread. The limbic system, which is responsible for emotions and memory, is where the NR2B subtype is primarily found. It is located in the olfactory bulb, the hippocampus, the amygdala, and the anterior region of the brain, specifically in the cingulate cortex. Additionally, the NR2B type contributes to the transmission of pain signals to the spinal cord, thalamus, and extrasynaptic regions, such as primary afferents. The cerebellum and spinal cord are both rich in NR2C and NR2D types, respectively. The NR2 subunit is essential for the spontaneous opening probability of the channel, which occurs regardless of ligands. The NR2A and NR2B subunits' N-terminal domains regulate the channel's opening. This extracellular component has the ability to bind allosteric inhibitors and regulates the receptor's sensitivity to endogenous inhibitors, particularly protons and zinc (Wong et al., 1996).

The process of activating NMDA receptors is quite intricate, involving the cooperation of several agonists and regulatory mechanisms that, on the other hand, support the closed state of the channel. The ABD region of the NR2 unit contains the glutamate binding site on NMDA receptors (Figure 5.3A). This is the location where N-methyl-D-aspartate selectively activates. One glycine molecule must simultaneously bind to a different location in the ABD region of the NR1 unit in order for the receptor to be activated. Thus, glutamate and glycine are referred to as the system's "coagonists" (Figure 5.3A).

Magnesium Channel Block:

The primary regulatory mechanism that impedes the channel's opening is the voltage-dependent magnesium block of the NMDA receptor. Even when glutamate and glycine, the coagonists, are bound to their respective sites, extracellular Mg^{2+} blocks the receptor-associated channel at the resting membrane potential (roughly 70 mV). On the intracellular channel side, the Mg^{2+} binding site is situated relatively low (Figure 5.3B). An exponential function of membrane voltage determines the magnesium dissociation constant. The cation is released when a neuron depolarizes because the negative electrostatic forces holding the ion Mg^{2+} at the NR2 subunit collapse. The coagonists' action causes the plug to be ejected, which permits a calcium influx related to the significance of depolarization (Figure 5.3C). While magnesium by itself does not appear to lessen postoperative pain, these phenomena may account for some of the antihyperalgesic effects of magnesium and the reduced amounts of propofol needed to induce narcosis. Additionally, there is a synergistic effect between magnesium and ketamine.

Receptor Phosphorylation:

An essential component of the NMDA receptor's activation is phosphorylation. The phosphorylation mechanisms underlie not only long-term potentiation but also the actions of morphine on NMDA receptors and hyperalgesia. Phosphatase protein type I (PP1) and cAMP-dependent protein kinase are two additional phosphoproteins that influence the NMDA receptor. Another anchor protein known as Yotiao connects these two regulatory proteins to the NR1 unit (Figure 5.3A). Many ion channels have this kind of control, which is the simultaneous presence of a kinase and a phosphatase that regulate the phosphorylation of a receptor (Dayton et al., 1983).

Allosteric Inhibitors:

Additionally, the allosteric sites of NR2 subunit permit either positive or negative modulation of the NMDA receptor's activity. Certain ions modify the spatial conformation of the receptor, which is a crucial part of their function in controlling channel opening. These are zinc ions (Zn^{2+}) and protons.

Strong non-competitive inhibitors of NMDA receptors are protons, or H+ ions. Although the exact location of the proton detector is unknown, it is known that protons function independently of membrane polarization by maintaining the closed state of the channel. Consequently, neuronal damage is decreased by tissue acidosis that follows ischemia or epileptic discharges. With an IC_{50} (concentration that inhibits 50% of the receptors) of 6.9 pH units, receptors made up of NR2A or NR1a subunits have an intermediate reactivity to pH, whereas NR2C units give the receptor virtual insensitivity. On the other hand, NR1a/NR2B or NR1a/NR2D dimer-based receptors are highly sensitive to pH. Their IC_{50} near pH 7.40 indicates that, in normal circumstances, half of these receptors are affected by a tonic inhibition of proton-mediated opening. This suggests that even slight pH variations can contribute to the opening of these NMDA channels, highlighting yet another negative feature of alkalosis.

The NTD domain of NR2A and NR2B subunits also plays an important role in NMDA receptor function modulation by selectively binding to non-competitive antagonists (Idwall et al., 1979).

As of right now, the only known ligand for NR2A and NR2B subunits is the zinc ion, which is frequently co-released with glutamate in synaptic vesicles (Figure 5.3A). With an IC_{50} of 15 nmol, Zn^{2+} binds to the NTD clam-shaped domain's opening area, causing it to close. The separation of the interface between the two ABD domains of the receptor results from this closure, which eases tension in the connections between the ABD and NTD domains. Stress applied to a membrane segment is relieved by this separation, and the channel can close thanks to the conformational shift and the bond to a proton. Thus, protons control the channel closure, which zinc amplifies. These mechanisms might account for a portion of the pathophysiology associated with near-death experiences (NDEs). When there is cerebral ischemia or hypoglycemia, neuronal depolarization opens the NMDA channel, which may be influenced by protons or zinc ions. Prodils that bind in the NTD domain, which partially overlaps with the zinc-binding site, such as ifenprodil, selectively inhibit NMDA receptors that contain the NR2B subunit. Traxoprodil, besonprodil, radiprodil, and other more recently described synthetic compounds that are highly selective for the NTD domain of NR2B subunits are used as pharmacological tools and may eventually be developed into therapeutic agents such as analgesics (including for chronic pain), neuroprotective agents, anticonvulsants, antidepressants, or treatments for Parkinson's disease and other neurodegenerative diseases. They encourage NMDA channel occlusion in response to protons in a manner similar to zinc. They show promise not only because they block the most common receptor implicated in pathological phenomena, but also because they become significantly more active when the channel has already been opened.

Polyamines: Endogenous Allosteric Activators:

Polyamines, putrescine, spermine, and spermidine are basic aliphatic amines, positively charged at normal pH. They are synthesized from ornithine, a metabolite in the urea cycle, and spread throughout the body. They are released in neurons in a calcium-dependent manner. Without being critical, they potentiate channel opening under the joint action of glutamate and glycine (Figure 5.3A). Polyamine deprivation has an analgesic effect in some animal models.

Other endogenous substances may allosterically modulate NMDA receptors, such as neurosteroids, such as pregnenolone sulfate. The release of these substances can be triggered by stress.

Consequences of the Opening of the N-Methyl-D-Aspartate Channel

The production of second and third messengers, prostaglandins and nitric oxide (NO), which facilitate the presynaptic release of glutamate and start the amplification of a vicious cycle, is triggered by an increase in intracellular calcium concentration.

Binding protein PSD-95 appears to be essential to the sequence, which links the increased synthesis of NO and calcium influx. The NR2 unit, rich in tyrosine residues on the cytoplasmic side, is linked to an intracellular tyrosine kinase of the Src family by means of the anchoring PSD-95 protein (Figure 5.3A). A major function of Src in the adult CNS is to regulate glutamatergic transmission and synaptic plasticity. PSD-95 is also linked to other intracellular enzymes, in particular NO-synthase (Thomson et al., 1988).

An elevation in intraneurial calcium leads to the secondary activation of kinases, which in turn control receptor activity and early gene expression downstream, such as c-fos. The transcriptional mechanisms involved facilitate long-term memory.

A neuronal NO-synthase is activated and NO is produced from L-arginine when the NMDA receptor is stimulated by glutamate released in the nociceptive afferents, resulting in an increase in intracellular calcium. Cyclic guanosine monophosphate 3′5′ (c-GMP) is synthesized in response to NO and is involved in the central transmission of pain signals, also known as "nitroxidergic" transmission. It has been shown that, following a peripheral inflammation, for instance, NO and c-GMPc contribute to the processes of central sensitization and hyperalgesia.

Mechanism of Action of Ketamine at the N-Methyl-D-Aspartate Receptor Level

The PCP site is an intrachannel location where ketamine and other NMDA receptor non-competitive antagonists (PCP, MK801, DXM, and memantine) are attached (Figure 5.3D). The intrachannel binding of ketamine shortens the duration of channel opening. Ketamine reduces the stimulus summation response to repeated stimulation, also known as "wind up," which is thought to be a basic type of central nervous system sensitization. In the event that glutamate fixation has previously opened the NMDA channel, the antagonism becomes more significant. The effective analgesic effects of ketamine in cases of significant or persistent pain can be explained by the "use dependence" theory.

The NMDA receptor's hydrophobic domain has a second site where ketamine can be fixed to reduce the frequency of channel opening. Additionally, ketamine is an allosteric antagonist of the receptor that exhibits a strong tropism for NR2B unity. It is specifically linked to the experiences of emotional perception and pain memory. Ketamine may have analgesic and anesthetic effects through direct inhibition of NO-synthase, even in the absence of its action on NMDA receptors.

S(+)-ketamine exhibits a strong analgesic and anesthetic effect, at least twice as strong as the racemic mixture, due to its affinity for the PCP site, which may be three times higher than that of R(−)-ketamine.

N-Methyl-D-Aspartate Receptors and Opioid-Induced Hyperalgesia

The way that ketamine inhibits pain is due to its interaction with NMDA receptors and opioids. The relationship between the opioid system and ketamine is not clear-cut. Morphine has a low affinity for NMDA receptors, on the one hand. In the cortex, morphine also reduces glutamatergic transmission. On the other hand, opioid-induced hyperalgesia—a phenomenon of acute and chronic tolerance—has been demonstrated in recent years to be favored by opioids. The CNS's NMDA receptors are involved in these effects, which are dose-dependent but not always present. The same cells have opioid and NMDA receptors on their surface, which interact with one another. Phosphorylation of the NMDA receptor inhibits the magnesium plug of the channel after opioid receptors and protein kinase C, particularly its γ isoform, are activated. This permits Ca^{2+} to enter the cell and initiates a series of events (activation of protein kinase C, prostaglandin and nitric oxide systems, transcriptional changes) that result in a down-regulation (underlying tolerance) and a blunted response of opioid receptors (underlying hyperalgesia). One of the most studied properties of ketamine for over a decade is its ability to prevent certain phenomena due to its antagonistic action on NMDA receptors (Thomson et al., 1988).

Excitotoxicity

NMDA receptors are involved in neuronal tissue physiology and synaptic plasticity, but in certain circumstances, also in acute or chronic neurotoxic effects. The concept of excitotoxicity, issued from the work of John Olney, confers to glutamate the status of "excitotoxin." While excitotoxicity could be mediated by any of the ionotropic receptors, the calcium conductance of the NMDA receptor makes it the privileged mediator of these phenomena. Indeed, a massive increase in calcium concentration inside the neuron is likely to produce a cascade of deleterious events, whose ultimate outcome is cell death. The cytoplasmic Ca^{2+} activates many enzymes such as protein kinase C (PKC), phospholipases A2 and C (PLA2 and PLC), protein kinase II Ca^{2+}, and calmodulin-dependent NO-synthase as well as proteases and endonucleases. This sequence of reactions has been proposed as a pathogenic model of cerebral ischemia and traumatic brain injury. In the case of hypoxia or ischemia, the collapse of the activity (or activity in reverse mode) of the high-affinity transporter, which normally removes glutamate from the synaptic cleft, provokes a significant increase in extracellular glutamate. The collapse of ATP-dependent ion pumps (Na/K-ATPase) increases extracellular potassium concentrations, which in turn causes a depolarization of neurons that terminates the magnesium block and reduces the effectiveness of high-affinity transporter glutamate, whose energy source is the transmembrane sodium gradient. In addition, potassium stimulates the secretion of glutamate and inhibits its glial capture. Finally, glutamate content of an injured cell is an important source of excitatory amino acids. A potassium current, independent of calcium, also intervenes in the apoptotic phenomena. Ischemia is finally associated with the stimulation of ornithine decarboxylase, which leads to the synthesis of polyamines. Thus, excitotoxicity is the efferent common pathway of pathological processes, all compromising cellular energy intake. The glutamatergic system would thus be involved in chronic neurological pathologies, such as amyotrophic lateral sclerosis and Huntington's, Alzheimer's, or Parkinson's diseases. NMDA antagonists experimentally have neuroprotective properties because they are able to reduce neuronal apoptosis or brain injury induced by hypoxia or brain trauma. There exists a window of opportunity with respect to the ischemic penumbra during the hours following cerebral infarction because the effectiveness of NMDA antagonists in this area is highly dependent on the precocity of their administration. Regarding neurodegenerative diseases, amantadine, originally used in the treatment of influenza, and its derivative memantine are NMDA antagonists, which improve the symptoms of Parkinson's disease. A recent study reported improved Parkinsonian symptoms (dyskinesia and tremor) in the minutes following the injection of low doses of ketamine (10 mg two bolus IV) (Pedraz et al., 1987).

Ketamine Neurotoxicity

It is well known from experiments that ketamine and NMDA antagonists have the potential to be neurotoxic and may encourage lesions caused by apoptosis in neurons. Conversely, ketamine does not cause neurotoxicity when used as an anesthetic in routine medical procedures. There are very few documented cases of possible but uncommon neurotoxicity. It is unknown what would happen if high doses were given more than once every 24 hours. Neurotoxic effects that are temporary may be associated with psychodysphoric effects. Chronic ketamine users frequently experience abnormalities in frontal white matter as well as cognitive disturbances. Numerous experimental studies conducted recently have suggested that the developing brain may be subject to neurotoxic effects. According to animal research, neonatal and early pediatric patients may have a long-term risk of neurodegeneration from anesthesia, which could lead to cognitive consequences. The available experimental evidence suggests that medications that enhance gamma-aminobutyric acid signal transduction, in addition to NMDA receptor antagonists, may be neurotoxic to the developing brain.

5.2.3 Dextromethorphan (DXM)

DXM is a widely used over-the-counter cough suppressant with dissociative and hallucinogenic properties when taken in high doses. In this essay, I'll explore DXM in detail, covering its history, pharmacology, medical uses, recreational use, effects, risks, and cultural impact (Pedraz et al., 1987).

History

DXM was first synthesized in the 1950s as a potential replacement for codeine, a widely used cough suppressant with addictive properties. It was introduced as a medication in the United States in the 1950s and has since become one of the most commonly used cough suppressants worldwide.

Pharmacology

DXM acts primarily as a non-selective serotonin reuptake inhibitor (SSRI) and NMDA receptor antagonist. At therapeutic doses, it suppresses cough by acting on the brainstem cough center. However, at higher doses, it produces dissociative and hallucinogenic effects by blocking NMDA receptors and increasing serotonin levels in the brain.

Medical Uses

DXM is primarily used as a cough suppressant in over-the-counter cough and cold medications. It is often combined with other ingredients such as antihistamines and decongestants to treat symptoms of the common cold and flu. Additionally, some research suggests potential uses for DXM in treating neuropathic pain and depression, although further studies are needed to confirm these effects.

Recreational Use

DXM is also used recreationally for its dissociative and hallucinogenic effects. In higher doses, typically above the therapeutic range, it can induce altered states of consciousness, hallucinations, and out-of-body experiences. Recreational users often refer to different "plateaus" of DXM intoxication, each associated with specific effects and doses (Clements et al., 1987).

Effects

The effects of DXM can vary depending on the dose and individual sensitivity, but common effects include:

- Euphoria
- Altered perception of time and space
- Dissociation from the body (feeling disconnected or out of body)
- Visual and auditory hallucinations
- Enhanced creativity and introspection
- Impaired motor coordination and judgment

Risks

While DXM is generally safe when used as directed, recreational use carries several risks, including:

- Overdose: High doses of DXM can lead to overdose, which may cause seizures, respiratory depression, and even death.
- Psychological dependence: Some individuals may develop a psychological dependence on DXM, leading to compulsive use despite negative consequences.
- Serotonin syndrome: Combining DXM with other serotonergic medications or substances can increase the risk of serotonin syndrome, a potentially life-threatening condition characterized by high levels of serotonin in the brain.
- Cognitive impairment: Chronic use of DXM, especially at high doses, may lead to cognitive impairment, memory problems, and difficulty concentrating.

Cultural Impact

DXM has gained popularity among certain subcultures, particularly among adolescents and young adults seeking altered states of consciousness. It has been referenced in popular culture, including music, literature, and film, often portraying its use in a recreational or illicit context. However, its recreational use is controversial, with concerns about its safety and potential for abuse.

Legal Status

DXM is legal and available over the counter in many countries for the treatment of cough and cold symptoms. However, some jurisdictions have placed restrictions on its sale to minors or require it to be sold behind the counter due to concerns about abuse. In some countries, pure DXM powder is regulated as a controlled substance.

5.2.4 Nitrous Oxide

Nitrous oxide, commonly known as laughing gas, is a dissociative drug with a long history of use in medicine, industry, and recreation. In this comprehensive overview, we'll explore nitrous oxide's origins, pharmacology, medical and recreational uses, effects, risks, and cultural impact within the context of dissociative drugs (Sigtermans et al., 2009).

History:

- Nitrous oxide was first synthesized in 1772 by English chemist Joseph Priestley.
- Its anesthetic properties were discovered by British chemist Humphry Davy in 1799, who noted its euphoric and analgesic effects.
- Nitrous oxide's medical use as a general anesthetic began in the 19th century, particularly during dental procedures and childbirth.

Pharmacology:

- Nitrous oxide acts as a non-competitive NMDA receptor antagonist and a potent agonist at the GABA-A receptor, leading to its dissociative effects.
- Its mechanisms of action involve the inhibition of excitatory neurotransmission and modulation of inhibitory neurotransmission in the central nervous system.

Medical uses:

- Nitrous oxide is commonly used in medical settings as an anesthetic agent, particularly in dentistry and minor surgical procedures.
- Its rapid onset and offset of action,

along with its relatively favorable safety profile, make it a popular choice for analgesia and sedation.

Recreational use:

- Nitrous oxide is also used recreationally for its dissociative and euphoric effects.
- It is typically inhaled from small metal canisters ("whippets") using a balloon or dispenser to capture the gas.
- Recreational users often experience brief but intense euphoria, altered perception, and dissociation from the body and surroundings.

Effects:

- Short-term effects of nitrous oxide inhalation include euphoria, dizziness, lightheadedness, and altered sensory perception.
- Some users report visual and auditory hallucinations, feelings of detachment from reality, and a sense of time distortion.
- Higher doses can lead to loss of consciousness, hypoxia, and potentially life-threatening complications.

Risks:

- Inhalation of nitrous oxide carries several risks, including hypoxia (oxygen deprivation) due to displacement of oxygen in the lungs.
- Prolonged or repeated use can lead to vitamin B12 deficiency, which can cause neurological symptoms such as numbness, tingling, and weakness.
- Chronic use may also lead to cognitive impairment, memory deficits, and psychiatric symptoms in some individuals.

Cultural impact:

- Nitrous oxide has a long history of use in various cultural and recreational contexts.
- It is commonly associated with music festivals, raves, and other events where it may be used as a recreational drug alongside other substances.
- The use of nitrous oxide has been portrayed in popular culture, including literature, music, and film, often depicting its euphoric and dissociative effects.

Regulation:

- In many countries, nitrous oxide is regulated as a prescription drug or controlled substance when used for medical purposes.
- However, its sale and possession for non-medical use are often less regulated, leading to concerns about its availability and misuse.

(Idwall et al., 1979)

A Closer Look

Effects of Hallucinogens

Hallucinogens encompass a diverse class of drugs known for their ability to alter perception, mood, and cognition. Their effects can vary widely depending on factors such as the specific substance, dosage, set (the individual's mindset and expectations), and setting (the physical and social environment). From classic psychedelics like LSD and psilocybin mushrooms to newer compounds such as MDMA and ketamine, each hallucinogen produces its own unique constellation of effects.

At a neurological level, hallucinogens primarily interact with serotonin receptors in the brain, particularly the 5-HT2A subtype. This interaction leads to profound changes in the brain's communication networks, resulting in alterations in sensory perception, thought patterns, and emotional experiences. Users may report seeing vivid visuals, experiencing synesthesia (the blending of senses), and feeling a heightened sense of connection to their surroundings or to others.

The psychological effects of hallucinogens can be wide-ranging and profound. Many users describe profound introspection and insights into their own thoughts, feelings, and behaviors. Some report experiencing ego dissolution, a temporary loss of the sense of self, which can lead to feelings of unity with the universe or a sense of interconnectedness with others. These experiences can be both awe-inspiring and potentially therapeutic, leading some researchers to investigate their potential for treating conditions such as depression, anxiety, and PTSD.

However, the effects of hallucinogens are not uniformly positive, and they can also be unpredictable and sometimes distressing. "Bad trips" characterized by anxiety, paranoia, or intense fear can occur, particularly in individuals predisposed to psychiatric disorders or in adverse environments. Additionally, hallucinogen use carries some risk of triggering psychosis or exacerbating underlying mental health conditions, although such instances are relatively rare.

Furthermore, hallucinogens are not without physical risks. While they are not considered addictive in the same way as drugs like opioids or stimulants, they can still pose dangers, particularly in high doses or when used in combination with other substances. Physiological effects can include increased heart rate and blood pressure, tremors, nausea, and in extreme cases, seizures or coma.

Summary

- Hallucinogens are a type of drug that changes a person's awareness of their surroundings. Also known as psychedelics, they alter a person's thoughts and feelings, as well. Some hallucinogens are synthetic, and some come from naturally occurring compounds found in certain plants and fungi (plural of fungus).
- Hallucinogenic drugs can cause hallucinations, which are sensations and images that seem real but aren't. People may hear, feel or see things that aren't really there. Some psychedelic drugs cause people to feel out of control or disconnected from their bodies and environment.
- The meaning of LSD is lysergic acid diethylamide. Made from lysergic acid, this drug is one of the strongest mind-altering chemicals. A fungus that grows on rye and other grains contains this chemical. LSD, or acid, looks like a clear or white material. People usually soak small squares of blotting paper in the LSD. Then, they swallow these acid tabs. LSD can also come as a tablet or capsule.
- Peyote is a small, spineless cactus in which the main active ingredient is mescaline. Mescaline is a naturally occurring substance found in the peyote cactus. The top of the peyote cactus also referred to as the crown, consists of disk-shaped buttons that people cut from the roots and dry. People generally chew the buttons or soak them in water to produce an intoxicating liquid.
- PCP stands for phenyl cyclohexyl piperidine, but you may also see the term phencyclidine. Other names for PCP include angel dust and killer weed. It comes in a variety of forms, including liquids, powders, tablets, and capsules. People usually swallow, sniff or inject the drug, but they can also smoke it.
- Ketamine is an anesthetic that healthcare providers use for surgery on humans and animals. Much of the ketamine people use is stolen from veterinary offices. People usually snort it as a powder or swallow it as a pill, but they can also inject it as a liquid.
- DMT stands for dimethyltryptamine. Some plants in the Amazon contain this naturally grown chemical. Ayahuasca is a type of tea made from these plants. As a tea, DMT is known as hoasca, aya or yagé.
- Nitrous oxide has a number of industrial uses and is used medically. When mixed with air (50/50 gas and air), it is used as an anaesthetic gas for pain relief in dentistry and childbirth. Because of its effects and how it is consumed through inhalation, nitrogen oxide is often categorised as a 'depressant', 'dissociative', or 'inhalant' type drug.
- A depressant drug slows the body down. A dissociative type of drug causes disconnect or detachment from yourself or your surroundings.

References

1. Johnstone M, Evans V, Baigel S. Sernyl (CI-395) in clinical anaesthesia. Br J Anaesth 1959;31:433–439.
2. Corssen G, Domino EF. Dissociative anesthesia: Further pharmacologic studies and first clinical experience with the phencyclidine derivative CI-581. Anesth Analg 1966;45:29–40.
3. Domino EF, Chodoff P, Corssen G. Pharmacologic effects of CI-581, a new dissociative anesthetic, in man. Clin Pharmacol Ther 1965;6:279–291.
4. Dayton PG, Stiller RL, Cook DR, Perel JM. The binding of ketamine to plasma proteins: Emphasis on human plasma. Eur J Clin Pharmacol 1983;24:825–831.
5. Schuttler J, Stanski DR, White PF, et al. Pharmacodynamic modeling of the EEG effects of ketamine and its enantiomers in man. J Pharmacokinet Biopharm 1987;15:241–253.
6. Grant IS, Nimmo WS, McNicol LR, Clements JA. Ketamine disposition in children and adults. Br J Anaesth 1983;55:1107–1111.
7. Noppers I, Olofsen E, Niesters M, al. Effect of Rifampicin on S-ketamine and S-norketamine Plasma Concentrations in Healthy Volunteers after Intravenous S-ketamine Administration. Anesthesiology 2011;114:1435–1445.
8. Park GR, Manara AR, Mendel L, Bateman PE. Ketamine infusion. Its use as a sedative, inotrope and bronchodilator in a critically ill patient. Anaesthesia 1987;42:980–983.
9. Edwards SR, Mather LE. Tissue uptake of ketamine and norketamine enantiomers in the rat: Indirect evidence for extrahepatic metabolic inversion. Life Sci 2001;69:2051–2066.
10. Domino EF, Domino SE, Smith RE, Domino LE, Goulet JR, Domino KE. Ketamine kinetics in unmedicated and diazepam premedicated subjects. Clin Pharmacol Ther 1984;36:645–653.
11. Sigtermans M, Dahan A, Mooren R, et al. S(+)-ketamine effect on experimental pain and cardiac output: A population pharmacokinetic-pharmacodynamic modeling study in healthy volunteers. Anesthesiology 2009;111:892–903.
12. Persson J, Hasselstrom J, Maurset A, et al. Pharmacokinetics and non-analgesic effects of S-and R-ketamine in healthy volunteers with normal and reduced metabolic capacity. Eur J Clin Pharmacol 2002;57:869–875.
13. Geisslinger G, Menzel-Soglowek S, Kamp HD, Brune K. Stereoselective high-performance liquid chromatographic determination of the enantiomers of ketamine and norketamine in plasma. J Chromatogr 1991;568:165–176.
14. Geisslinger G, Hering W, Kamp HD, Vollmers KO. Pharmacokinetics of ketamine enantiomers. Br J Anaesth 1995;75:506–507.
15. Kharasch ED, Labroo R. Metabolism of ketamine stereoisomers by human liver microsomes. Anesthesiology 1992;77:1201–1207.
16. Ihmsen H, Geisslinger G, Schuttler J. Stereoselective pharmacokinetics of ketamine: R(−)-ketamine inhibits the elimination of S(+)-ketamine. Clin Pharmacol Ther 2001;70:431–438.
17. Noppers I, Niesters M, Aarts L, Smith T, Sarton E, Dahan A. Ketamine for the treatment of chronic non-cancer pain. Expert Opin Pharmacother 2010;11:2417–2429.

18. Henthorn TK, Krejcie TC, Niemann CU, Enders-Klein C, Shanks CA, Avram MJ. Ketamine distribution described by a recirculatory pharmacokinetic model is not stereoselective. Anesthesiology 1999;91:1733–1743.

19. White PF, Schuttler J, Shafer A, Stanski DR, Horai Y, Trevor AJ. Comparative pharmacology of the ketamine isomers. Studies in volunteers. Br J Anaesth 1985;57:197–203.

20. Malinovsky JM, Servin F, Cozian A, Lepage JY, Pinaud M. Ketamine and norketamine plasma concentrations after IV, nasal and rectal administration in children. Br J Anaesth 1996;77:203–207.

21. Wieber J, Gugler R, Hengstmann JH, Dengler HJ. Pharmacokinetics of ketamine in man. Anaesthesist 1975;24:260–263.

22. Idwall J, Ahlgren I, Aronsen KR, Stenberg P. Ketamine infusions: Pharmacokinetics and clinical effects. Br J Anaesth 1979;51:1167–1173.

23. Clements JA, Nimmo WS. The pharmacokinetics and analgesic effect of ketamine in man. Br J Anaesth 1981;53:27–30.

24. Pedraz JL, Lanao JM, Calvo MB, Muriel C, Hernandez-Arbeiza J, Dominguez-Gil A. Pharmacokinetic and clinical evaluation of ketamine administered by IV and epidural routes. Int J Clin Pharmacol Ther Tox 1987;25:77–80.

25. Wong CS, Liaw WJ, Tung CS, Su YF, Ho ST. Ketaminepotentiates analgesic effect of morphine in postoperative epidural pain control. Reg Anesth 1996;21:534–541.

26. Thomson IA, Fitch W, Campbell D, Watson R. Effects of ketamine on liver blood flow and hepatic oxygen consumption. Studies in the anaesthetised greyhound. Acta Anaesthesiol Scand 1988;32:10–14.

27. White PF, Way WL, Trevor AJ. Ketamine its pharmacology and therapeutic uses. Anesthesiology 1982;56:119–136.

28. Rogers R, Wise RG, Painter DJ, Longe SE, Tracey I. An investigation to dissociate the analgesic and anesthetic properties of ketamine using functional magnetic resonance imaging. Anesthesiology 2004;100:292–301.

29. Sprenger T, Valet M, Woltmann R, et al. Imaging pain modulation by subanesthetic S-(+)-ketamine. Anesth Analg 2006;103:729–737.

30. Honey GD, Honey RA, O'Loughlin C, et al. Ketamine disrupts frontal and hippocampal contribution to encoding and retrieval of episodic memory: An fMRI study. Cereb Cortex 2005;15:749–759.

Chapter

SYNTHETIC CANNABINOIDS

6

Contents

Introduction

A class of chemical medications known as synthetic cannabinoids (SCBs) is sprayed on plant material and then smoked. Even though these medications act on the brain's cannabinoid receptors, their effects are far more unpredictable and harmful than THC's.

You can feel pleasantly sleepy and extremely "out of it" when using SCBs. They may also induce vertigo, nausea, anxiety, and loss of consciousness. The type of synthetic cannabinoid you have and how it was sprayed on the plant material can affect how strong the effects are.

Some people may use SCBs—also referred to as "synthetic marijuana," "Spice," or "K2"—as an alternative to marijuana. These tiny, seemingly harmless packets of "fake weed" can have major adverse effects that are considerably dissimilar from those of marijuana.

Products containing SCBs may be harmful. Smokers of these products may, therefore, experience agitation, confusion, vomiting, rapid heartbeat, and hallucinations. Some people need to receive assistance from emergency medical services, as well as from hospital emergency rooms or intensive care units.

Orientation and Directional Terms

Term	Definition	Illustration
Endocannabinoids	Endocannabinoids are a new class of lipid mediators, which include amides, esters, and ethers of long-chain polyunsaturated fatty acids.	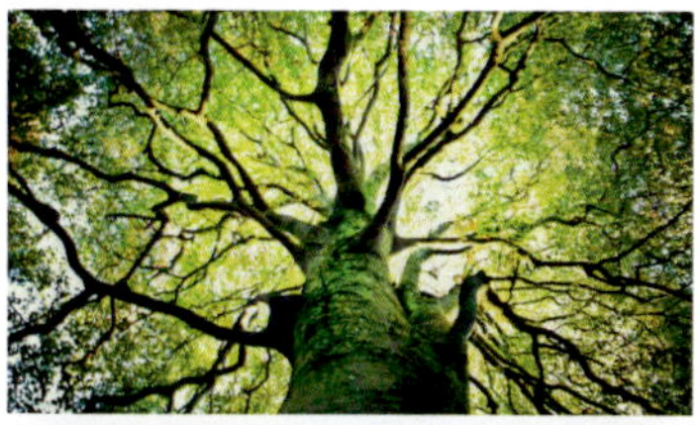
Serotonin syndrome	Serotonin syndrome is a potentially life-threatening condition precipitated by the use of serotonergic drugs.	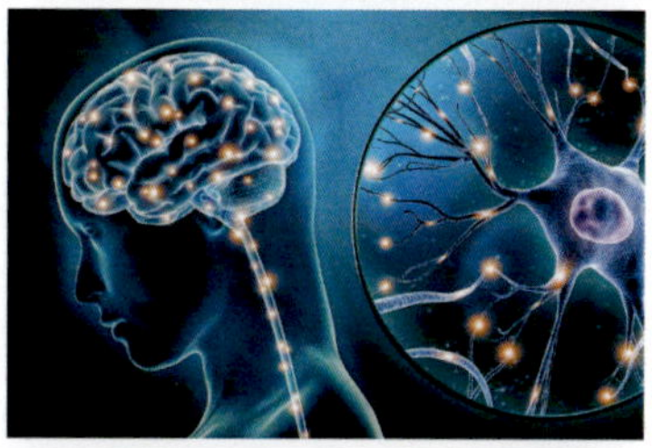
Marijuana	Marijuana refers to the dried leaves, flowers, stems, and seeds from the hemp plant, *Cannabis sativ*a.	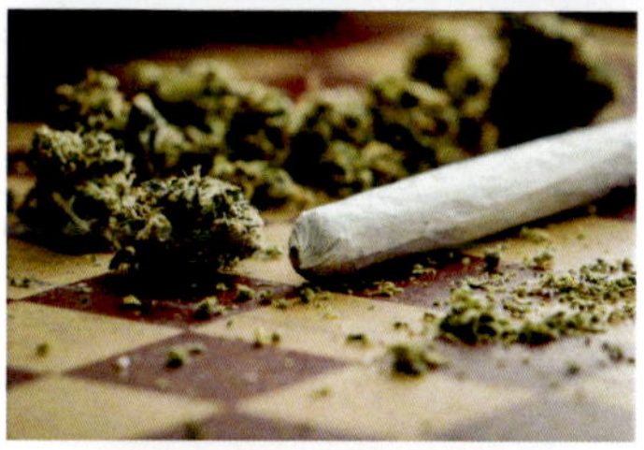
JWH-018	JWH-018 is an analgesic chemical from the naphthoylindole family that acts as a full agonist at both the CB_1 and CB_2 cannabinoid receptors, with some selectivity for CB_2.	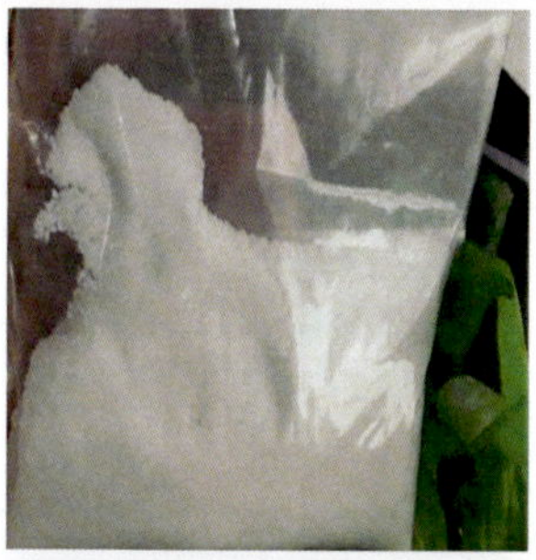
Cannabinoids	Cannabinoids are a class of biological compounds that bind to cannabinoid receptors.	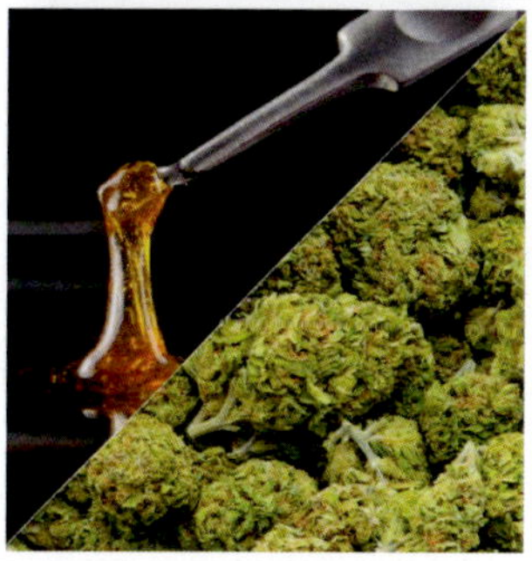

6.1 Overview of Synthetic Cannabinoids

Spice, also known as synthetic cannabis, is a cheap, easily accessible, and becoming more and more well-liked kind of designer drug. Although the SCBs resemble cannabis in many ways, they are more potent and can cause seizures, vomiting, tachycardia, chest pain, and serotonin syndrome because important chemical components have been changed to get around legal restrictions. Very little is known about how to treat acute drug intoxication or abuse.

Chemicals known as SCBs are created in labs to replicate the biological effects of THC, or delta-9-tetrahydrocannabinol, the primary psychoactive component of marijuana. A limited quantity of these compounds were first created in the 1980s for scientific study, mainly to look into the biologic workings of the cannabinoid system and to create new treatments for different medical ailments. In the middle of the 1990s, more SCBs were created for scientific research in order to examine how the cannabinoid system interacts with drugs through receptors.

Before being discovered in the US in late 2008, SCBs were sold as "herbal incense" in a number of European nations. Law enforcement interactions describing SCBs laced on plant material and being abused for their psychoactive properties marked the beginning of their use in the United States in 2009. Numerous variations in the kind and quantity of synthetic cannabinoid applied to the plant material were found by forensic analysis.

Most SCBs come from overseas, mainly from China and other Southeast Asian nations. Large quantities of drugs are brought into the country illegally and end up in covert operations that produce designer drug products in garages, warehouses, and other similar locations across the country. SCBs in powder form are usually dissolved in solvents (e.g., acetone) prior to being dissolved in a propellant meant for use in e-cigarette devices or applied to green plant material.

Synthetic Cannabinoid Drug Facts	
Street names	K2, Spice, Aroma, Barely Legal, Black Mamba, Bliss, Bombay Blue, Bonsai, Dream, Fake Weed, Fake Pot, Fire, Fusion Galaxy, Genie, Gorilla, Incense, K3, Legal High, Moon Rocks, Pep Spice, Skunk, Smacked, Yucatan, Zohai, 50-state Legal
Commercial names	No commercial uses
Common forms	Dried, shredded plant material that looks like potpourri and is sometimes sold as "incense"
Common ways taken	Smoked, swallowed (brewed as tea)
DEA schedule	Schedule I

Source: National Institute on Drug Abuse, 2015b.

The majority of "spice" by weight is made up of pharmacologically inert vegetable matter that has been sprayed with SCBs. Users smoke these substances, which are purportedly derived from plants. In most cases, the ingredients listed on the package are inaccurate or incomplete. The amount of synthetic cannabinoids in one gram of "spice" can vary greatly from package to package. Customers are unaware of the type of active ingredient or dosage they are taking. Large amounts of tocopherol (vitamin E), possibly added to avoid detection, and the β2-mimetic substance clenbuterol, which may be responsible for the sympathomimetic manifestations of "spice" intoxication (tachycardia, hypokalemia), are other ingredients that are frequently added to the vegetable matter.

6.1.1 Pharmacology

Delta-9-tetrahydrocannabinol, or Δ9-THC, is the main cannabinoid found in cannabis. It is a partial agonist of the CB1 receptor. The human body is full of CB1 receptors, particularly in the central nervous system. When used recreationally, SCBs can function as full or partial CB1 agonists. Products that contain SCBs and are used recreationally include single synthetic cannabinoid compounds or combinations of them sprayed on virtually unknown amounts of psychoactively inert pulverized plant material. When added to herbal mixtures, the active ingredient can have potencies hundreds of times greater than those of cannabis and be very hard to find.

There is a wide range of compounds referred to as SCBs, and their names can be confusing. The JWH series (a set of analogs developed in 1994 by Dr. John W.) contains hundreds of compounds. Huffman for research on cannabinoid receptors), even though a large number of them haven't been classified as addictive substances yet. In addition, 32 related metabolites and 43 JWH compounds of known toxicologic significance are known to exist. There are various classifications even within the JWH series, such as naphthoylindoles (e.g., JWH-018), methylindoles (e.g., JWH-175), as well as phenylacetylindoles (e.g. , JWH-201). The AM, UR, RCS, and XLR series are a few more groups of SCBs; some of these have close relationships with the compounds in the JWH series.

Despite being sold as "natural" herbal blends, these products are typically laced with a variety of SCBs, the majority of which are JWH family aminoalkylindoles. 2008 saw the discovery of these and other SCBs in "natural" herbal blends, including HU-210, CP-47, and 497. JWH-018 is one aminoalkylindole in particular that is present in many different K2 product batches and brands.

When these drugs were initially introduced to the European market, it was stated that only organic plant ingredients could have produced the drug's psychotropic effects. The real active ingredient was found in 2009 when Volker Auwärter and colleagues at the University of Freiburg in Germany found undeclared synthetic cannabinoid receptor agonists.

Cannabinoid receptor agonists are classified according to their chemical structure, as follows:

- Classic cannabinoids
  - delta-9-tetrahydrocannabinol (THC) from the cannabis plant (*Cannabis sativa*)
  - the approved anti-emetic nabilone, and
  - HU cannabinoids, which closely resemble THC
- Non-classic cannabinoids, such as the cyclohexylphenol (CP) cannabinoids
- Aminoalkylindoles: the JWH series, synthesized by the chemist J. W. Huffman, contains many CB ligands
- Eicosanoids, such as the endocannabinoid anandamide

Regardless of branding, all products containing SCBs are now commonly referred to as "Spice.". SCBs have the potential to be more toxic than THC due to their potency, effectiveness as CB1 agonists, and potential longer half-life. The risk of toxicity may also be increased by the significant compositional variability and broad concentration ranges of SCBs.

6.1.2 Acute Effects of Cannabinoids

SCBs can be taken orally or intranasally, but they are usually smoked through a joint, bowl, or water pipe. Acute effects such as tachycardia, conjunctival injection, and mood alteration are similar to those of cannabis. Most effects seem to fade 2 to 6 hours after use, with some reports stating that effects begin as soon as 10 minutes after inhalation. On the other hand, acute effects may be linked to clinical symptoms such as hypertension, agitation, hallucinations, psychosis, seizures, and panic attacks that are not typically associated with marijuana use. Generally speaking, using synthetic cannabis has far more severe side effects than using marijuana.

Regular abuse of synthetic cannabis can lead to serious withdrawal and dependency issues. The use of SCBs has been directly linked to at least one fatal overdose and is suspected to have played a role in several other deaths, leading to over 2,500 calls to poison control centers in just one year. Additionally, there have been numerous visits to emergency departments in both the United States and Europe due to the negative effects of synthetic cannabis.

Adverse psychological effects are frequent and can include delusions, agitation, anxiety, difficulty thinking clearly, and paranoia. SCBs have been shown to exacerbate pre-existing chronic psychotic disorders and induce acute psychosis, which is more likely in users with underlying biological vulnerability due to a family history of psychosis. In documented cases, psychotic symptoms have been known to last anywhere from one week to five months.

Some chronic cannabis users may switch to synthetic cannabinoid to ease the symptoms of cannabis withdrawal; this is probably a sign of cross-tolerance between synthetic cannabinoid and THC. It also seems that SCBs are an adequate cannabis replacement, particularly in situations where cannabis is not accessible. Case studies have shown that using synthetic cannabinoid products can cause withdrawal symptoms as well as a dependence syndrome that is comparable to cannabis use.

Headache, dizziness, and dry mouth are physiological side effects. Additional undesirable adverse physiological effects encompass dystonia, dyspnea, tremors, and diaphoresis. Instead of being the result of a direct sympathetic effect, tachycardia is frequently experienced by users of SCBs (similar to those who use cannabis). This is possibly because of decreased peripheral vascular resistance and the ensuing need to maintain cardiac output by raising the heart rate. There may be severe chest pain, hypertension, and tachycardia. There has also been one case report of severe bradycardia accompanied by chest pain.

Cannabinoid hyperemesis syndrome, a chronic disorder initially observed in chronic cannabis users, has been linked to several synthetic cannabinoid compounds (JWH-018, JWH-073, and AM-2201). The syndrome is characterized by cyclic episodes of vomiting and abdominal pain that are relieved by bathing or showering in hot water. Hyperemesis syndrome associated with cannabis is uncommon, though. Such symptoms may help distinguish between intoxication and nausea, to the extent that SCBs may be more likely to induce them.

There have been cases of severe synthetic cannabinoid-related toxicity that required immediate medical attention, including myocardial infarction, seizures, and acute renal failure. SCBs have been linked to fatalities in cases of cardiac ischemia and severe anxiety leading to suicidal thoughts.

Studies on the long-term effects of SCBs are lacking. Some sources advise vaporization over smoking as a method of delivering SCBs because smoking them usually involves inhaling burned, unknown plant material in addition to the synthetic cannabinoid, which may have negative effects on the pulmonary system. JWH-018 might also be carcinogenic. Anecdotal evidence suggests that prolonged use can lead to the development of tolerance and withdrawal syndrome.

Legislative and public health officials have taken notice of these observations and the U.S. For a minimum of one year, the Drug Enforcement Administration (DEA) will utilize its emergency authority to designate JWH-018 and four additional SCBs as Schedule I substances. They pose an immediate risk to public safety. On July 9, 2012, these compounds were permanently classified as Schedule I substances due to the Synthetic Drug Abuse Prevention Act of 2012.

In most nations across the world, SCBs remain available and lawful despite proactive legislative efforts to the contrary. It is obvious that there is a serious risk to the public's health associated with the rapidly rising use of SCBs among young people, their present inability to be identified by common drug urine tests, and the ongoing introduction of new structurally similar products with unknown contents. Both the pharmacologic and toxicologic profiles of these products and the mechanisms underlying the numerous negative effects linked to the use of SCBs are essentially unknown.

6.2 Natural and Synthetic Cannabinoids

Cannabis (*C. sativa*, commonly known as marijuana) and cannabinoids are legal for non-medical use in some countries (or states within the United States), and they have recognized medical indications in some jurisdictions. As more states establish medical and recreational cannabis programs, new prescription cannabinoid products are approved, and the consumer market for cannabidiol (CBD) grows, the use of natural cannabinoids is becoming more and more common in the US.

The primary plant components of cannabis, referred to as cannabinoids or phytocannabinoids, have the ability to interact with the human body's nonECS pathways or the endocannabinoid system (ECS) to produce both desired and undesired effects. In an attempt to mimic the desired euphoric effects of cannabis, SCBs may produce compounds with a higher potential for abuse and serious toxicities. The pharmacology and epidemiology of both natural and SCBs need to be taken into account.

This narrative review aims to provide an overview of the current state of cannabis use, both naturally occurring and synthetically produced, in the US and around the world. The fact that cannabinoids are used for both medical and non-medical purposes complicates this review. This avoids talking about the chemistry, pharmacology, and potential adverse drug events (ADEs) associated with using cannabis and cannabinoids for medicinal and recreational purposes. The evidence supporting medical cannabis and cannabinoids will also be compiled in this review, along with an assessment of potential drug-drug interactions (DDIs) and special populations that may be encountered in clinical practice.

6.2.1 The Endocannabinoid System

Numerous synthetic and natural cannabinoids can be categorized based on their pharmacologic effects on the endocrine system. The best reviews of the extracellular cholinergic system (ECS), particular enzyme and receptor distributions and activities, and biological effects can be found in earlier research examining particular anatomic systems or diseases, such as pain, psychiatric disorders, gastrointestinal disorders, inflammation, and neurologic disease.

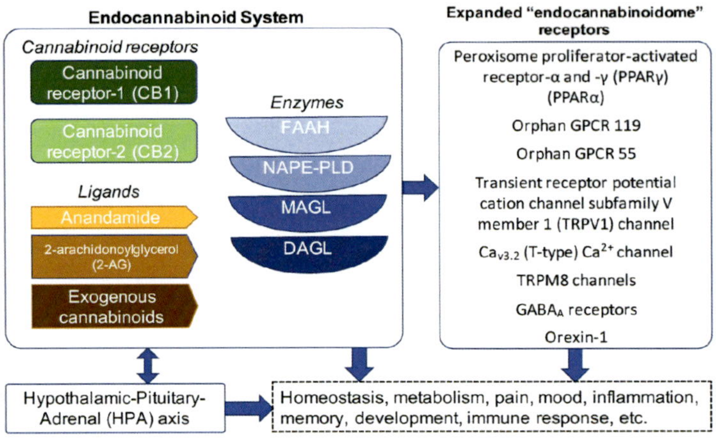

Figure 6.1. Receptors, enzymes, and ligands that make up the endocannabinoid system and the expanded endocannabinoidome. Complex interplays between these systems modulate many biological processes, therapeutic benefits, and adverse effects of cannabis and cannabinoids.DAGL, diacylglycerol lipase; FAAH, fatty acid amide hydrolase; GABA, gammaaminobutyric acid; GPCR, G-protein coupled receptor; MAGL, monoacylglycerollipase; NAPEPLD, N-acyl phosphatidylethanolamine phospholipase D.

Source. https://accp1.onlinelibrary.wiley.com/doi/pdf/10.1002/jcph.1871

In summary, the endogenous lipid-based retrograde neurotransmitters that bind to cannabinoid receptors and other protein targets expressed by vertebrates make up the ECS. It controls a number of immune system functions, appetite, pain, mood, memory, and reproductive, prenatal, and postnatal development processes. To control these functions, the ECS also communicates with the hypothalamic-pituitary-adrenal axis.

CB1 and CB2 cannabinoid receptors were initially identified as the targets of THC in the human brain. However, further research revealed the existence of endogenous ligands known as endocannabinoids, such as anandamide and 2-AG, which have a strong affinity for CB1 and CB2 receptors. While CB1 is primarily found in the central nervous system and is linked to the negative effects of cannabis, CB2 is mainly found in the peripheral system and is believed to have anti-inflammatory and immunomodulating properties useful for certain medical conditions. The endocannabinoidome, which includes enzymes involved in the production and breakdown of endocannabinoids, is a wider network that affects the effects of both endogenous and exogenous cannabinoids on various receptors. This complex system presents challenges for developing cannabinoid-based therapies and predicting adverse drug reactions.

6.2.2 Cannabinoid Chemistry and Pharmacology

More than 100 natural cannabinoids have been identified in the cannabis plant. While other non-cannabis cannabinoids have been reported, natural cannabinoids are found in or can be extracted from the cannabis plant. In this review, directly synthesized cannabinoids that are equivalent to naturally occurring cannabinoids (e.g., dronabinol) shall be regarded as organic. The effects of synthetic or semi SCBs include modulating one or more ECS targets. Other substances found in cannabis plants include terpenes, amides, alkaloids, flavonoids, fatty acids, and noncannabinoid phenols. Some of these substances give cannabis its characteristic color and smell, and they may also have pharmacological effects of their own or alter the effects of cannabinoids. i.e., the effect of entourage). More than 400 naturally occurring phytochemicals have been identified in cannabis plants, and more than 2000 more are produced during the pyrolysis process during smoking or vaping.

A lipophilic side chain, a northern aliphatic hydroxyl, a southern aliphatic hydroxyl, a phenolic hydroxyl, and other essential components of the cannabinoid structure all function as pharmacophores.

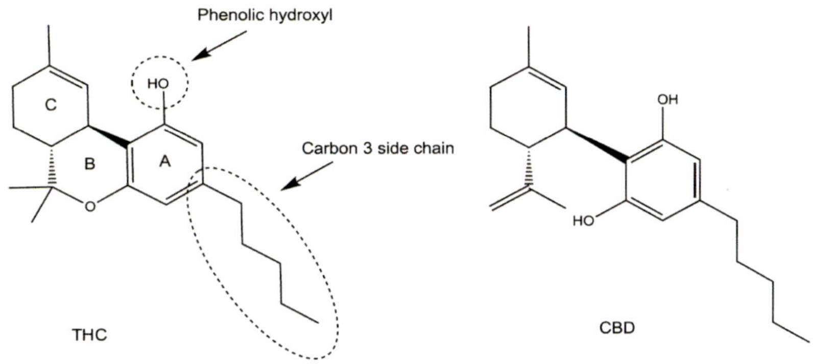

Figure 6.2. Structural features of the primary cannabinoids trans-9-tetrahydrocannabinol (THC) and cannabidiol (CBD). Most cannabinoids are naturally derived from cannabigerolic-acid (CBGA). Typical features of THC include a phenolic hydroxy, aromatic ring (A), pyran ring (B), and cyclohexenyl (C). CBD is formed by a separate biosynthesis pathway and lacks a B-ring.

Source. https://accp1.onlinelibrary.wiley.com/doi/pdf/10.1002/jcph.1871

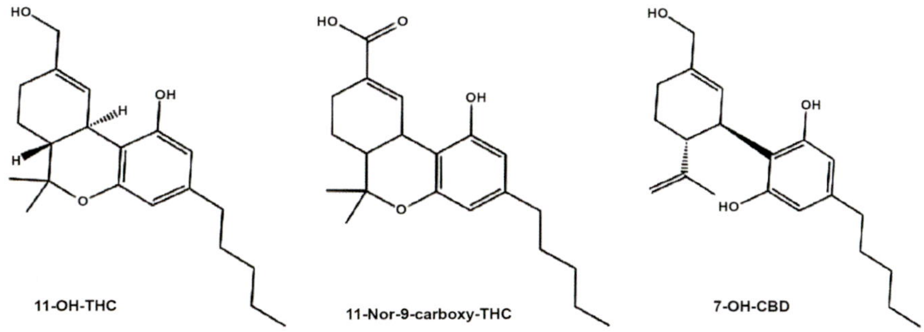

Figure 6.3. Structures of active metabolites of tetrahydrocannabinol (THC) and cannabidiol (CBD). 11-Hydroxy-THC (11-OH-THC) is formed by oxidation by liver enzymes and further converted to 11-Nor-9-carboxy-THC (THC-COOH or 11-COOH-THC). 11-OH-THC retains psychoactive properties, whereas THC-COOH has other effects. 7-OH-CBD is understudied but believed to have similar effects as CBD.

Source. https://accp1.onlinelibrary.wiley.com/doi/pdf/10.1002/jcph.1871

For instance, THC has three side chains made of carbon, a phenolic hydroxyl, and three rings made of aromatic A, pyran B, and cyclohexenyl C rings. Modifications to THC's base structure, like extending the alkyl side chain, can improve the drug's selectivity and affinity for receptor targets. This is also the basis for many of the SCBs that will be covered later.

As a partial agonist of CB receptors, THC causes these targets to be downregulated, which eventually results in tolerance and decreased efficacy. After extended exposure, THC may induce COX-2 and inhibit COX enzymes. Other non-CB receptor activity of THC has pharmacological effects that are not entirely clear. The effects of antiemetic medication and appetite enhancement are influenced by antagonist activity on 5-HT3A receptors as well as other serotonergic system effects. The active metabolites 11-hydroxy-THC and 11-Nor-9-carboxy-THC are produced from THC.

Through first-pass metabolism, 11-hydroxy-THC may be more potent and anecdotally associated with a stronger euphoric and psychoactive effect felt with edible products. Other naturally occurring cannabinoids, such as cannabinol and cannabinodiol, are also known to have psychoactive effects akin to those of THC. THC breaks down to produce cannabinol, which is more prevalent in dried goods.

CBD is another naturally occurring cannabinoid that is widely used. Since CBD doesn't have the same psychoactive effects as THC, it can be used medicinally without having negative side effects that limit dosage. Due to its low affinity for CB receptors, CBD may act as an inverse agonist of CB2, which could have anti-inflammatory and other effects on the immune system. Activation of the peroxisome proliferator-activity receptor-γ, inhibition of anandamide uptake, several ion channel effects, antagonist activity on α1-adrenergic and μ-opioid receptors, agonist activity at 5-HT1A/2A/3A and vanilloid receptors, and inhibition of synaptosomal uptake of noradrenaline, dopamine, serotonin, and γ -aminobutyric acid are among the other known targets of CBD.

Both in the central nervous system and the peripheral nervous system, SCBs directly or indirectly stimulate or inhibit the ECS. They are used for non-medical purposes now, but they were originally developed as pharmacologic tools to probe the ECS or for therapeutic use. Numerous SCBs are known to exist; they all have distinct structural features and can bind to either one or both CB receptors. SCBs have been shown to interact with non-CB receptors like serotonergic or vanilloid receptors, just like natural cannabinoids do.

Products containing SCBs are referred to as "Spice," "K2," fake weed, and legal highs on the black market. These products vary greatly in terms of their precise makeup and toxicology; typically, they contain multiple SCBs in different mixtures to avoid legal repercussions. Lipid-soluble, nonpolar, and highly volatile SCBs that have the potential to be abused are substances that mimic the chemistry and pharmacologic effects of THC, particularly on the CB1 receptor. According to data, SCBs have a higher affinity and potency for CB receptors than THC, leading to effects that are comparable to THC intoxication. CB1 agonists, like nabilone, mimic the effects of THC in medicine to treat pain, nausea and vomiting brought on by chemotherapy, and HIV/AIDS-related anorexia and weight loss. Though no other products than nabilone are currently on the market, more indications for CB1 agonists are presently being investigated.

Potential treatments include SCBs that inhibit fatty acid amide hydrolase (FAAH), act as CB1 and CB2 agonists, and all three. Postoperative pain, atopic dermatitis, and a number of other indications have been studied for CB2 agonists; however, no CB2 agonists are presently on the market. CB1 antagonists are marketed for the treatment of obesity, weight loss, and nicotine addiction (e.g., through late-phase clinical trials). e.g. rimonabant). The marketing and clinical trials of the first-generation CB1 antagonists were stopped due to severe mental events. The development of peripherally restricted CB1 antagonists for the treatment of obesity and other disorders is still of interest. Certain antagonists of CB1 (i.e. drinabant and surinabant) are being researched as remedies for sudden overdoses of cannabis.

The breakdown of endogenous cannabinoids is caused by FAAH. FAAH inhibitors raise endocannabinoid concentrations and have been shown to be safe but with limited efficacy, despite the fact that they are not cannabinoids.

The synthetic cannabinoid family known as "JWH," after John W., is the most well-known. Huffman. These compounds, which have more than 60 known compounds, are aminoalkylindoles and are the predominant components found in Spice/K2. One such substance, JWH-018, is readily synthesized, has potent pharmacologic effects, and is utilized to create other SCBs with different properties and CB receptor affinities. Figure 6.3 illustrates the corresponding substitutions to the core structure that led to the formation of JWH-018. JWH-073, MAM-2201, and AM2201 are a few more examples of compounds that belong to the JWH or aminoalkylindoles family (Sobolevsky et al., 2012).

The "HUs" and "CPs" are two other popular synthetic cannabinoid families in addition to the JWH family. Hebrew University (HU) compounds are classified as classical cannabinoids, while Pfizer developed cannabimimetics, or cannabis-like substances, as early as the 1970s. Both classes have no acknowledged medicinal applications, were never commercialized, and are frequently listed as illicit goods in numerous nations (e.g., the United States' Schedule 1). Although more potent, HU-210 shares a structure with THC and is difficult to synthesize. It is also uncommon to find HU-210 in products sold on black markets. Indazole-based compounds like 5F-ADB (5F-MDMB-PINACA), which was the most frequently detected synthetic cannabinoid found in US Drug Enforcement Agency seizures as recently as 2016, are examples of more recent SCBs. The wide range of SCBs ' pharmacokinetic and pharmacologic activities is still mostly unknown. SCBs, in contrast to THC and CBD, have not been thoroughly investigated, and it is difficult to comprehend the class as a whole due to the abundance of compounds and shifting epidemiology.

6.2.3 Product Availability, Legality, and Composition

Worldwide, at least four prescription products containing natural cannabinoids and one containing synthetic cannabinoids have received approval. These include the THC and CBD-only extract Epidiolex, the isomeric, synthetic forms of THC known as dronabinol Marinol and Syndros, and the THC-only extract Sativex (nabiximols), which is not authorized in the US. Currently available only as a prescription drug, cesamet (generic name: nabilone) is the only known synthetic cannabinoid. These products are prescribed for a number of conditions, such as pain from cancer, nausea and vomiting brought on by chemotherapy, pain from multiple sclerosis, severe seizures, and anorexia related to HIV/AIDS. The availability of medical marijuana and cannabinoid products varies by state. States with medical cannabis programs in the US may only include low-THC products (Seely et al., 2011). Certain state cannabis programs are classified as "comprehensive medical cannabis programs," which allow products with higher THC concentrations.

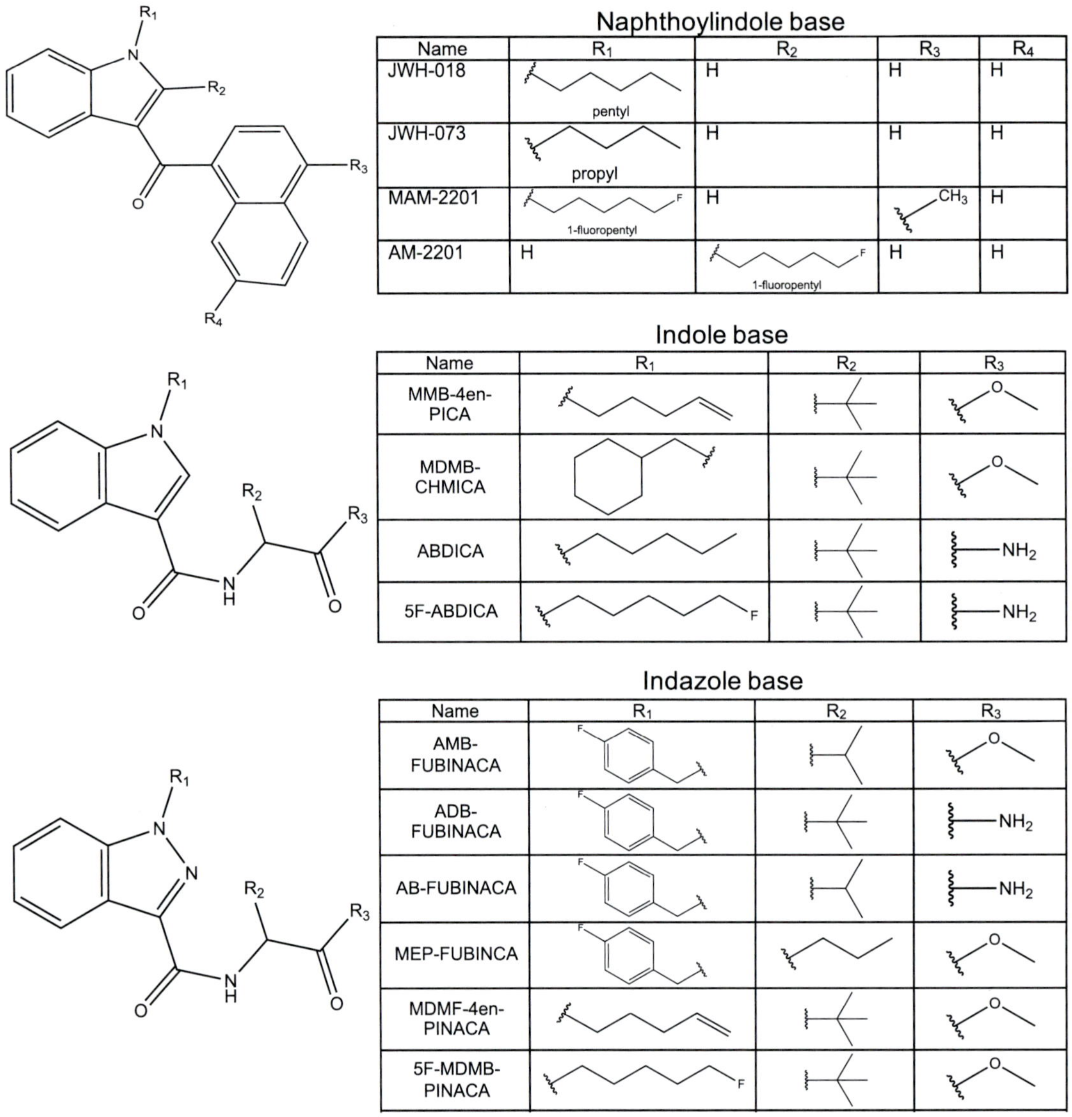

Figure 6.4. Structures of select synthetic cannabinoids (SCBs). Classes of SCBs share a parent structure with substitutions made in various locations.

Source. https://accp1.onlinelibrary.wiley.com/doi/pdf/10.1002/jcph.1871

Products, even within these programs, differ and can be categorized as full-spectrum (containing THC, CBD, and other cannabinoids), broad-spectrum (containing CBD along with other cannabinoids), or purified (containing only CBD) (Ashton et al., 2001).

Since the 2018 "Farm Bill" was passed, which authorized the cultivation of low-THC hemp, CBD possession and sales are regarded as lawful nationwide. According to the Farm Bill, hemp contains less than 0.3 % THC. Plants and products with THC concentrations higher than these would be classified as cannabis and be subject to tighter laws (e.g., a controlled substance on Schedule 1. After the prescription drug Epidiolex was descheduled, marketing CBD-based consumer goods became more feasible; however, this descheduling did not specifically apply to other products containing CBD. In the consumer market, CBD products can be found in lip balms, vaporizers, edibles, topicals, essential oils, pet food, and tinctures and oils for medical use (Franklin et al., 2013). The US Food and Drug Administration (FDA) said that claims of therapeutic effects are still within its jurisdiction when it comes to consumer goods and that no food products containing cannabinoids are allowed to be sold across state lines or be classified as dietary supplements or food additives. The agency has sent numerous warning letters to retailers and manufacturers regarding packaging, labeling, and marketing claims of safety and medical benefits,.

Recreational cannabis use is permitted as of March 2021 in a select few nations, including Uruguay, Canada, Georgia, South Africa, and some areas of the United States. While many Asian and Middle Eastern nations have strict prohibitions in place, recreational cannabis use is still illegal in other parts of Europe, Central America, and South America, but is either not enforced or decriminalized (Gaoni et al., 1964).

Table 6.1. Product information for cannabis-derived pharmaceutical products that contain natural or synthetic cannabinoids

Product (Approval Date)	Active Ingredient(s)	Dosage Form	Route	Recommended Dose	Indication(s)
Sativex[a] (2011-12)	THC and CBD; *nabiximols*	Solution, spray	Buccal spray	Titrated up to 12 sprays per day (patient median is 4-8 sprays); 2.7 mg THC and 2.5 mg CBD per spray	Adjunctive treatment of spasticity and neuropathic pain in MS Adjunctive analgesic for moderate to severe pain in advanced cancer
Marinol (1985)	Dronabinol[b]	Capsules	Oral	2.5 mg 2× daily; max 5 mg 2× daily 5 mg/m^2 4-6× daily; max 15 mg/m^2 4-6× daily	Anorexia associated with AIDS Nausea and vomiting with chemotherapy in patients who failed conventional treatment
Syndros (1985)	Dronabinol[b]	Solution	Oral	2.1 mg 2× daily; max 8.4 mg daily 4.2 mg/m^2 4-6× per day; max 12.6 mg/m^2 4-6× per day	Anorexia associated with AIDS Nausea and vomiting with chemotherapy in patients who failed conventional treatment
Epidiolex (2018)	CBD	Solution	Oral	2.5 mg/kg 2× daily; maintenance 5 mg/kg 2× daily; max 10 mg/kg 2× daily	Seizures associated with Lennox-Gastaut or Dravet syndrome
Cesamet (1985)[c]	Nabilone	Capsules	Oral	1-2 mg 2× daily in 1 mg capsules; max 6 mg daily	Nausea and vomiting with chemotherapy in patients who failed conventional treatment

CBD, cannabidiol; MS, multiple sclerosis; THC, tetrahydrocannabinol.

[a]Sativex is not approved in the United States but was approved in other countries between 2011 and 2012. It is currently in phase 3 clinical trials in the United States.

[b]Dronabinol is a synthetic form of THC and is not extracted from cannabis.

[c]Nabilone is a synthetic cannabinoid with cannabimimetic activity.

Source. https://accp1.onlinelibrary.wiley.com/doi/pdf/10.1002/jcph.1871

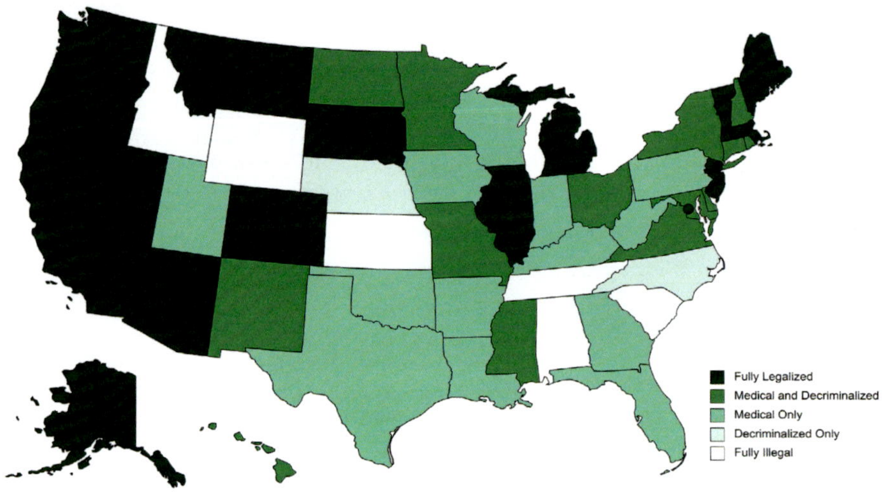

Figure 6.5. US state-based regulation of recreational and medical cannabis.

Source. https://accp1.onlinelibrary.wiley.com/doi/pdf/10.1002/jcph.1871

Currently, 16 states in the US have fully legalized cannabis for recreational use along with medical programs, 14 states have decriminalized recreational use along with medical programs, 13 states only have medical programs, 2 states have decriminalized cannabis use without any medical programs, and 6 states still prohibit cannabis use in any form (Ghisleni et al., 2008).

Cannabidiol (CBD) products: "hemp," <0.3% THC. Legalized via 2018 "Farm Bill" allowing cultivation of hemp. Used in:
- Medical cannabis programs: oils and tinctures for sublingual or oromucosal sprays; edibles
- Available in consumer and animal products including topicals, edibles, etc. Consumer products are not regulated.

Full spectrum cannabis products: Contain tetrahydrocannabinol (THC) and other cannabinoids. Available on street (illicit) markets, recreational, and medical programs. Typical products include:
- Dry flower – "bud," smokable part of cannabis plant. Smoked, vaporized. Cannabinoid content dependent on strain.
- Concentrates – "crumble, badder, budder, shatter, Rick Simpson Oil, dabs, wax, etc." Smoked or vaporized. Highly concentrated THC (40%-80%) and other cannabinoids dependent on strain. Reserved for experienced users of THC.
- Other concentrates – "dry sift, kief, hash, bubble hash, rosin." Concentrated using mechanical, heat, pressure, or water methods without solvents. Smoked or vaped.
- Oils, tinctures, distillates – used for vaporizing or added to edibles, topicals, oral sprays
- Recreational or homemade food products such as cannabutter and cooking oil

Synthetic cannabinoids: Marketed as natural products containing various plants or crystalline media and labeled "not for human consumption." Synthetic cannabinoids are added and unlabeled usually containing more than one synthetic cannabinoid and possible other drugs, medications, or contaminants. Products are smoked or vaporized.

Figure 6.6. Characteristics and terminology of medical and recreational cannabis and cannabinoid products.

Source. https://accp1.onlinelibrary.wiley.com/doi/pdf/10.1002/jcph.1871

Many THC-based cannabis products, both medical and recreational, are still federally categorized as Schedule 1 in the United States. Dried flowers, concentrates, and other processed cannabis products are examples of possible products. The specific strain profile that is used has a significant impact on the effects of these products. Solvents are used to extract concentrates, which include substances marketed under the names crumble, badder, budder, shatter, butane honey oil, black glass, "710," wax, and Rick Simpson Oil, among many others. Other concentrated products such as dry sift, kief, hash, rosin, and bubble hash are mechanical, pressure, or heat processed without using solvents (Fantegrossi et al., 2008).

Concentrate contents are determined by the quality of the extraction method, the solvents utilized, and the composition of the plant used in the extractions. Smoking concentrates is the most popular method (e. g. vaporized, "dabbing"), or incorporated into food items. These concentrated products, which are only recommended for experienced users, can contain up to 40–80% THC by weight. When smoked, they produce quick, potent highs. Concentrates, like distillates, are the building blocks for topical and edible products and can be used to create additional tinctures and oils. Food items made at home or sold recreationally, like cooking oil and cannabutter (infused butter), are also popular (Gamaleddin et al., 2012).

In the US, authorized medical applications for cannabis (i.e., state laws differ regarding the list of ailments or symptoms that each state defines as qualifying a patient for medical cannabis. Chronic pain (including pain from cancer), nausea and vomiting, muscle spasms, inflammatory diseases (such as Crohn's disease and rheumatism), seizures, and HIV/AIDS are the most common medical conditions. Certain conditions are more common in the elderly, while others have their roots in illnesses that children had (e.g., autism). Certain states also permit the use of cannabis to treat mental health issues like anxiety and PTSD (ElSohly et al., 2011). Consequently, there is a greater chance of ADEs due to the growing number of medical cannabis approvals, which show a shift in the user base from one that generally uses cannabis and cannabinoids with little medical supervision to one that may have more complex physical and mental health profiles. Prioritizing public health messaging and clinician knowledge of these potential ADEs is crucial for the growth of cannabis and cannabinoids as therapeutics, particularly for special populations. SCBs are commonly referred to as "legal highs" or "synthetic marijuana" and are typically sold as "incense" in street markets or semilegal retail settings. Common names for these compounds include "K2" and "spice.". Even though they might be marked "not for human consumption," some synthetic cannabinoid products pass for "natural products" when they are sold in retail settings because they do contain plant material. Most frequently, SCBs are added to this plant material by spraying them on or finding them in other crystalline forms (Gunderson et al., 2012; Gunderson et al., 2014). After that, spice pouches are smoked (e.g., vaporized, rolled into a joint, or used with a pipe.

A large number of products containing SCBs originate from Chinese laboratories, where exports of research chemicals are not strictly regulated. The majority of US states and other nations have criminalized the sale of SCBs, outlawed their use in certain situations, and prohibited them entirely through a variety of administrative measures, prosecution tactics, and laws. These goods are still in demand, and one can find and purchase both high- and low-quality goods in a variety of retail establishments and on the black market.

6.2.4 Evidence for Cannabis and Cannabinoid Efficacy for Select Indications

There is conflicting data supporting the effectiveness of medical cannabis and cannabinoids as adjuvant therapies or treatments for a variety of illnesses and symptoms. The National Academies of Sciences, Engineering, and Medicine have identified and summarized clinical evidence through 2016, providing the most thorough review of the available data to date. There is limited evidence to support the use of cannabis as adjuvant therapy or as a treatment for conditions other than multiple sclerosis, chronic pain, and seizure disorders like epilepsy (Howlett et al., 1990; Haj-Dahmane et al., 2011).

Two recent meta-analyses on epilepsy corroborate previous results from randomized clinical trials showing cannabis effectively lowers the frequency and duration of seizures in some seizure disorders. In 2018, the United States approved Epidiolex, an oral solution containing pure CBD derived from cannabis, to treat severe seizure disorders such as Lennox-Gastaut syndrome, Dravet syndrome, or tuberous sclerosis complex.

For chronic pain that is not related to cancer, the evidence is strongest. Cannabis has been shown in numerous recent meta-analyses to be useful in reducing pain associated with a range of conditions. There is not as much evidence to support treating pain in cancer patients specifically. A 2017 meta-analysis that included cancer as a subgroup discovered a reduction in pain associated with the disease. Two additional recent meta-analyses found no evidence of a clear benefit from cannabinoids for palliative care or for cancer-related pain in general (Huffman et al., 2011; Huffman et al., 2008). Numerous outcomes have been evaluated for possible medicinal applications of cannabis in multiple sclerosis. For patients with multiple sclerosis, there is moderate to strong evidence supporting the use of cannabis as adjuvant therapy to improve bladder function and reduce spasticity or frequency of spasms. For other conditions, the evidence base is still shaky or contradictory. Clinical evidence currently available has several drawbacks, such as small sample sizes, heterogeneous products (cannabis vs. cannabinoids; differing strengths and contents), and a high risk of bias.

SCBs, with the exception of nabilone, have no established medical applications. Many are still being investigated for potential therapeutic benefits, while others have had their development or commercialization halted because of unfavorable side effects or insufficient efficacy.

6.2.5 Adverse Drug Events with Natural and Synthetic Cannabinoids

For the majority of cannabis preparations and indications, efficacy data is comparatively weak, but the possibility of ADEs is more clear. The pooled risk of ADEs was three times higher with cannabis and cannabinoid therapies when compared to placebo, according to a recent meta-analysis analyzing the results of clinical trials involving these substances. This result held true for all indications. The fact that THC was either present alone or in combination with CBD in every product under study is noteworthy, though (Iseger et al., 2015; Jankovics et al., 2012).

Practically speaking, the main emphasis for ADE prevention should be on the effects of THC and SCBs that are CB1 agonists. Unless used in very high doses for antiseizure activity, CBD is unlikely to cause clinically significant adverse events when taken by itself. Certain adverse drug reactions (ADEs), such as transaminase elevations, sedation, somnolence, lethargy, decreased appetite, and sleep disturbances, were linked to CBD in clinical trials for seizure disorders. On the other hand, although these effects differ amongst studies, CBD may even reduce the incidence of ADEs caused by THC in recreational or medicinal cannabis products. Although there are other SCBs with different CB receptor activities, there isn't enough information or accessibility to talk about ADEs for these substances.

The main psychoactive component of cannabis, THC, is known to be even more pharmacologically complex and may cause both DDIs and ADEs. The most prevalent ADEs are cardiac problems, cognitive impairments, and mental and neurological illnesses. The most often reported adverse effects (ADEs) and the main causes of treatment discontinuation are the euphoric and dissociative effects of THC (Hutter et al., 2012). According to pooled data from clinical trials, THC-containing products were associated with 3–5 times higher levels of dizziness, euphoria, disorientation, drowsiness, and confusion than placebo. Mania, depression, and schizophrenia exacerbations have been linked to THC and other CB1 agonists. Prescription cannabis products with FDA-approved labeling advise screening to stop suicidal thoughts and behaviors, which these mental health issues may make worse. The use of any THC or THC mimetic product, such as SCBs, medical cannabis, and cannabinoid extracts, should be covered by this screening recommendation for psychiatric disorders and suicide risk. In the case of the latter, the consequences are frequently far more severe and may result in medical emergencies (Kacinko et al., 2011). Synergistic effects may make synthetic cannabinoid mixtures even more potent.

The main justification for the use of medical cannabis and other cannabinoids is pain relief, which is generally believed to be caused by the cognitive effects of THC, including euphoria, sedation, and dissociative effects. But there's also evidence linking long-term memory impairments to THC use. Intractable nausea and vomiting brought on by cannabis use is known as cannabis hyperemesis syndrome, a less common and underdiagnosed cannabis-related illness. 86 Cannabis hyperemesis syndrome is linked to long-term, continuous use of high-THC products and is believed to be related to cannabis effects on CB1 receptors or elsewhere on the ECS (Huffman et al., 2005). One explanation for the anecdotal evidence of the CBD-to-THC ratio (CBD:THC) is the coadministration of THC with CBD, which may reduce cognitive and neuropsychiatric adverse effects. Although there is some evidence that CBD reduces the short-term effects of THC, there is little evidence in favor of standardization due to the variability of CBD:THC in studies. Furthermore, there are negative correlations between the cognitive and neuropsychiatric effects of THC and previous cannabis use (Huestis et al., 2005). This suggests that users are making their own decisions based on their positive experiences with cannabis, their ability to tolerate it, or both. This provides more evidence in favor of the advice to "start low and go slow" when using cannabis and, whenever feasible, to more explicitly titrate THC dosages slowly or stay away from THC-based products.

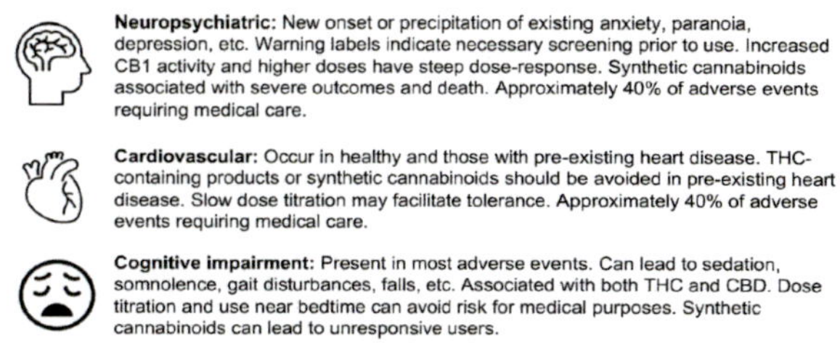

Figure 6.7. Most common adverse drug events associated with tetrahydrocannabinol (THC) and other cannabinoid receptor type 1 (CB1) agonists. These reactions are dose-limiting and the primary reasons for treatment discontinuation. These reactions are associated with medical emergencies when precipitated by synthetic cannabinoids, which are more potent at CB1.

Source. https://accp1.onlinelibrary.wiley.com/doi/pdf/10.1002/jcph.1871

Patients who use cannabis and cannabinoids are becoming increasingly concerned about cardiovascular side effects. Angina can result from smoking and vaping because they raise the body's need for oxygen and reduce its supply (Kochanowski and Kala, 2005; Loeffler et al., 2016). Moreover, epidemiological research connects cannabis use to heart failure, stroke, and myocardial infarction. Some people think that THC is sympathomimetic, which means that it affects blood pressure and heart rhythm. On cardiac tissue, CB1 receptors may exacerbate vasodilation, fibrosis, inflammation, and cardiac stress. There have been reports of bradycardia, tachycardia, and hypotension linked to cannabis use. International labeling for Sativex (nabiximols; containing both THC and CBD) includes a contraindication for preexisting cardiovascular diseases, such as hypertension, coronary heart disease, heart failure, and prior stroke, even though the medication is not yet approved in the United States (Moran et al., 2011).

Additional toxicities and severity brought on by either occasional or continuous use are shown in ADE reports involving SCBs. It has been documented that coagulopathies, renal failure, neurologic and psychiatric emergencies, and cardiac abnormalities can occur. Along with these side effects, SCBs can cause agitation, psychosis, seizures, and strokes. Medical attention is limited to supportive care for ADEs associated with SCBs. Because of the lack of product standardization and unknown content, even among seasoned users of synthetic cannabinoid products, the risk of adverse effects is consistently high.

Contrary to popular belief, approved medication labels advise against using THC and other CB1 agonists in people with SUDs due to the possibility of dependency. Chronic use leads to the downregulation of CB1 receptors, which results in tolerance and fewer side effects (Lapoint et al., 2011; Lindigkeit et al., 2009). Withdrawal symptoms usually go away after 30 days and can include anxiety, irritability, depression, sleep disturbances, and decreased appetite. The prevalence of cannabis use disorder increased to 50% of daily users who met diagnostic criteria. Cannabis has an addictive potential that is correlated with younger users, lower CBD doses, and higher THC doses. Cannabis should always be used carefully, even for acceptable purposes, and medical use does not prevent users from developing use disorders.

Understanding the effects of natural or SCBs is further complicated by the presence of common contaminants that raise ADEs. Different substances and microorganisms, such as bacteria, heavy metals, pesticides or other toxins, preservatives, additives, or prescription drugs (e.g., opioids). While some of those ingredients are naturally present or added during processing, chemical synthesis, or growing, others may be added on purpose in an effort to produce a more pronounced psychoactive effect. Consumer CBD products fall under the jurisdiction of the US Department of Agriculture rather than the FDA if they are not promoted or claimed to be dietary supplements or medical products. This may have a detrimental effect on the final products' quality (Watanabe et al., 2007; Sobolevsky et al., 2010).

Natural cannabinoids contain microbial contaminants that pose a particular risk to immunocompromised and pediatric populations that use cannabis medicinally. It is also problematic when metals found in cannabis-based products are present. Cannabis contains a number of metals, including copper, lead, magnesium, mercury, and cadmium. Certain products containing both natural and SCBs frequently contain trace levels of pesticides. For instance, an outbreak of coagulopathies and five fatalities occurred in one US state as a result of contamination with rodenticides, which are vitamin K antagonists comparable to warfarin (Sobolevsky et al., 2012; Wiley et al., 2011).

Both medicinal and recreational extracts that are vaporized may include harmful substances such as vitamin E, medium-chain triglycerides, or other lipids that have been connected to lung damage. Seldom do products have as much cannabinoids as stated on the label. Case studies have also shown that consumer CBD products contain unreported SCBs, significantly raising the risk profile. Many other factors, such as the particular dispensary, manufacturer, farm, batch, patient-level factors (physiology, genetics), and route of administration, can also contribute to ADE variability between products containing cannabis or specific cannabinoids. Within 15 to 30 minutes, smoking and vaporization reach their peak concentrations, and during this time, acute intoxication or ADEs can be observed. These concentrations and effects can differ significantly between people and even between uses in the same person. Maximum concentrations can be reached up to 3–5 hours after ingestion through oral administration routes, which include capsules, sublingual, buccal, and inhalation products. These routes also exhibit less variability than inhalation products. Compared to oral products, edibles have significantly less predictable absorption profiles that vary depending on the medium (e.g., brownies, lollipops, gummy bears, and so on), with a gradual start and lingering effects (Winstock et al., 2015; Winstock et al., 2013).

6.2.6 Drug-Drug Interactions with Cannabinoids

There have been descriptions of the DDI potential of the main natural cannabinoids, with implications for ADEs. Though their potential is unknown, given their similar chemical structures, other naturally occurring and SCBs may, in many cases, have properties similar to these primary cannabinoids. THC is an inhibitor and substrate of the enzymes that break down drugs. As previously indicated, the main active metabolites of THC are THC-carboxylic acid and 11-hydroxy-THC (11-OH-THC). The former may account for the greater "high" felt after oral administration since it is just as active, if not more so, at CB1 receptors than THC. In the gastrointestinal tract and liver, oxidation is mediated by the cytochrome P450 (CYP) system, which includes subtypes CYP2C9, CYP2C19, and CYP3A4. Specifically, significant effects on THC bioavailability have been linked to CYP2C9 polymorphisms (prevalence up to 35 % in White people), which in clinical studies increased THC exposure by two to three times. Although they are glucuronidated, THC and its metabolites do not seem to be substrates of the P-glycoprotein transporter (Zhang et al., 2006).

When combined with the CYP3A4 and CYP2C19 inducer rifampicin, THC exposure dropped 36%, and 11-OH-THC exposure dropped 87%. THC rose by 27% and 11-OH-THC by 204% when combined with the CYP3A inhibitor ketoconazole; all the healthy adult participants experienced severe psychiatric events. Therefore, CYP3A and CYP2C subfamily strong to moderate inhibitors and inducers may cause changes in THC concentrations that are clinically significant. THC bioavailability may be increased, and ADEs may worsen if combined with inhibitors such as protease inhibitors (found in HIV/AIDS medications), "azole" antifungals, amiodarone, proton pump inhibitors, fluoxetine, verapamil, and cimetidine. THC effects are reduced when combined with enzyme-inducing drugs like phenytoin, carbamazepine, and rifampin. This combination may result in lower clinical efficacy when THC is used therapeutically (Zhang et al., 2002; Zhang et al., 2004).

THC has been shown to interact with enzymes such as CYP3A4, CYP2C9, CYP2C19, CYP2D6, and carboxylesterase, which can lead to significant drug interactions. By understanding which common medications interact with these enzymes, healthcare providers can focus on key characteristics to prevent ADEs. It is important to consider factors such as protein binding and therapeutic indices when assessing the potential for DDIs with THC. By taking into account metabolic interactions, protein binding, outcome severity, and pharmacodynamic overlap, strategies can be developed to minimize the risk of severe DDIs. For instance, medications that overlap in multiple areas with THC should be used with caution when used together to reduce the likelihood of harmful interactions (Zimmermann et al., 2009).

CBD and THC both affect the same metabolic enzymes. Recent research on CBD's potential for interacting with these enzymes involved using high doses for managing seizures. However, the typical exposure to CBD in recreational or medical cannabis products is much lower than in prescription products. It is less likely to cause DDI at these lower doses. Nonetheless, caution should be taken when combining CBD with medications that are metabolized by specific enzymes and have a narrow therapeutic range (Weinstein et al., 2017; Yamamoto et al., 1987). There is no evidence to suggest that medications affecting CBD concentrations increase adverse effects related to CBD.

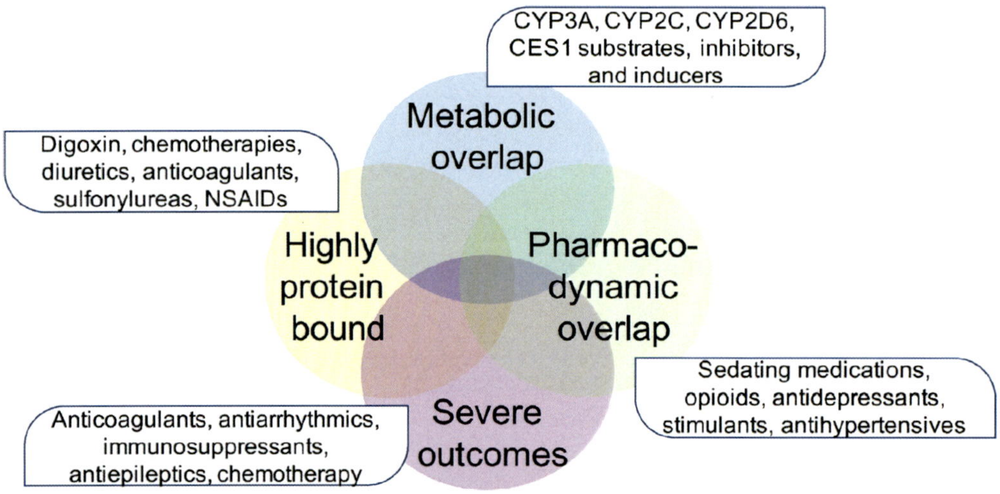

Figure 6.8. Key characteristics contributing to drug-drug interactions with cannabinoids and example medications. Medications with 2 or more categories of overlap should be used with caution, as these could lead to severe acute outcomes.

Source. https://accp1.onlinelibrary.wiley.com/doi/pdf/10.1002/jcph.1871

It should be used caution when distinguishing between inactivated and activated medications (i.e. prodrugs) by means of these enzymes. One enzyme that metabolizes certain medications, for instance, is CES1. e.g. methylphenidate) but stimulates other substances (e.g., dabigatran etexilate) and figuring out how to forecast ADEs from these DDIs requires knowledge of these dynamics (Sim-Selley et al., 2006).

Pharmacodynamic interactions are possible in addition to these pharmacokinetic or metabolic interactions. THC-related side effects, particularly those that are psychiatric, cognitive, and cardiovascular, are the main issues surrounding cannabinoids. Combinations with drugs or other illegal substances like cocaine or stimulants can intensify psychological side effects like anxiety, depression, and suicidal thoughts and behavior. Examples of medications that may pharmacodynamically exacerbate depression or other mood disorders linked to THC or SCBs include beta blockers, opioids, and benzodiazepines. Debilitating illnesses are linked to higher rates of depression and other psychiatric disorders. Patients who use medical cannabis for these conditions may, therefore, already have more severe neuropsychiatric adverse effects, which puts them at risk of exacerbations (Klein et al., 2003; Patton et al., 2013).

Combining cannabis with sedative drugs like opioids and benzodiazepines can worsen cognitive impairment. Overdosing on sedatives can interfere with driving and cause disruptions to regular activities or work. Avoiding coadministration and offering the right kind of patient counseling are important. The best advice is to save THC (and other sedative medications) close to bedtime and to use continued caution upon waking if cannabinoids must be used alone or in combination with other sedatives. Anticholinergic medications may exacerbate common side effects like dry mouth and cognitive impairments, especially in older adults who use cannabis and cannabinoids (Paine et al., 2006).

As previously stated, THC can affect the cardiovascular system and should not be taken with medications that have similar effects. It is recommended to avoid using THC in individuals with existing heart conditions. Mixing THC with stimulants can increase the risk of tachycardia, while combining it with antihypertensive medications may cause dangerous drops in blood pressure and orthostatic hypotension. Prescription products containing THC are not recommended for individuals with heart disease (Moller et al., 2011).

SCBs that activate the CB1 receptor are anticipated to exhibit adverse drug event profiles comparable to THC. As a result, it is anticipated that SCBs will have comparable, yet more potent, pharmacodynamic interactions with the medication classes mentioned above (Patel et al., 2010).

As the use of cannabis and cannabinoids for medical purposes continues to grow, the concern for potential DDIs is also increasing. Individuals using these products range in age, from younger to older, and may have more complex medical needs. These individuals may not receive the same level of patient counseling and DDI screening as they would for other medications. It is important for medication reconciliation, patient education, and DDI screening tools to include cannabinoids in a similar manner as vitamins and herbal supplements.

6.3 Synthetic and Non-Synthetic Cannabinoid Drugs and Their Adverse Effects

The most accessible and commonly used drug in the world is cannabis. Approximately 4 % of adult people worldwide have used cannabis at some point in their lives, according to the United Nations Office on Drugs and Crime (UNODC, 2016). Eleven percent (36 million) of adults in the United States of America (USA) alone reported having used cannabis at least once in the past. Furthermore, the medical application of cannabis and its derivatives is growing and has been tested for a number of ailments, such as multiple sclerosis, pain, anorexia, chemotherapy side effects, and muscle spasms. Tetra-hydro-cannabinol, or THC, is the main psychoactive ingredient in cannabis (Seely et al., 2012). It interacts with CB1 and CB2 receptors to produce its main effects. Recently, there has been an increase in the recreational use of Novel Psychoactive Substances (NPS) containing SCBs, particularly among young adults. It looks that the number of SC users is rising in contrast to the decrease in the use of many NPSs, such as piperazines and cathinones. While SC medications have similar psychotropic effects to cannabis, they also have more severe and unpredictable side effects. Even though research on the medicinal potential of cannabinoid-based drugs is becoming more and more interesting, repeated exposure to organic or synthetic cannabinoid agonists is linked to negative psychological and physiological effects. Mental disorders such as affective disorders, schizophrenia, and psychotic states are the most well-known psychological side effects. The current review's objective is to outline what is currently known about the acute and chronic use of both synthetic and organic cannabis products, as well as the negative effects they may have on public health (Seelyet al., 2011).

6.3.1 Epidemiology and Pattern of Use of Cannabinoids

The general population's lifetime prevalence of using SC is estimated to be between 0.2 and 4 % based on national and regional representative surveys. In contrast, a higher percentage of people—between 25% and 33%—use cannabis over the course of their lifetime. However, according to Winstock and Barratt, SC products are very well-liked by cannabis users who use the drug recreationally. With the exception of cannabis, the annual prevalence of SC usage among high school seniors in the USA was higher than that of any other drug (Tournebize et al., 2017). Research gathered from multiple surveys indicates that 6–17% of American college students have used SC drugs at least once while they were enrolled in school. Apart from that, teens and young adults used SC relatively frequently. One percent of Europeans aged 14 to 18 years reported using SC drugs at least once in their lifetime. This is particularly significant because research, both clinical and preclinical, suggests that adolescent exposure to THC and SC increases the likelihood of developing schizophrenia in later life (Spaderna et al., 2013).

Due to the concerning rise of synthetic cannabinoid (SC) drugs, many countries have implemented legal measures to regulate their distribution. For instance, the United Kingdom passed laws to control first generation SCs in 2009 and introduced additional regulations in 2013 for second generation SCs. However, despite these efforts, new variants of SCs have emerged that are not yet covered by UK laws (Tournebize et al., 2017). This trend is also seen in other countries, as manufacturers exploit legal loopholes to create new, legal versions of SCs for sale. A study by Waugh et al. in 2011 revealed a significant increase in SC drug use, indicating that current legislation alone is not sufficient to address the issue. It is clear that more comprehensive prevention strategies are needed to effectively combat the distribution and use of SC drugs.

Naive consumers usually report using stem cells (SCs) for a variety of reasons, including affordability, ease of use, high availability, and curiosity compared to cannabis (Uchiyama et al., 2013). Since SCs are largely imperceptible by a straightforward urine test, one of the main reasons people use SC drugs is to get "cannabis-like" effects without running the risk of being caught. The low cost and comparatively high availability of SCs are additional reasons to use them. Unlike cannabis, these synthetic medications are usually not meant to be combined with tobacco, presumably in order to produce the strongest effects.

Table 6.2. Summary of acute and long-term clinical side-effects of cannabinoid-based drugs

Symptoms	**Type of effect**[+]	**Type of drug**	
		Synthetic Cannabinoids	**Cannabis**
Neuropsychiatric	Acute	Severe psychotic symptoms including; agitation , aggression, catatonia, paranoia, auditory and visual hallucinations, perceptual alterations, and persistent psychosis episode.	Perceptual alterations including; hallucinations and distortion of spatial perception are typical effects. Paranoia, aggressiveness, and prolonged psychosis were observed in vulnerable users and are dose-related.
	Long-term	Chronic use may increase the risk for developing psychotic disorders.	An increased risk of psychotic disorders in vulnerable individuals and naïve users.
Affect	Acute	Negative mood, panic attacks, manic behavior , depression, and suicidal ideation.	Anxiety and panic attacks; especially in naïve users.
	Long-term	Depression, irritability and persistent anxiety.	An increased risk for developing anxiety, and mood disorders.
Cognitive	Acute	Severe cognitive impairments including; memory alteration, attention difficulties, and amnesia.	Wide range of dose-related cognitive deficits including; attention, working-memory, cognitive inhibition, and psychomotor function.
	Long-term	Executive function deficits of working memory and attention	Impairments of set-shifting, verbal learning, attention, short-term memory and psychomotor functions .
Cardiovascular	Acute	Tachycardia, hypertension, myocardial infraction, arrhythmias, chest pain, and palpitations.	An increase of cardiovascular activity, increase heart rate, and decrease blood pressure.
	Long-term	Prolong use may increase risk of cardiovascular disease.	An increased risk of cardiovascular disease after prolong use.
Neurologic	Acute	Dizziness, somnolence, seizures, hypertonicity, hyperflexion, hyperextension, sensation changes, and fasciculations.	Dizziness, somnolence, and muscle tension.
	Long-term	Preliminary evidence for structural and functional central nervous system alterations.	Structural and functional abnormalities in a range of brain areas including the hippocampus and amygdala.
Gastrointestinal	Acute	Nausea, emesis, and appetite change.	Hyperemesis, and increase appetite.
	Long-term	Severe weight-loss after prolong use.	Low body weight among regular users.

Other	Acute	Acute kidney injury, abdominal pain, miosis, mydriasis, xerostomia, hyperthermia, fatigue, rhabdomyolysis, cough, deficits of driving ability.	Bronchodilation, impairments of driving ability.
	Long-term	Kidney diseases, insomnia, nightmares, dependency, tolerance, and withdrawal.	An increased risk of obstructive lung disease including lung-cancer, an increased risk of cancers of the oral cavity, pharynx and esophagus, cannabis addiction, tolerance, and withdrawal.

Source. https://www.ncbi.nlm.nih.gov/pmc/articles/PMC5999798/

6.3.2 Adverse Health Effects of Cannabinoids

Acute Effects of Cannabinoids

Cannabis users describe the intoxicating effects of the drug as mild euphoria, relaxation, and an overall pleasant feeling. It is thought that the presence of THC is connected to these desired psychotropic effects. Cannabis and THC cause dose-related impairment in a number of laboratory settings, including executive function and motor coordination.

Additional unwanted symptoms like anxiety, panic attacks, and psychotic episodes have been linked to cannabis intoxication, especially in inexperienced users and those who are susceptible. Similarly, the use of SCBs can also lead to effects such as relaxation, euphoria, changes in perception, distorted sense of time, and slight cognitive impairments (Rajasekaran et al., 2013; Volkow et al., 2016).

When people who use cannabis or SC drive while intoxicated, their cognitive changes make them more likely to be involved in car accidents. Cannabis is the most often detected illicit drug in drivers involved in fatal traffic accidents or stopped for driving dangerously, according to epidemiological evidence (1). Consequently, there is a link between drivers who use cannabis and a higher chance of getting into a car accident. Although the link between SC drugs and auto accidents is not well-documented in epidemiological studies, driving while under the influence of SCs has been shown in a number of case studies (Tai and Fantegrossi, 2014). Musshoff and associates eight drivers in Germany were reportedly stopped by police for driving recklessly. All suspected serum samples contained multiple types of SCs; drivers also exhibited delayed reactions, delayed movements, and impaired fine motor skills. Twelve incidents of driving while under the influence of SCs were reported by Yeakel and Logan; in each case, the drivers had generally poor motor coordination. In a seven-week study carried out in Norway, 2.2 % of the 726 blood samples taken from drivers suspected of driving under the influence of drugs tested positive for SCBs, and most of the drivers were involved in car accidents. When considered collectively, it appears that driving after SCs may raise the risk of getting into a car accident, just like driving while high on cannabis (Watanabe et al., 1995).

Notwithstanding these similarities, the range and strength of the effects of cannabis and SC medications differ significantly. Case report studies reveal a broad spectrum of undesirable somatic effects, from mild symptoms like nausea to more severe ones like palpitations, diaphoresis, and psychomotor agitation. Even with large doses of organic cannabis, some symptoms, like agitation, hypotension, emesis, seizures, and hypokalemia, are indicative of SC intoxication and do not occur (Wintermeyer et al., 2010; Xi et al., 2011).

The psychotropic effects of excessive SC intoxication differ greatly. While some users report feeling sedentary, others claim to be agitated, tired, or flushed. This variation might be the result of varying SC concentrations across various brands. SCs have a shorter duration and peak earlier than the intoxication caused by organic cannabis products, which have a slow effect that fades over time. For instance, JWH-018's effects last for about one to two hours, whereas CP-47,497's effects last for about five to six hours. Additionally, after using SC products, some side effects, like anxiety, hallucinations, insomnia, and psychotic episodes, may persist for days or weeks (Aung et al., 2000; Beuck et al., 2011).

Chronic Effects of Cannabinoids

Numerous studies show a link between chronic cannabis use and long-term cognitive decline as well as an elevated risk of various mental health issues. These consist of schizophrenia, depression, anxiety, and bipolar disorder. There is mounting evidence linking SC drugs to serious adverse medical and mental health outcomes. According to this data, repeated exposure to SCs causes general adverse side effects that are worse and last longer than those associated with THC (Morgan et al., 2013).

Most recently, Cohen et al. demonstrates deficits in a range of higher-order cognitive abilities, such as working memory, attention, and recall, that are seen in SC users as opposed to recreational cannabis users. According to a different study, patients taking SC drugs and developing acute psychotic disorder exhibit cognitive deficits akin to those experienced by individuals with schizophrenia. These findings are in line with data from rodent studies that demonstrate repeated exposure to SCs causes long-lasting behavioral and cognitive deficits that mimic schizophrenia in rodent models (Hoffman et al., 2016).

There is proof that cannabis has a negative impact on cardiovascular health. Research indicates that the consumption of cannabis may heighten the likelihood of grave cardiovascular conditions, such as myocardial infarction, vasospasm, and artery thrombosis. THC and other cannabinoid agonists both raise heart rate in a dose-dependent way (1). Therefore, it is likely that the increase in catecholamines brought on by cannabinoid agonists, along with an increased cardiac workload and a decreased oxygen supply, mediate these effects. Since the psychoactive ingredients in SC drugs have a much higher affinity for CB1 receptors, it is not surprising that a number of reports link SC use to major cardiovascular issues like tachycardia and myocardial infarction in both adults and adolescents (Fattore et al., 2011; Hall et al., 2009).

Cannabinoids and Psychosis

Although the link between cannabis and psychosis has been documented and is widely acknowledged, a casual relationship between the two variables has not been proven. Nonetheless, accumulating data indicates that cannabis use may have the ability to cause psychosis. Unlike natural cannabis, SC products don't contain any CBD and instead contain substances that function as extremely strong full agonists for CB1 and CB2. Owing to the psychoactive properties of the ingredients in SC drugs, it is not surprising that many reports exist of healthy and susceptible people experiencing recurrent psychosis following acute or repeated SC drug use. According to recent reports from Europe, 15% of SC users who visit emergency rooms exhibit symptoms of psychosis (Grigoryev et al., 2011a; Grigoryev et al., 2011b).

Effects of Cannabinoids on the Central Nervous System (CNS)

Numerous recent studies show a variety of anatomical and functional neuronal abnormalities linked to regular cannabis use. Users of cannabis typically exhibit structural, gray matter, and volumetric changes in the brain, especially in the limbic and prefrontal regions. Furthermore, pharmacological research links cannabis use to changes in dopamine synthesis. Increased THC dosage and an earlier age of onset are linked to these changes in the neurons (Frost et al., 2010).

There are fewer brain imaging studies investigating the neural correlates of SC use than there are for cannabis. Nurmedov along with others. found that when 20 males who used SC products were compared to 20 healthy control participants, the thalamus and cerebellum of the SC users had smaller gray-matter volumes (de Jager et al., 2012). Lately, Zorlu and associates discovered that people who use SC had smaller white matter volumes in a number of brain regions, including the subcortical structures and the left temporal lobe. A young SC user described experiencing severe symptoms after choosing to voluntarily stop using SC drugs in a different case study. When compared to healthy control participants, the patient's striatum and extra-striatal regions had less availability of dopamine D2 and D3 receptors during abstinence; however, these receptors were restored following treatment. Although these are preliminary studies, they do show some neurotoxic potential for SC products. There needs to be more research done (Griffin et al., 1998; Hirvonen et al., 2012).

Health Hazards and Withdrawal

Unlike cannabis, the use of SC has been linked to fatalities as well as extremely dangerous health effects on a number of systems. In the UK, there have been 510 reports of SC use during the previous eight years that called for immediate medical attention. In the United States, in 2014, there were 37,500 documented cases of seizures and 3,682 cases of poisonings associated with the use of SC. Furthermore, although there isn't any record of a cannabis-related overdose death (1), there are several accounts of fatalities that happen after using SC drugs. Tait and associates. determined that at least 26 cases of people who used SC products and had fatal side-effect complications have been documented (Chin et al., 1999). Acute kidney injury, respiratory depression, pulmonary complications, and cardiovascular events were the main side effects. Serious withdrawal symptoms, such as agitation, irritability, anxiety, and mood swings, are linked to long-term SC use. While some of these symptoms are comparable to those of cannabis, the variations in how they manifest could be due to the high affinity of these SCs as well as the presence of extraneous psychoactive substances like stimulants that resemble amphetamines.

6.4 Health Risks by Synthetic Cannabinoid

The consumption of cannabis has experienced a significant shift, moving beyond the conventional use of natural cannabinoids to include synthetic variations like Delta-8 and Delta-10. Even though these artificial substances provide users with an interesting alternate experience, more research is necessary to fully understand the possible health risks and issues related to their use (Cohen et al., 2017; Cohen and Weinstein, 2018).

6.4.1 The Rise of Synthetic Cannabinoids

Two well-known SCBs that have attracted a lot of interest in the cannabis community are Delta-8 and Delta-10. Due to their similar psychoactive effects to those of Delta-9 THC, the main psychoactive ingredient in natural cannabis, these compounds have become more and more well-known. The important difference, though, is that they are artificial; rather than coming straight from the cannabis plant, they are chemically created (Chimalakonda et al., 2011).

6.4.2 Health Risks and Concerns

There are a lot of issues with consuming SCBs. First off, there is a dearth of thorough studies on the long-term impacts of these substances on human health. In contrast to naturally occurring cannabinoids, which have been thoroughly studied by science, SCBs have not been subjected to the same level of scrutiny in order to determine their effects (Fan et al., 1994; Pertwee, 2005).

Furthermore, there is an element of unpredictability associated with the manufacturing process of SCBs. Variations in potency levels caused by production inconsistencies can present problems for users who might unintentionally take larger concentrations than they meant to. In addition, users may be exposed to substances with unanticipated health effects if unknown additives are present in synthetic cannabinoid products, which begs the question of possible interactions or side effects.

Moreover, SCBs may have higher potencies than their natural counterparts, which increases the possibility of negative side effects, especially in people with reduced tolerance or inexperience with potency levels. The consumption of SCBs may carry risks, as evidenced by reports of increased anxiety, paranoia, and other negative psychological effects among users. The possible effects on respiratory and cardiovascular health have also drawn criticism (Dowling and Regan, 2011; Whiting et al., 2015).

6.4.3 Regulatory Challenges

The dynamic characteristics of SCBs pose significant obstacles for regulatory bodies. Requirements for regulatory frameworks are growing more and more quickly as chemists work to create new compounds that mimic the effects of naturally occurring cannabinoids by constantly modifying their chemical structures. The challenge of guaranteeing consumer safety is made more difficult by the absence of regulations and standardized testing (Villares, 2007).

The production, distribution, and use of goods containing synthetic cannabinoid receptor agonists—more colloquially, "synthetic cannabinoids"—have increased significantly in recent years. With 169 SCBs detected between 2008 and 2016, these constitute "the largest group of substances currently monitored by the EU Early Warning System.". Products containing SCBs have become popular as replacements for cannabis with the goal of simulating its effects. SCBs, which are usually sprayed onto a smokable herbal mixture, work similarly to THC, the active component of cannabis, by binding to the same cannabinoid receptors in the brain (Atwood et al., 2010; Atwood et al., 2011).

Many products sold under more consumer-friendly names like "Spice" and "K-2" contain SCBs like JWH-018, JWH-073, and CP47,497-C6 as their active ingredients. The early 2010s saw a rise in the variety and popularity of these products, primarily because they provided a legal substitute for cannabis that was widely accessible (but largely unregulated) through high-street and internet retailers (Onaivi et al., 2008).

Despite the fact that many SCBs are currently illegal under UN drug conventions, drug control organizations have not been able to keep up with the volume and speed at which new variants are emerging. National drug control laws also forbid the use of many SCBs. In an effort to prevent new variations from undermining successive bans, a "catch-all" blanket prohibition on all psychoactive substances has been imposed in certain places, including the UK, Poland, and Ireland (Celofiga et al., 2014).

6.4.4 Risk Profile

While the pharmacology and toxicology of cannabis and THC are well-established, the pharmacology and toxicology of SCBs and the products containing them are far less well-documented. While many formal human studies have been conducted, there is compelling evidence that SCBs pose a greater risk than cannabis or THC. SCBs "may be more potent at the cannabinoid receptors and in turn have greater toxicities," according to a 2019 review. This means there is a far higher risk of overdose and acute adverse events than with cannabis, especially considering the wide range of synthetic cannabinoid products regarding the kind and amount of substances present (Borgelt et al., 2013). Generalizations become more difficult because different SCBs have varied risk profiles.

6.4.5 Prevalence of Use

There is limited information available on the use of SCBs, with most countries, especially in Europe, reporting low prevalence rates. However, in the US, particularly among young people, the use of SCBs appears to be relatively high but is declining. For example, the 2020 US Monitoring the Future survey showed a decrease in prevalence among 17- to 18-year-olds from 5.8% in 2014 to 2.4% in 2020. In contrast, the UK Crime Survey for England and Wales found that only 0.5% of adults reported using NPSs, including SCBs, in the past year. Despite their availability, many individuals prefer natural cannabis over SCBs due to the former producing more pleasant effects. However, SCBs have found a market among vulnerable populations engaged in high-risk or dependent drug use, offering a potent and relatively inexpensive alternative to other drugs (Dresen et al., 2010).

6.4.6 Regulatory Response

Many SCBs are currently prohibited by national drug laws, and their legal status would not change if cannabis were to be regulated legally. In fact, we suggest that no new, functionally equivalent synthetic substance be made lawfully available for retail sale within the confines of a legal regulatory framework to control cannabis. Though it seems unlikely, regulators might reconsider this stance and possibly allow certain synthetic cannabinoid products to be sold in retail settings if they can later show a level of risk comparable to or lower than that of conventional cannabis products.

Equivalent penalties for unauthorised production or supply would still be in place, even though all penalties for possessing and using such products would be eliminated. Since cannabis would be sold through a market that is legally regulated, it makes sense to forbid the manufacture or retail sale of any products containing SCBs. The management of SCBs would be based on a harm reduction model, which is intended for preparations of stimulants with higher potential risks (Pavanello et al., 2012).

In New Zealand, a regulatory framework has been established that permits producers of NPS, such as SCBs, to lawfully sell them under restricted circumstances, provided they can prove that the substances fulfill specific low risk requirements. This kind of regulation, which evolved from previous attempts to control the synthetic stimulant BZP, aims to safeguard drug users by directing them toward safer products whose risks have been adequately established. Though this regulatory framework is still in effect in theory, it has encountered political resistance and several technical difficulties, most notably the question of how to determine thresholds for "low-risk" harm without resorting to animal testing, which is expressly forbidden (Chimalakonda et al., 2011; Chimalakonda et al., 2012).

As a result, although New Zealand is the only nation in the world having comprehensive legislation governing NPS for non-medical use (though some SCBs are thought to be the most likely initial candidates for review), in actuality, no NPS are currently covered by the system.

Although New Zealand has made efforts to address the demand for SCBs through a practical approach and established markets, the need for regulated supply will decrease once cannabis is legalized. The demand for synthetic cannabis is currently low and would likely decrease even more as consumers would prefer to purchase legal cannabis over synthetic products (Franklin et al., 2013).

The small population of people with heavy or dependent patterns of use who are not interested in switching back to cannabis, as well as use in prisons and for probationers subject to testing (since SCBs are not consistently identified by conventional testing regimes), are likely to present the biggest obstacles going forward. While synthetic cannabinoid use gradually declines over time, a targeted harm reduction model will help lessen these harms while addressing problematic or high-risk use, including among the homeless (Bornheim et al., 1992; Castaneto et al., 2014).

Above all, it is critical to recognize that SCBs and other NPS initially emerged as a result of the prohibitionist legal environment that exists today. SCBs were initially more appealing for their legal status than for their actual effects, as this gave them a competitive edge over cannabis. For instance, it is noteworthy that, in the Netherlands, where cannabis is de facto legal, no sizable market for SCBs has developed (Brents et al., 2011).

The inevitable outlawing of SCBs did nothing but spur the development of more, frequently riskier, products with slight molecular differences. Though this was not the intended outcome of the bans, more extensive "crackdowns" or universal NPS prohibitions may have positively shifted some present or potential users back toward less hazardous traditional cannabis. However, even though the market for SCBs is currently contracting (either as a result of prohibitions or because cannabis is now available under legal, regulated conditions), the prohibition of cannabis has allowed over 100 dangerous synthetic cannabis imitators to enter the market, and the entrenchment of their problematic use among important vulnerable populations suggests that there is no simple solution (Brents et al., 2012; Brents et al., 2013).

A Closer Look

Delta-9-Tetrahydrocannabinol

One type of cannabinoid present in cannabis is delta-9-tetrahydrocannabinol (THC) (*Cannabis sativa*). THC is primarily responsible for cannabis's intoxicating effects.

Although *C. sativa* contains over 80 different cannabinoids, the most researched are THC and cannabidiol (CBD). THC acts by attaching itself to particular locations on the brain and nerves. The plant's leaves and flowers contain the greatest concentration of it.

THC is frequently used recreationally. In addition, many other conditions such as alcohol use disorder, multiple sclerosis, nerve pain, nausea and vomiting from chemotherapy, and many others are treated with THC, although these uses lack strong scientific backing. Furthermore, there is insufficient proof to back up the use of THC for COVID-19.

THC should not be confused with other cannabinoids that are present in cannabis, such as delta-8-THC, tetrahydrocannabivarin (THCV), cannabichromene (CBC), CBD, cannabidivarin (CBDV), cannabigerol (CBG), cannabinol (CBN), or cannabichromene (CBC). Additionally, it should not be confused with artificial cannabinoids like K2/Spice or plants that contain THC like hemp or cannabis. They're not the same thing. In the US, THC is prohibited at the federal level. Cannabis is categorized as a Schedule I controlled substance because of its THC content. However, some states have made recreational use legal or decriminalized.

Summary

- Synthetic cannabinoids are a group of chemical drugs that are sprayed onto plant material and then smoked.
- Synthetic cannabis (spice, K2) is a widely available, cheap, and increasingly popular type of designer drug.
- The primary cannabinoid in cannabis is delta-9-tetrahydrocannabinol (Δ9-THC), a partial CB1 receptor agonist.
- Chronic abuse of synthetic cannabis may result in a severe withdrawal and dependence syndrome. The use of synthetic cannabinoids has even been causally linked to at least one death by overdose and has been implicated for likely involvement in several other fatalities, resulting in over 2,500 calls to poison control
- Synthetic cannabinoids are synthesized to replicate the desired euphoric effects of cannabis but may result in compounds with greater abuse potential and severe toxicities.
- The cannabinoid receptors 1 and 2 (CB1 and CB2) were researched as the target of tetrahydrocannabinol (often referred to as trans-9-tetrahydrocannabinol [THC]) in the human brain.
- The intoxication effects of cannabis are characterized by cannabis users as; mild euphoria, relaxation, and a general pleasant feeling.
- Delta-8 and Delta-10 represent two prominent synthetic cannabinoids that have garnered significant attention within the cannabis community.
- Many synthetic cannabinoids are currently banned under domestic drug laws, and under a system of legal cannabis regulation their legal status would not automatically change.

References

1. Amato L, Minozzi S, Mitrova Z, Parmelli E, Saulle R, Cruciani F, et al.. Systematic review of safeness and therapeutic efficacy of cannabis in patients with multiple sclerosis, neuropathic pain, and in oncological patients treated with chemotherapy. *Epidemiol Preven.* (2017) 41:279–93. 10.19191/EP17.5-6.AD01. 069
2. Ashton CH. Pharmacology and effects of cannabis: a brief review. *Br J Psychiatry* (2001) 178:101–6. 10.1192/bjp.178.2.101
3. Atwood BK, Huffman J, Straiker A, Mackie K. JWH018, a common constituent of 'Spice' herbal blends, is a potent and efficacious cannabinoid CB receptor agonist. *Br J Pharmacol.* 2010;160:585–593.
4. Atwood BK, Lee D, Straiker A, Widlanski TS, Mackie K. CP47, 497-C8 and JWH073, commonly found in 'Spice' herbal blends, are potent and efficacious CB(1) cannabinoid receptor agonists. *Eur J Pharmacol.* 2011;659:139–145.
5. Aung MM, Griffin G, Huffman JW, Wu M, Keel C, Yang B, Showalter VM, Abood ME, Martin BR. Influence of the N-1 alkyl chain length of cannabimimetic indoles upon CB (1) and CB(2) receptor binding. *Drug Alcohol Depend.* 2000;60:133–140.

6. Beuck S, Moller I, Thomas A, Klose A, Schlorer N, Schanzer W, Thevis M. Structure characterisation of urinary metabolites of the cannabimimetic JWH-018 using chemically synthesised reference material for the support of LC-MS/MS-based drug testing. *Anal Bioanal Chem.* 2011;401:493–505.
7. Borgelt LM, Franson KL, Nussbaum AM, Wang GS. The pharmacologic and clinical effects of medical cannabis. *Pharmacotherapy* (2013) 33:195–209. 10.1002/phar.1187
8. Bornheim LM, Lasker JM, Raucy JL. Human hepatic microsomal metabolism of delta 1-tetrahydrocannabinol. *Drug Metab Dispos.* 1992;20:241–246.
9. Brents LK, Gallus-Zawada A, Radominska-Pandya A, Vasiljevik T, Prisinzano TE, Fantegrossi WE, Moran JH, Prather PL. Monohydroxylated metabolites of the K2 synthetic cannabinoid JWH-073 retain intermediate to high cannabinoid 1 receptor (CB1R) affinity and exhibit neutral antagonist to partial agonist activity. *Biochem Pharmacol.* 2012;83:952–961.
10. Brents LK, Reichard EE, Zimmerman SM, Moran JH, Fantegrossi WE, Prather PL. Phase I hydroxylated metabolites of the K2 synthetic cannabinoid JWH-018 retain in vitro and in vivo cannabinoid 1 receptor affinity and activity. *PLoS One.* 2011;6:e21917.
11. Brents LK, Zimmerman SM, Saffell AR, Prather PL, Fantegrossi WE. Differential drug-drug interactions of the synthetic cannabinoids JWH-018 and JWH-073: implications for drug abuse liability and pain therapy. *J Pharmacol Exp Ther.* 2013;346:350–361.
12. Castaneto MS, Gorelick DA, Desrosiers NA, Hartman RL, Pirard S, Huestis MA. Synthetic cannabinoids: epidemiology, pharmacodynamics, and clinical implications. *Drug Alcohol Depend.* (2014) 144:12–41. 10.1016/j.drugalcdep.2014.08.005
13. Celofiga A, Koprivsek J, Klavz J. Use of synthetic cannabinoids in patients with psychotic disorders: case series. *J Dual Diagn.* 2014;10(3):168–173.
14. Chimalakonda KC, Bratton SM, Le VH, Yiew KH, Dineva A, Moran CL, James LP, Moran JH, Radominska-Pandya A. Conjugation of synthetic cannabinoids JWH-018 and JWH-073, metabolites by human UDP-glucuronosyltransferases. *Drug Metab Dispos.* 2011;39:1967–1976.
15. Chimalakonda KC, Moran CL, Kennedy PD, Endres GW, Uzieblo A, Dobrowolski PJ, Fifer EK, Lapoint J, Nelson LS, Hoffman RS, James LP, Radominska-Pandya A, Moran JH. Solid-phase extraction and quantitative measurement of omega and omega-1 metabolites of JWH-018 and JWH-073 in human urine. *Anal Chem.* 2011;83:6381–6388.
16. Chimalakonda KC, Seely KA, Bratton SM, Brents LK, Moran CL, Endres GW, James LP, Hollenberg PF, Prather PL, Radominska-Pandya A, Moran JH. Cytochrome P450-mediated oxidative metabolism of abused synthetic cannabinoids found in K2/Spice: identification of novel cannabinoid receptor ligands. *Drug Metab Dispos.* 2012;40:2174–2184.
17. Chin CN, Murphy JW, Huffman JW, Kendall DA. The third transmembrane helix of the cannabinoid receptor plays a role in the selectivity of aminoalkylindoles for CB2, peripheral cannabinoid receptor. *J Pharmacol Exp Ther.* 1999;291:837–844.
18. Cohen K, Kapitány-Fövény M, Mama Y, Arieli M, Rosca P, Demetrovics Z, et al.. The effects of synthetic cannabinoids on executive function. *Psychopharmacology* (2017) 234:1121–34. 10.1007/s00213-017-4546-4
19. Cohen K, Weinstein A. The effects of cannabinoids on executive functions: evidence from cannabis and synthetic cannabinoids—a systematic review. *Brain Sci.* (2018) 8:40. 10.3390/brainsci8030040

20. de Jager AD, Warner JV, Henman M, Ferguson W, Hall A. LC-MS/MS method for the quantitation of metabolites of eight commonly-used synthetic cannabinoids in human urine – an Australian perspective. *J Chromatogr B Analyt Technol Biomed Life Sci.* 2012;897:22–31.

21. Dowling G, Regan L. A method for CP 47, 497 a synthetic non-traditional cannabinoid in human urine using liquid chromatography tandem mass spectrometry. *J Chromatogr B Analyt Technol Biomed Life Sci.* 2011;879:253–259.

22. Dresen S, Ferreiros N, Putz M, Westphal F, Zimmermann R, Auwarter V. Monitoring of herbal mixtures potentially containing synthetic cannabinoids as psychoactive compounds. *J Mass Spectrom.* 2010;45:1186–1194.

23. ElSohly MA, Gul W, Elsohly KM, Murphy TP, Madgula VL, Khan SI. Liquid chromatography-tandem mass spectrometry analysis of urine specimens for K2 (JWH-018) metabolites. *J Anal Toxicol.* 2011;35:487–495.

24. Fan F, Compton DR, Ward S, Melvin L, Martin BR. Development of cross-tolerance between delta-9-tetrahydrocannabinol, CP 55,940 and WIN 55,212. *J Pharmacol Exp Ther.* 1994;271:1383–1390.

25. Fantegrossi WE, Murnane KS, Reissig CJ. The behavioral pharmacology of hallucinogens. *Biochem Pharmacol.* 2008;75:17–33.

26. Fattore L, Fratta W. Beyond THC: the new generation of cannabinoid designer drugs. *Front Behav Neurosci.* 2011;5:60.

27. Franklin JM, Carrasco GA. G-protein receptor kinase 5 regulates the cannabinoid receptor 2-induced up-regulation of serotonin 2A receptors. *J Biol Chem.* 2013;288:15712–15724.

28. Franklin JM, Vasiljevik T, Prisinzano TE, Carrasco GA. Cannabinoid 2 receptor- and beta arrestin 2-dependent upregulation of serotonin 2A receptors. *Eur Neuropsychopharmacol.* 2013;23:760–767.

29. Frost JM, Dart MJ, Tietje KR, Garrison TR, Grayson GK, Daza AV, El-Kouhen OF, Yao BB, Hsieh GC, Pai M, Zhu CZ, Chandran P, Meyer MD. Indol-3-ylcycloalkyl ketones: effects of N1 substituted indole side chain variations on CB(2) cannabinoid receptor activity. *J Med Chem.* 2010;53:295–315.

30. Gamaleddin I, Zvonok A, Makriyannis A, Goldberg SR, Le Foll B. Effects of a selective cannabinoid CB2 agonist and antagonist on intravenous nicotine self administration and reinstatement of nicotine seeking. *PLoS One.* 2012;7:e29900.

31. Gaoni Y, Mechoulam R. Isolation, structure, and partial synthesis of an active constituent of hashish. *J Am Chem Soc.* (1964) 86:1646–7. 10.1021/ja01062a046

32. Ghisleni G, Kazlauckas V, Both FL, Pagnussat N, Mioranzza S, Rocha JB, Souza DO, Porciuncula LO. Diphenyl diselenide exerts anxiolytic-like effect in Wistar rats: putative roles of GABAA and 5HT receptors. *Prog Neuropsychopharmacol Biol Psychiatry.* 2008;32:1508–1515.

33. Griffin G, Atkinson PJ, Showalter VM, Martin BR, Abood ME. Evaluation of canna-binoid receptor agonists and antagonists using the guanosine-5□-O-(3-[35S]thio)-triphosphate binding assay in rat cerebellar membranes. *J Pharmacol Exp Ther.* 1998;285:553–560.

34. Grigoryev A, Melnik A, Savchuk S, Simonov A, Rozhanets V. Gas and liquid chromatography-mass spectrometry studies on the metabolism of the synthetic phenylacetylindole cannabimimetic

JWH-250, the psychoactive component of smoking mixtures. *J Chromatogr B Analyt Technol Biomed Life Sci.* 2011;879:2519–2526.

35. Grigoryev A, Savchuk S, Melnik A, Moskaleva N, Dzhurko J, Ershov M, Nosyrev A, Vedenin A, Izotov B, Zabirova I, Rozhanets V. Chromatography-mass spectrometry studies on the metabolism of synthetic cannabinoids JWH-018 and JWH-073, psychoactive components of smoking mixtures. *J Chromatogr B Analyt Technol Biomed Life Sci.* 2011;879:1126–1136.
36. Gunderson EW, Haughey HM, Ait-Daoud N, Joshi AS, Hart CL. "Spice" and "K2" herbal highs: a case series and systematic review of the clinical effects and biopsychosocial implications of synthetic cannabinoid use in humans. *Am J Addict.* 2012;21:320–326.
37. Gunderson EW, Haughey HM, Ait-Daoud N, Joshi AS, Hart CL. A survey of synthetic cannabinoid consumption by current cannabis users. *Subst Abuse* (2014) 35:184–9. 10.1080/08897077.2013.846288
38. Haj-Dahmane S, Shen RY. Modulation of the serotonin system by endocannabinoid signaling. *Neuropharmacology.* 2011;61:414–420.
39. Hall W, Degenhardt L. Adverse health effects of non-medical cannabis use. *Lancet* (2009) 374:1383–91. 10.1016/S0140-6736(09)61037-0
40. Hirvonen J, Goodwin RS, Li CT, Terry GE, Zoghbi SS, Morse C, Pike VW, Volkow ND, Huestis MA, Innis RB. Reversible and regionally selective downregulation of brain cannabinoid CB1 receptors in chronic daily cannabis smokers. *Mol Psychiatry.* 2012;17:642–649.
41. Hoffman AF, Lycas MD, Kaczmarzyk JR, Spivak CE, Baumann MH, Lupica CR. Disruption of hippocampal synaptic transmission and long-term potentiation by psychoactive synthetic cannabinoid 'Spice' compounds: comparison with Δ9-tetrahydrocannabinol. *Addict Biol.* 2016 in press.
42. Howlett AC, Champion TM, Wilken GH, Mechoulam R. Stereochemical effects of 11-OH-delta 8-tetrahydrocannabinol-dimethylheptyl to inhibit adenylate cyclase and bind to the cannabinoid receptor. *Neuropharmacology.* 1990;29:161–165.
43. Huestis MA. Pharmacokinetics and metabolism of the plant cannabinoids, delta9-tetrahydrocannabinol, cannabidiol and cannabinol. *Handb Exp Pharmacol.* 2005;(168):657–690.
44. Huffman JW, Padgett LW. Recent developments in the medicinal chemistry of can-nabimimetic indoles, pyrroles and indenes. *Curr Med Chem.* 2005;12:1395–1411.
45. Huffman JW, Szklennik PV, Almond A, Bushell K, Selley DE, He H, Cassidy MP, Wiley JL, Martin BR. 1-Pentyl-3-phenylacetylindoles, a new class of cannabimimetic indoles. *Bioorg Med Chem Lett.* 2005;15:4110–4113.
46. Huffman JW, Thompson AL, Wiley JL, Martin BR. Synthesis and pharmacology of 1-deoxy analogs of CP-47,497 and CP-55,940. *Bioorg Med Chem.* 2008;16:322–335.
47. Hutter M, Broecker S, Kneisel S, Auwarter V. Identification of the major urinary metabolites in man of seven synthetic cannabinoids of the aminoalkylindole type present as adulterants in 'herbal mixtures' using LC-MS/MS techniques. *J Mass Spectrom.* 2012;47:54–65.
48. Iseger TA, Bossong MG. A systematic review of the antipsychotic properties of cannabidiol in humans. *Schizophr Res.* (2015) 162:153–61. 10.1016/j.schres.2015.01.033

49. Jankovics P, Varadi A, Tolgyesi L, Lohner S, Nemeth-Palotas J, Balla J. Detection and identification of the new potential synthetic cannabinoids 1-pentyl-3-(2-iodobenzoyl)indole and 1-pentyl-3-(1-adamantoyl)indole in seized bulk powders in Hungary. *Forensic Sci Int.* 2012;214:27–32.

50. Kacinko SL, Xu A, Homan JW, McMullin MM, Warrington DM, Logan BK. Development and validation of a liquid chromatography-tandem mass spectrometry method for the identification and quantification of JWH-018, JWH-073, JWH-019, and JWH-250 in human whole blood. *J Anal Toxicol.* 2011;35:386–393.

51. Klein TW, Newton C, Larsen K, Lu L, Perkins I, Nong L, Friedman H. The cannabinoid system and immune modulation. *J Leukoc Biol.* 2003;74:486–496.

52. Kochanowski M, Kala M. Tetrahydrocannabinols in clinical and forensic toxicology. *Przegl Lek.* 2005;62:576–580.

53. Lapoint J, James LP, Moran CL, Nelson LS, Hoffman RS, Moran JH. Severe toxicity following synthetic cannabinoid ingestion. *Clin Toxicol.* 2011;49:760–764.

54. Lindigkeit R, Boehme A, Eiserloh I, Luebbecke M, Wiggermann M, Ernst L, Beuerle T. Spice: a never ending story? *Forensic Sci Int.* 2009;191:58–63.

55. Loeffler G, Delaney E, Hann M. International trends in spice use: prevalence, motivation for use, relationship to other substances, and perception of use and safety for synthetic cannabinoids. *Brain Res Bull.* (2016) 126:8–28. 10.1016/j.brainresbull.2016.04.013

56. Moller I, Wintermeyer A, Bender K, Jubner M, Thomas A, Krug O, Schanzer W, Thevis M. Screening for the synthetic cannabinoid JWH-018 and its major metabolites in human doping controls. *Drug Test Anal.* 2011;3:609–620.

57. Moran CL, Le VH, Chimalakonda KC, Smedley AL, Lackey FD, Owen SN, Kennedy PD, Endres GW, Ciske FL, Kramer JB, Kornilov AM, Bratton LD, Dobrowolski PJ, Wessinger WD, Fantegrossi WE, Prather PL, James LP, Radominska-Pandya A, Moran JH. Quantitative measurement of JWH-018 and JWH-073 metabolites excreted in human urine. *Anal Chem.* 2011;83:4228–4236.

58. Morgan D, Kondabolu K, Kuipers A, Sakhuja R, Robertson KL, Rowland NE, Booth RG. Molecular and behavioral pharmacology of two novel orally-active 5HT2 modulators: potential utility as antipsychotic medications. *Neuropharmacology.* 2013;72:274–281.

59. Onaivi ES, Ishiguro H, Gong JP, Patel S, Meozzi PA, Myers L, Perchuk A, Mora Z, Tagliaferro PA, Gardner E, Brusco A, Akinshola BE, Hope B, Lujilde J, Inada T, Iwasaki S, Macharia D, Teasenfitz L, Arinami T, Uhl GR. Brain neuronal CB2 cannabinoid receptors in drug abuse and depression: from mice to human subjects. *PLoS One.* 2008;3:e1640.

60. Paine MF, Hart HL, Ludington SS, Haining RL, Rettie AE, Zeldin DC. The human intestinal cytochrome P450 "pie" *Drug Metab Dispos.* 2006;34:880–886.

61. Patel KD, Davison JS, Pittman QJ, Sharkey KA. Cannabinoid CB(2) receptors in health and disease. *Curr Med Chem.* 2010;17:1393–1410.

62. Patton AL, Chimalakonda KC, Moran CL, McCain KR, Radominska-Pandya A, James LP, Kokes C, Moran JH. K2 toxicity: fatal case of psychiatric complications following AM2201 exposure. *J Forensic Sci.* 2013;58:1676–1680.

63. Pavanello S, Fedeli U, Mastrangelo G, Rota F, Overvad K, Raaschou-Nielsen O, Tjonneland A, Vogel U. Role of CYP1A2 polymorphisms on lung cancer risk in a prospective study. *Cancer Genet.* 2012;205:278–284.

64. Pertwee RG. Pharmacological actions of cannabinoids. In Pertwee R. G. editor. *Handbook of Experimental Pharmacology*, Vol. 168 New York, NY: Springer; (2005). p. 1–51.

65. Rajasekaran M, Brents LK, Franks LN, Moran JH, Prather PL. Human metabolites of synthetic cannabinoids JWH-018 and JWH-073 bind with high affinity and act as potent agonists at cannabinoid type-2 receptors. *Toxicol Appl Pharmacol.* 2013;269:100–108.

66. Seely KA, Brents LK, Radominska-Pandya A, Endres GW, Keyes GS, Moran JH, Prather PL. A major glucuronidated metabolite of JWH-018 is a neutral antagonist at CB1 receptors. *Chem Res Toxicol.* 2012;25:825–827.

67. Seely KA, Lapoint J, Moran JH, Fattore L. Spice drugs are more than harmless herbal blends: a review of the pharmacology and toxicology of synthetic cannabinoids. *Prog Neuropsychopharmacol Biol Psychiatry.* 2012;39:234–243.

68. Seely KA, Prather PL, James LP, Moran JH. Marijuana-based drugs: innovative therapeutics or designer drugs of abuse? *Mol Interv.* 2011;11:36–51.

69. Sim-Selley LJ, Schechter NS, Rorrer WK, Dalton GD, Hernandez J, Martin BR, Selley DE. Prolonged recovery rate of CB1 receptor adaptation after cessation of long-term cannabinoid administration. *Mol Pharmacol.* 2006;70:986–996.

70. Sobolevsky T, Prasolov I, Rodchenkov G. Detection of JWH-018 metabolites in smoking mixture post-administration urine. *Forensic Sci Int.* 2010;200:141–147.

71. Sobolevsky T, Prasolov I, Rodchenkov G. Detection of urinary metabolites of AM-2201 and UR-144, two novel synthetic cannabinoids. *Drug Test Anal.* 2012;4:745–753.

72. Spaderna M, Addy PH, D'Souza DC. Spicing things up: synthetic cannabinoids. *Psychopharmacology* (2013) 228:525–40. 10.1007/s00213-013-3188-4

73. Tai S, Fantegrossi W. Synthetic cannabinoids: pharmacology, behavioral effects, and abuse potential. *Curr Addict Rep.* 2014:1–8.

74. Tournebize J, Gibaja V, Kahn JP. Acute effects of synthetic cannabinoids: update 2015. *Subst Abuse* (2017) 38:344–66. 10.1080/08897077.2016.1219438

75. Uchiyama N, Kawamura M, Kikura-Hanajiri R, Goda Y. URB-754: a new class of designer drug and 12 synthetic cannabinoids detected in illegal products. *Forensic Sci Int.* 2013;227:21–32.

76. UNDOC *World Drug Report 2015*. Vienna: United Nation Office on Drugs and Crime 2016; (2016).

77. Villares J. Chronic use of marijuana decreases cannabinoid receptor binding and mRNA expression in the human brain. *Neuroscience.* 2007;145:323–334.

78. Volkow ND, Swanson JM, Evins AE, DeLisi LE, Meier MH, Gonzalez R, et al.. Effects of cannabis use on human behavior, including cognition, motivation, and psychosis: a review. *JAMA Psychiatry* (2016) 73:292–7. 10.1001/jamapsychiatry.2015.3278

79. Watanabe K, Matsunaga T, Yamamoto I, Funae Y, Yoshimura H. Involvement of CYP2C in the metabolism of cannabinoids by human hepatic microsomes from an old woman. *Biol Pharm Bull.* 1995;18:1138–1141.

80. Watanabe K, Yamaori S, Funahashi T, Kimura T, Yamamoto I. Cytochrome P450 enzymes involved in the metabolism of tetrahydrocannabinols and cannabinol by human hepatic microsomes. *Life Sci.* 2007;80:1415–1419.

81. Weinstein AM, Rosca P, Fattore L, London ED. Synthetic cathinone and cannabinoid designer drugs pose a major risk for public health. *Front Psychiatry* (2017) 8:156. 10.3389/fpsyt.2017.00156

82. Whiting PF, Wolff RF, Deshpande S, Di Nisio M, Duffy S, Hernandez AV, et al.. Cannabinoids for medical use: a systematic review and meta-analysis. *JAMA* (2015) 313:2456–73. 10.1001/jama.2015.6358

83. Wiley JL, Marusich JA, Huffman JW, Balster RL, Thomas BF. Hijacking of basic research: the case of synthetic cannabinoids. *Methods Rep RTI Press.* 2011;2011:17971.

84. Winstock A, Lynskey M, Borschmann R, Waldron J. Risk of emergency medical treatment following consumption of cannabis or synthetic cannabinoids in a large global sample. *J Psychopharmacol.* (2015) 29:698–703. 10.1177/0269881115574493

85. Winstock AR, Barratt MJ. Synthetic cannabis: a comparison of patterns of use and effect profile with natural cannabis in a large global sample. *Drug Alcohol Depend.* (2013) 131:106–11. 10.1016/j.drugalcdep.2012.12.011

86. Wintermeyer A, Moller I, Thevis M, Jubner M, Beike J, Rothschild MA, Bender K. In vitro phase I metabolism of the synthetic cannabimimetic JWH-018. *Anal Bioanal Chem.* 2010;398:2141–2153.

87. Xi ZX, Peng XQ, Li X, Song R, Zhang HY, Liu QR, Yang HJ, Bi GH, Li J, Gardner EL. Brain cannabinoid CB(2) receptors modulate cocaine's actions in mice. *Nat Neurosci.* 2011;14:1160–1166.

88. Yamamoto I, Watanabe K, Kuzuoka K, Narimatsu S, Yoshimura H. The pharmacological activity of cannabinol and its major metabolite, 11-hydroxycannabinol. *Chem Pharm Bull.* 1987;35:2144–2147.

89. Zhang Q, Ma P, Cole RB, Wang G. Identification of in vitro metabolites of JWH-015, an aminoalkylindole agonist for the peripheral cannabinoid receptor (CB2) by HPLC-MS/MS. *Anal Bioanal Chem.* 2006;386:1345–1355.

90. Zhang Q, Ma P, Iszard M, Cole RB, Wang W, Wang G. In vitro metabolism of R(+)-[2,3-dihydro-5-methyl-3-[(morpholinyl)methyl]pyrrolo [1,2,3-de]1,4-benzoxazinyl]-(1-naphtha-lenyl) methanone mesylate, a cannabinoid receptor agonist. *Drug Metab Dispos.* 2002;30:1077–1086.

91. Zhang Q, Ma P, Wang W, Cole RB, Wang G. Characterization of rat liver microso-mal metabolites of AM-630, a potent cannabinoid receptor antagonist, by high-performance liquid chromatography/electrospray ionization tandem mass spectrometry. *J Mass Spectrom.* 2004;39:672–681.

92. Zimmermann US, Winkelmann PR, Pilhatsch M, Nees JA, Spanagel R, Schulz K. Withdrawal phenomena and dependence syndrome after the consumption of "spice gold" *Dtsch Arztebl Int.* 2009;106:464–467.

Chapter 7

OPIOIDS: SYNTHETIC ANALGESICS AND ANALOGS

Contents

Introduction

The natural substances, or "opiates," that are extracted from the opium poppy plant (*Papaver somniferum*), as well as their synthetic and semi-synthetic derivatives, are referred to as "opioids." They all interact with the opioid receptors in the human body to produce a variety of physiological effects, and their biochemical profiles are comparatively similar. They have long been used medicinally for their sedative and analgesic properties and to treat severe and chronic pain. They have also been used recreationally and non-medically to induce feelings of well-being, relaxation, and euphoria. The emergence of a new synthetic opioid illegal market over the past ten years has led to a significant rise in drug-related deaths and unintentional overdoses, making it a major global public health concern. Fentanyl, its analogs, and newly developed non-fentanyl opioids are examples of synthetic opioids. Their popularity is due to several factors, including shifts in the criminal market, affordability, potency, availability in comparison to traditional opioids, ease of use and transportation, quick effects, and lack of detection by traditional testing methods.

Orientation and Directional Terms

Term	Definition	Illustration
Codeine	Codeine is an opioid pain reliever used to treat mild to moderately severe pain. It is also used, usually in combination with other medications, to reduce coughing.	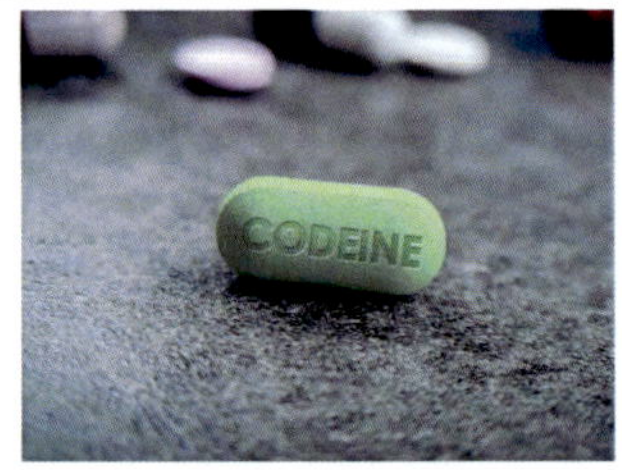
Enkephalin	An enkephalin is a pentapeptide involved in regulating nociception (pain sensation) in the body. The enkephalins are termed endogenous ligands, as they are internally derived and bind to the body's opioid receptors. Discovered in 1975, two forms of enkephalin have been found, one containing leucine ("leu"), and the other containing methionine ("met").	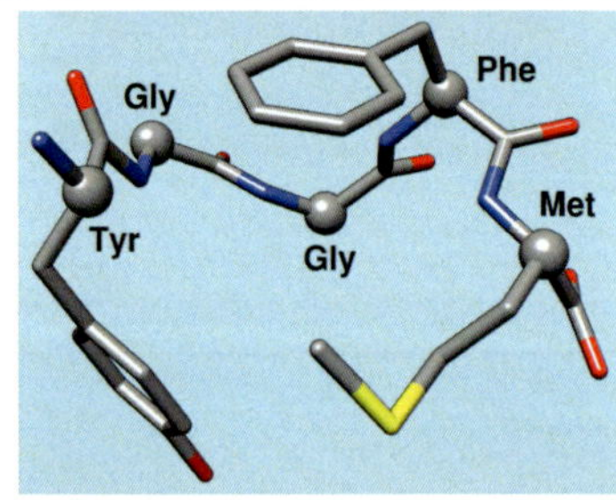
Fentanyl	Fentanyl is a potent synthetic opioid drug approved by the Food and Drug Administration for use as an analgesic (pain relief) and anesthetic. It is approximately 100 times more potent than morphine and 50 times more potent than heroin as an analgesic.	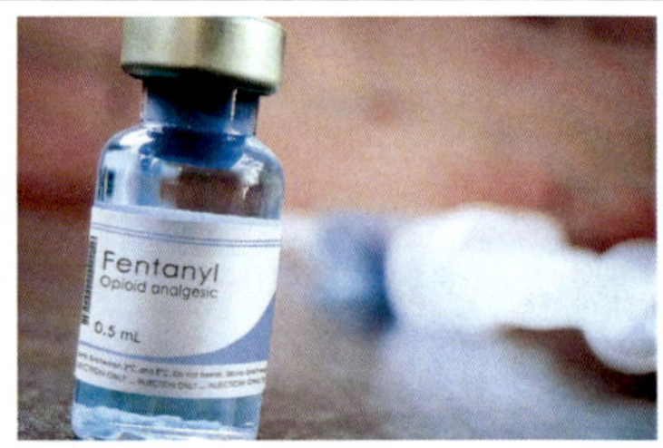
Hydrocodone	Hydrocodone is primarily used to treat severe chronic pain that requires opioid analgesia and is not effectively treated by nonopioid alternatives. Hydrocodone is used in combination formulations to treat nonproductive cough in adults and has antitussive properties.	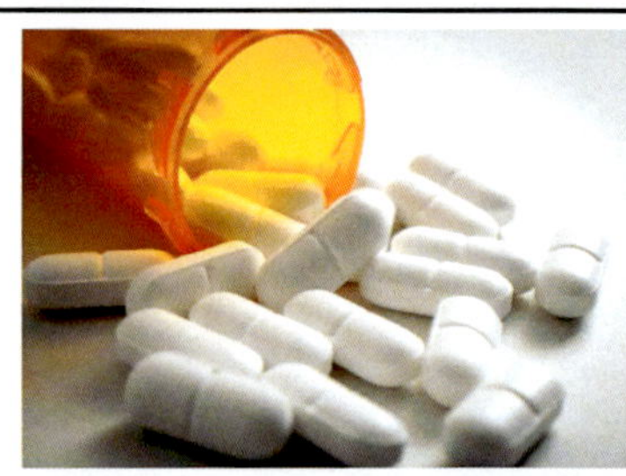
Intractable pain	Intractable pain, also known as intractable pain syndrome, is a severe, constant, and debilitating pain that is incurable and cannot be managed with normal pain management techniques. It is a subgroup of chronic pain, which is defined as pain that lasts more than three months.	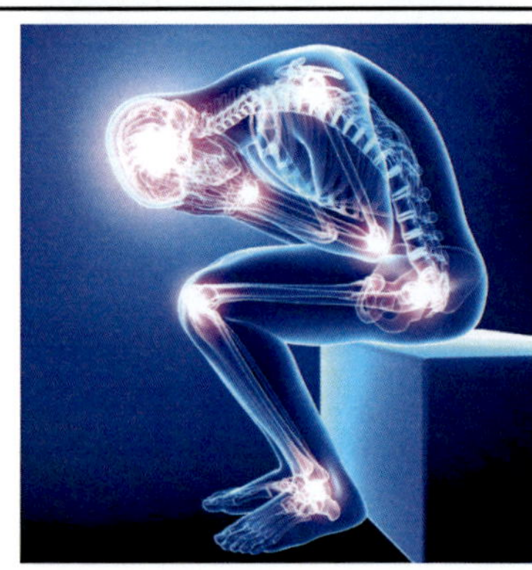

7.1 Opioid Pharmacology

In clinical practice, a class of analgesic drugs known as opioids is frequently employed. The novel NOP receptor is thought to represent a non-opioid branch of the opioid receptor family, whereas the three classical opioid receptors include DOP, KOP, and mu opioid peptide (MOP). Opioids can function as partial agonists, antagonists, or agonists at these receptors. G-protein coupled receptors are occupied by opioid agonists, which results in cellular hyperpolarization. In order to produce analgesia, the majority of clinically relevant opioid analgesics bind in an agonistic fashion to MOP receptors in the central and peripheral nervous systems. Alkaloids, semi-synthetic, and synthetic compounds are the other categories into which opioids can be divided based on how they are made.

Most people agree that morphine is the standard opioid analgesic and that it is the drug that all other painkillers are measured against. Evidence suggests that the opium poppy, *P. somniferum*, was cultivated for its active ingredients as early as 3000 BC. However, modern opioid pharmacology did not fully emerge until Sertürner separated morphine from opium in 1806. The more exact and extensive clinical use of morphine resulted from the derivation of its chemical formula in 1847 and the development of the hypodermic needle in 1853 (Manchikanti et al., 2018).

7.1.1 Opioids

For thousands of years, people have used opioids to treat pain. Opium was used as a pain reliever, according to papyrus records from ancient Egypt. When graduate student Candace Pert used radioactive morphine in 1973 to assess the drug's site of action, she discovered—surprisingly—that the drug bound to very particular brain regions known as "morphine receptors." This discovery led to a hunt for the chemical that would endogenously stimulate that receptor because mice would not have a "need" for a receptor for an alien alkaloid of the poppy plant. John Hughes and Hans Kosterlitz eventually discovered "endogenous morphines," or "endorphins," in 1975. Since most clinically significant opioids primarily act on the initial "morphine receptor" or "mu receptors," they are referred to as "mu agonists."

The pharmacokinetic parameters of opioids, such as half-life, clearance, and volume of distribution, have been well-established for some time (Manchikanti et al., 2018). Despite this, the metabolism of opioids has only recently started to be better understood. There is now a growing interest in how metabolites play a role in altering the pharmacodynamic response in patients, particularly in terms of both pain relief and potential negative effects. This new understanding is starting to shed light on certain perplexing clinical observations.

7.1.2 Opioid Structure

The benzene ring of morphine, the classic opioid, has hydroxyl groups from phenol at position 3 and alcohol at position 6, as well as at the nitrogen atom (Fig. 7.1). It is possible to transform both hydroxyl groups into ethers or esters. For instance, heroin is morphine that is O-acetylated at positions 3 and 6 (diacetyl morphine), whereas codeine is morphine that is O-methylated at position 3. Since the quaternary form of nitrogen cannot enter the CNS, it significantly reduces the analgesic effects of morphine, suggesting that the tertiary form of nitrogen is essential to its analgesic effects. Alterations to the nitrogen's methyl group also reduce analgesia, leading to the creation of antagonists like nalorphine. Only the levorotatory isomer of morphine has analgesic properties; the other is optically active.

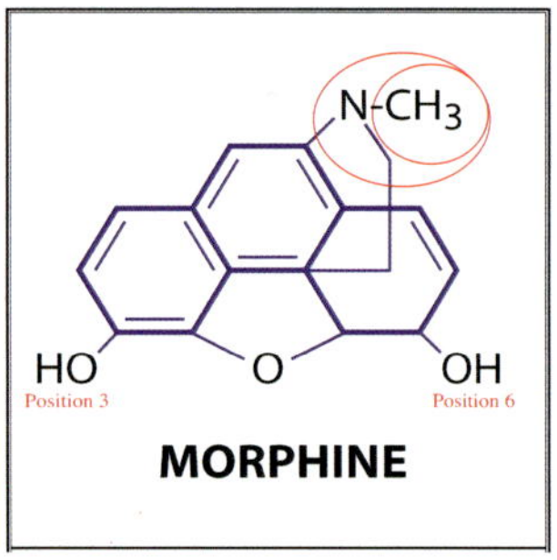

Figure 7.1: Structure of morphine.

Source: Andrea M. Trescot, Sukdeb Datta, Marion Lee, and Hans Hansen. Opioid Pharmacology. Pain Physician 2008: Opioid Special Issue: 11: S133-S153. ISSN 1533-3159. https://www.painphysicianjournal.com/current/pdf?article=OTg3&journal=42

7.1.3 Opioid History

In Mesopotamia, opium poppies were first grown as early as 3400 BC. A combination of alkaloids from the poppy seed is referred to as opium. Opiates are alkaloids that are found in nature, like codeine or morphine. All drugs that act at the opioid receptors are collectively referred to as opioids. The word "narcotic" (derived from the Greek word "stupidity") was first used to refer to sleep aids, then to opioids, and currently it refers to prescription drugs that have been abused (Pardo et al., 2020).

7.1.4 Classification

Even though the most well-known *P. somniferum* extract is morphine, it is possible to separate four naturally occurring alkaloids (amines derived from plants) from it: thebaine, morphine, codeine, and papaverine. After morphine was identified by Sertürner as the primary constituent of the opium poppy, a variety of semi-synthetic opioids that are beneficial in clinical medicine were produced by straightforward chemical manipulations of these fundamental opiate alkaloids (agents such as diamorphine, dihydrocodeine, buprenorphine, nalbuphine, naloxone, and oxycodone). Many synthetic opioids were also created in the 20th century, either on purpose or by accident. The morphinan derivatives (levorphanol, butorphanol), the diphenylheptane derivatives (methadone, propoxyphene), the benzomorphan derivatives (pentazocine, phenazocine), and the phenylpiperidine derivatives (pethidine, alfentanil, fentanyl, sufentanil, and remifentanil) are the four chemical groups into which these synthetic compounds can be categorized (Table 7.1).

Table 7.1: Classification of opioids by synthetic process.

Naturally occurring compounds	Semi-synthetic compounds	Synthetic compounds
Morphine	Diamorphine (heroin)	Pethidine
Codeine	Dihydromorphone	Fentanyl
Thebaine	Buprenorphine	Methadone
Papaverine	Oxycodone	Alfentanil
		Remifentanil
		Tapentadol

Source: Hasan Pathan and John Williams. Basic opioid pharmacology: an update. British Journal of Pain. Sage Journals. https://journals.sagepub.com/doi/10.1177/2049463712438493

Another way to categorize opioids is based on how they interact with opioid receptors. Opioids can thus be classified as antagonists, partial agonists, and agonists. Agonists work with a receptor to maximize its response; one example of this is analgesia after morphine is administered. On the other hand, antagonists block agonists from binding to the same receptor (naloxone) while also binding to the receptor itself without eliciting a functional response. No matter how much drug is given, partial agonists (like buprenorphine) bind to receptors but only produce a partial functional response (Suzuki et al., 2017).

7.1.5 Opioid Receptors

Opioid receptors are present in both peripheral tissues and the CNS. Endogenous peptides (endorphins, enkephalins, and dynorphins) generated in reaction to noxious stimulation typically stimulate these receptors. Based on their prototype agonists, the opioid receptors are named in Greek letters (Table 7.2).

- ***Mu (μ) (agonist morphine)***: Mu receptors are mainly located in the medial thalamus and brainstem. Supraspinal analgesia, euphoria, sedation, reduced gastrointestinal motility, and physical dependence are all brought on by mu receptors. Mu1 and Mu2 are subtypes; Mu1 is associated with analgesia, euphoria, and tranquility, whereas Mu2 is associated with pruritus, respiratory depression, prolactin release, dependence, anorexia, and sedation. These are sometimes referred to as MOR (morphine opioid receptors) or OP3.
- ***Kappa (κ) (agonist ketocyclazocine)***: Spinal analgesia, sedation, dyspnea, dependence, dysphoria, and respiratory depression are caused by kappa receptors, which are located in the brain stem, spinal cord, limbic and other diencephalic areas, and spinal cord itself. These are sometimes referred to as KORs (kappa opioid receptors) or OP2.
- ***Delta (δ) (agonist delta-alanine-delta-leucine-enkephalin)***: The majority of delta receptors are found in the brain, and little is known about their effects. They could be in charge of dysphoric and psychomimetic effects. They go by the names DOR (delta opioid receptors) and OP1.
- ***Sigma (σ) (agonist N-allylnormetazocine)***: Depression brought on by stress, dysphoria, and psychomimetic effects are all caused by sigma receptors. They are now the target sites for phencyclidine (PCP) and its analogs rather than opioid receptors.

The three main opioid receptors are controlled by distinct genes. An intracellular C-terminus, three extracellular and intracellular loops, seven transmembrane helical twists, and an extracellular N-terminus make up each receptor (Fig. 7.2). A portion of the G protein is released by the activated receptor and diffuses through the membrane until it reaches the target, which could be an ion channel or an enzyme. These targets change protein phosphorylation by inhibiting cyclic AMP (cAMP), which functions as a second messenger in the cell and activates gene transcription proteins and/or protein kinases (long-term effects) and/or short-term effects (short-term effects) (Fig. 7.3). When an opioid agonist activates the opioid receptors on the presynaptic terminals of the nociceptive C-fibers and A-delta fibers, it indirectly inhibits these voltage-dependent calcium channels, lowering cAMP levels and preventing the release of pain neurotransmitters from the nociceptive fibers, including glutamate, substance P, and calcitonin gene-related peptide, which causes analgesia (Fig. 7.4) (Prekupec et al., 2017).

Table 7.2: Analgesic effects at opioid receptors.

	Mu (μ)	Delta (δ)	Kappa (κ)
	• Mu 1 – Analgesia • Mu 2 – Sedation, vomiting, respiratory depression, pruritus, euphoria, anorexia, urinary retention, physical dependence	• Analgesia, spinal analgesia	• Analgesia, sedation, dyspnea, psychomimetic effects, miosis, respiratory depression, euphoria, dysphoria, dyspnea
Endogenous Peptides			
Enkephalins	Agonist	Agonist	
β-Endorphin	Agonist	Agonist	
Dynorphin A	Agonist		Agonist
Agonists			
Morphine	Agonist		Weak agonist
Codeine	Weak agonist	Weak agonist	
Fentanyl	Agonist		
Meperidine	Agonist	Agonist	
Methadone	Agonist		
Antagonists			
Naloxone	Antagonist	Weak Antagonist	Antagonist
Naltrexone	Antagonist	Weak Antagonist	Antagonist

Source: Andrea M. Trescot, Sukdeb Datta, Marion Lee, and Hans Hansen. Opioid Pharmacology. Pain Physician 2008: Opioid Special Issue: 11: S133-S153. ISSN 1533-3159. https://www.painphysicianjournal.com/current/pdf?article=OTg3&journal=42

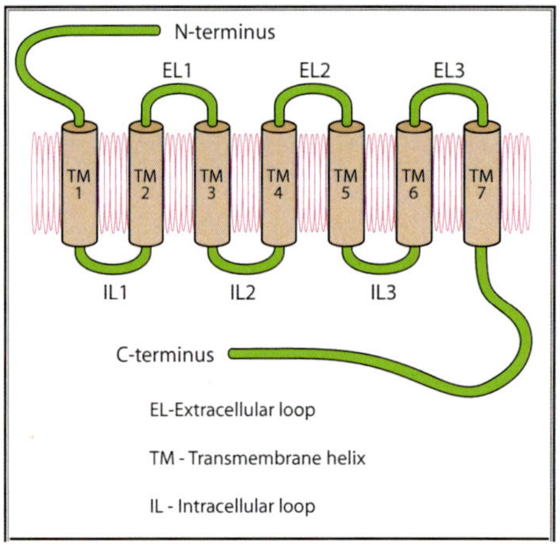

Figure 7.2: Opioid receptor structure.

Source: Andrea M. Trescot, Sukdeb Datta, Marion Lee, and Hans Hansen. Opioid Pharmacology. Pain Physician 2008: Opioid Special Issue: 11: S133-S153. ISSN 1533-3159. https://www.painphysicianjournal.com/current/pdf?article=OTg3&journal=42

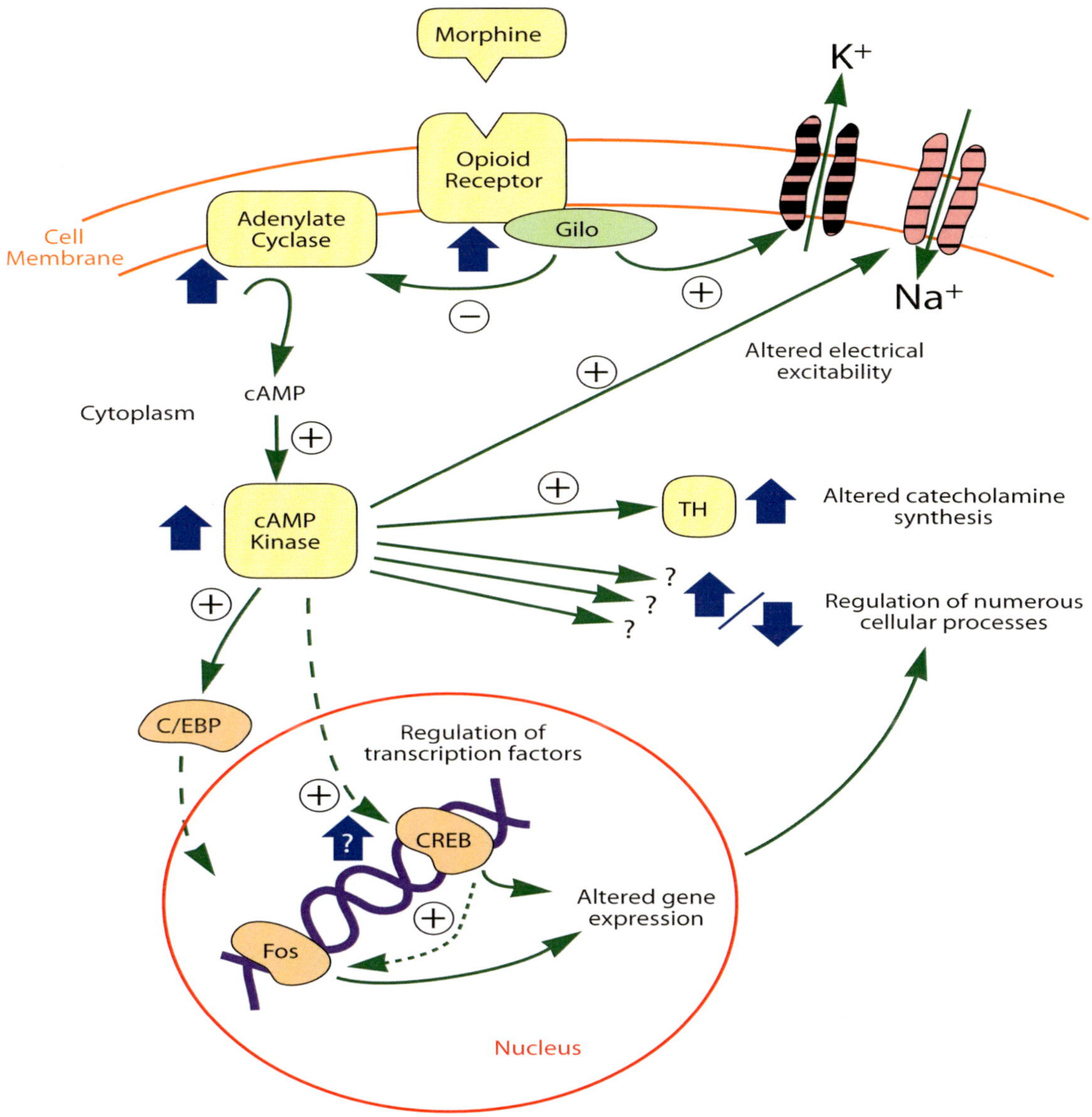

Figure 7.3: Opioid action.

Source: Andrea M. Trescot, Sukdeb Datta, Marion Lee, and Hans Hansen. Opioid Pharmacology. Pain Physician 2008: Opioid Special Issue: 11: S133-S153. ISSN 1533-3159. https://www.painphysicianjournal.com/current/pdf?article=OTg3&journal=42

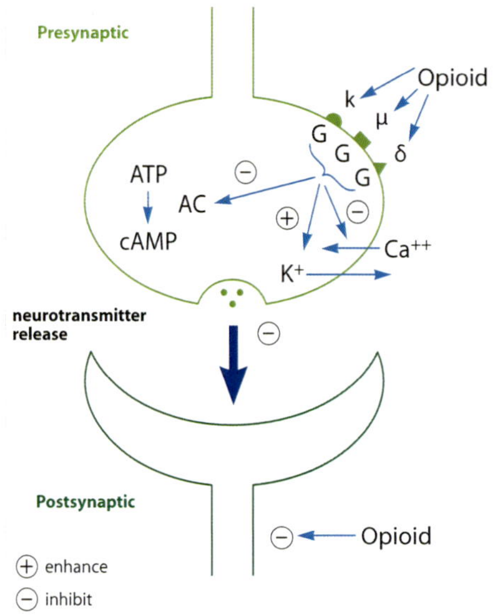

Figure 7.4: Opioid receptor locations.

Source: Andrea M. Trescot, Sukdeb Datta, Marion Lee, and Hans Hansen. Opioid Pharmacology. Pain Physician 2008: Opioid Special Issue: 11: S133-S153. ISSN 1533-3159. https://www.painphysicianjournal.com/current/pdf?article=OTg3&journal=42

Presynaptic receptors on gamma amino butyric acid (GABA) neurons are activated by opioids and endogenous opioids, which prevents GABA from being released in the ventral tegmental area (Fig. 7.5). Dopaminergic neurons can fire more quickly when GABA is inhibited, and the extra dopamine in the nucleus accumbens produces a highly pleasurable feeling. So, different opioids may have different degrees of affinity for different receptors, which could explain why opioids have different effects.

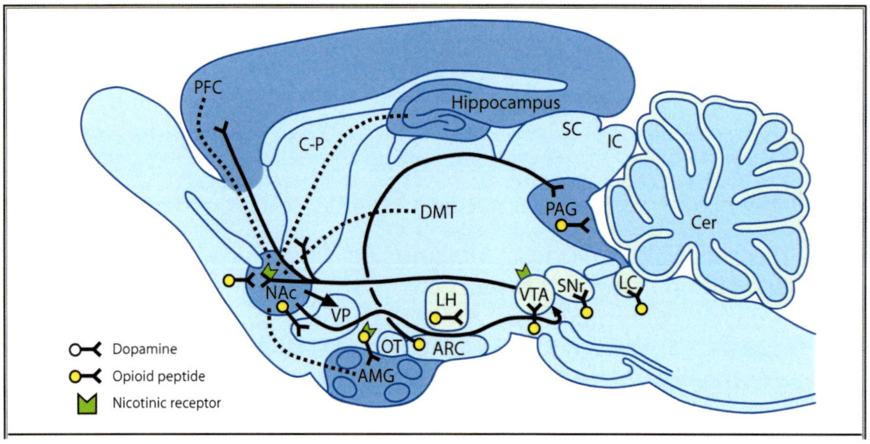

Figure 7.5: Locations of opioid and abused medications site of action.

Source: Andrea M. Trescot, Sukdeb Datta, Marion Lee, and Hans Hansen. Opioid Pharmacology. Pain Physician 2008: Opioid Special Issue: 11: S133-S153. ISSN 1533-3159. https://www.painphysicianjournal.com/current/pdf?article=OTg3&journal=42

Opioids have the potential to activate the descending serotonin and noradrenaline pain pathways from the brain stem by antagonistically binding to N-methyl-D-aspartate (NMDA) receptors to varying degrees. Neuropathic pain and the emergence of tolerance may be brought upon by stimulation of these same NMDA receptors.

The first endogenous opioid, enkephalin, was identified in 1975. The location of endogenous opioids, also known as endorphins, in the CNS opioid receptors, was discovered in 1973. They can act as neurotransmitters because of their location in the CNS, and might also be involved in the release of hormones, thermoregulation, and cardiovascular control (Prekupec et al., 2017).

- Enkephalins are derived from pro-enkephalin and are relatively selective δ ligands.
- Endorphins are derived from pro-opiomelanocortin (also the precursor for ACTH and MSH) and bind to the μ receptor.
- Dynorphins are derived from pro-dynorphins and are highly selective at the μ receptor.
- Nociceptins (nociceptin/orphaninFQ [N/OFQ]) (orphanin), identified in 1995, may have potent hyperalgesic effects. They have little affinity for the μ, δ, or κ receptors, and their receptors are now being called ORL1 ("opioid-receptor-like"). Nociceptin antagonists may be antidepressants and analgesics.

Pure opioid agonists (e.g., morphine, hydromorphone, and fentanyl) stimulate μ receptors and are the most potent analgesics. As the dose is increased, analgesia theoretically occurs in a log-linear fashion; the degree of analgesia induced is limited only by intolerable dose-related adverse effects. On the other hand, there is a ceiling effect on the level of analgesia that opioid agonists/antagonists and opioid partial agonists (buprenorphine, pentazocine, nalbuphine, butorphanol, nalorphine) can produce. Opiate withdrawal reactions can be triggered by partial agonists and agonist/antagonist combinations. Naloxone does not totally undo the partial agonists' respiratory depressant effects (Ghelardini et al., 2015).

7.1.6 Opioid Categories

The Drug Enforcement Agency (DEA) classifies opioids into schedules, as illustrated in Table 7.3 and Table 7.4.

Table 7.3: DEA schedules of controlled drugs.

Schedule	Criteria	Examples
I	No medical use; high addiction potential	Heroin, marijuana, PCP
II	Medical use; high addiction potential	Morphine, oxycodone, methadone, fentanyl, amphetamines
III	Medical use; moderate addiction potential	Hydrocodone, codeine, anabolic steroids
IV	Medical use; low abuse potential	Benzodiazepines, meprobamate, butorphanol, pentazocine, propoxyphene
V	Medical use; low abuse potential	Buprenex, Phenergan with codeine

Source: Andrea M. Trescot, Sukdeb Datta, Marion Lee, and Hans Hansen. Opioid Pharmacology. Pain Physician 2008: Opioid Special Issue: 11: S133-S153. ISSN 1533-3159. https://www.painphysicianjournal.com/current/pdf?article=OTg3&journal=42

Table 7.4: Drug Enforcement Agency schedules of common medications (may vary by State).

	Schedule I	Schedule II	Schedule III	Schedule IV	Schedule V
Opioid Agonists	Benzylmorphine Dihydromorphinone Heroin Ketobemidone Levomoramide Morphine-methylsulfonate Nicocodeine Nicomorphine Racemoramide	Codeine various Fentanyl Sublimaze® Hydrocodone Hydromorphone Dilaudid® Meperidine Demerol® Methadone Morphine Oxycodone Endocet® OxyContin® Percocet® Oxymorphone Numorphan®	Buprenorphine Buprenex® Subutex® Codeine compounds Tylenol #3® Hydrocodone compounds Lorcet® Lortab® Tussionex® Vicodin®	Propoxyphene Darvon® Darvocet®	Opium preparations Donnagel PG® Kapectolin®
Mixed Agonist-Antagonists			Buprenorphine + naloxone Suboxone®	Pentazocine naloxone Talwin-Nx®	
Stimulants	N-methyl-amphetamine 3,4-methylenedioxy amphetamine MDMA, Ecstasy	Amphetamine Adderall® Cocaine Dextro amphetamine Dexedrine® Methamphetamine Desoxyn® Methylphenidate Concerta® Metadate® Ritalin® Phenmetrazine Fastin® Preludin®	Benzphetamine Didrex® Pemoline Cylert® Phendimetrazine Plegine®	Diethylpropion Tenuate® Fenfluramine Phentermine Fastin®	1-deoxy-ephedrine Vicks Inhaler®
Hallucinogens, Other	Lysergic acid diamine LSD Marijuana Mescaline Peyote Phencyclidine PCP Psilocybin Tetrahydro-cannabinols		Dronabinol Marinol®		
Sedative-Hypnotics	Methaqualone Quaalude® Gamma-hydroxy butyrate GHB	Amobarbital Amytal® Glutethimide Doriden® Pentobarbital Nembutal® Secobarbital Seconal®	Butabarbital Butisol® Butalbital Fiorecet® Fiorinal® Methyprylon Noludar®	Alprazolam Xanax® Chlordiazepoxide Librium® Chloral betaine Chloral hydrate Noctec® Clonazepam Klonopin® Clorazepate Tranxene® Diazepam Valium® Estazolam Prosom® Ethchlorvynol Placidyl® Ethinamate Flurazepam Dalmane® Halazepam Paxipam® Lorazepam Ativan® Mazindol® Sanorex® Mephobarbital Mebaral® Meprobamate Equanil® Methohexital Brevital Sodium® Methyl-phenobarbital Midazolam Versed® Oxazepam Serax® Paraldehyde Paral® Phenobarbital Luminal® Prazepam Centrax® Temazepam Restoril® Triazolam Halcion® Zaleplon Sonata® Zolpidem Ambien®	Diphenoxylate preparations Lomotil®

Source: Andrea M. Trescot, Sukdeb Datta, Marion Lee, and Hans Hansen. Opioid Pharmacology. Pain Physician 2008: Opioid Special Issue: 11: S133-S153. ISSN 1533-3159. https://www.painphysicianjournal.com/current/pdf?article=OTg3&journal=42

There are 4 chemical classes of opioids (Fig. 7.6):

- *Phenanthrenes* are the prototypical opioids. The presence of a 6-hydroxyl may be associated with a higher incidence of nausea and hallucinations. For example, morphine and codeine (both with 6-hydroxyl groups) are associated with more nausea than hydromorphone and oxycodone (which do not have 6-hydroxyl groups). Opioids in this group include morphine, codeine, hydromorphone, levorphanol, oxycodone, hydrocodone, oxymorphone, buprenorphine, nalbuphine, and butorphanol.
- *Benzomorphans* have only pentazocine as a member of this class. It is an agonist/antagonist with a high incidence of dysphoria.
- *Phenylpiperidines* include fentanyl, alfentanil, sufentanil, and meperidine. Fentanyl has the highest affinity for the mu receptor.
- *Diphenylheptanes* include propoxyphene and methadone.
- *Tramadol* does not fit in the standard opioid classes. A unique analgesic, tramadol is an atypical opioid, a 4-phenyl-piperidine analog of codeine, with partial mu agonist activity in addition to central GABA, catecholamine, and serotonergic activities.

Opioids can also be categorized as an antagonist, partial agonist, agonist/antagonist, or agonist. It is possible for compounds to exhibit both intrinsic affinity and efficacy at receptors. The affinity of a compound is defined as the "strength of interaction" when it binds to its receptor, while its efficacy is the degree of activity or effect that results from this binding.

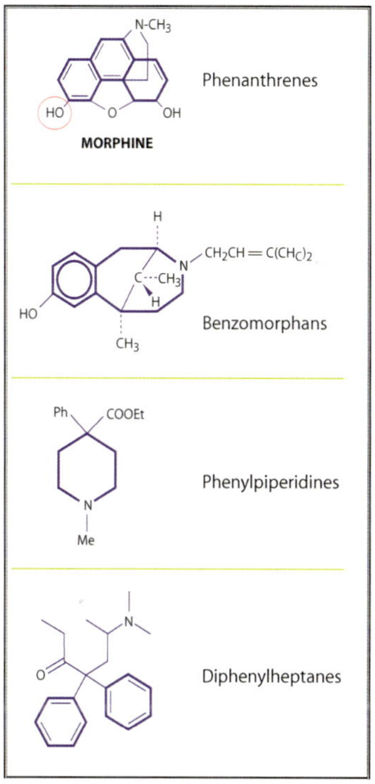

Figure 7.6: Opioid chemical classification.

Source: Andrea M. Trescot, Sukdeb Datta, Marion Lee, and Hans Hansen. Opioid Pharmacology. Pain Physician 2008: Opioid Special Issue: 11: S133-S153. ISSN 1533-3159. https://www.painphysicianjournal.com/current/pdf?article=OTg3&journal=42

An antagonist has affinity but no efficacy, a partial agonist has affinity but only partial efficacy, and an agonist possesses both affinity and efficacy. The mu, kappa, and delta receptors are the relevant receptors in relation to opioids. Different compounds may be more or less effective and affinistic at these different receptors (Ghelardini et al., 2015).

Opioid Agonists

The majority of widely used opioids function as agonists, stimulating the opioid receptors to produce their desired effects. It appears that variations in the relative stimulation of the different opioid receptors (mu, kappa, etc.) account for differences in efficacy and activity.) in addition to variations in opioid receptor sensitivity caused by genetics.

Opioid Partial Agonists

One category for buprenorphine is partial agonist. It has a strong affinity for the mu receptor, where it binds with low efficacy and produces a partial effect. However, it also exhibits kappa receptor antagonist activity, which makes it useful not only as an analgesic but also in detoxification, maintenance, and deterrent treatments for opioid abuse. Buprenorphine's first-pass effect by the liver is extensive, and its bioavailability is low.

While these drugs have a limited analgesic effect, taking more of them will only increase the negative effects of opioids. Nevertheless, they can be used as analgesics. Unwanted dysesthesias can result from kappa receptor stimulation, as in the case of pentazocine (Talwin®). Due to their strong mu affinity, both types of opioid partial agonists/antagonists have the ability to reduce opioid mu activity and may even cause withdrawal symptoms in those who are opioid-dependent.

With a significant first-pass hepatic effect, buprenorphine (Suboxone®, Subutex®) has a low bioavailability. However, due to its high solubility in lipids, it has a great sublingual bioavailability. For maintenance therapy, a single daily dosage is administered. Sedation, nausea, vomiting, headaches, dizziness, and respiratory depression are among the common side effects of buprenorphine.

Opioid Agonists-Antagonists

Opioids that are categorized as agonist-antagonists have low efficacy at the mu-opioid receptor, which means they can function as mu-opioid receptor antagonists while also exhibiting kappa agonistic characteristics. Pentazocine, nalbuphine, and butorphanol are examples of partial agonist-antagonists that have partial kappa agonist activity in addition to partial mu agonist activity. These compounds share a high mu affinity but little mu efficacy because they are partial mu agonists that can also act as mu-opioid receptor antagonists. Although these substances have a limited or partial analgesic effect, increasing the dosage beyond a certain point will only result in more severe opioid side effects and may, therefore, reduce the likelihood of abuse (Benyamin et al., 2008). Unwanted dysesthesias may result from kappa receptor stimulation. It is important to keep in mind that their antagonistic qualities could hasten withdrawal.

Opioid Antagonists

Naloxone and naltrexone, two opioid receptor antagonists, have a strong affinity for the mu receptor but no mu receptor efficacy. They are competitive antagonists at the mu, kappa, and delta receptors. Though they have different pharmacokinetic profiles that favor different therapeutic uses, naltrexone and naloxone have similar central and peripheral actions. Although naloxone is not very bioavailable when taken orally, it acts quickly when administered parenterally to reverse the effects of acute opioid overuse. Due to the possibility of "re-narcotization," its brief duration of action does not offer sufficient duration of effect coverage for long-acting opioid maintenance or deterrent therapy. Because of its prolonged duration of action when taken orally, naltrexone is helpful in detoxification, maintenance, and abuse-deterrent treatment modalities. In the United States, nalmefene, a mu-opioid receptor antagonist, is a water-soluble derivative of naltrexone with a longer half-life than naloxone that can be used to reverse the effects of opioid drugs. It is possible to combine partial or mu agonists with naloxone and naltrexone. In order to stop intravenous buprenorphine abuse, naloxone is used in conjunction with sublingual buprenorphine (Suboxone®). The same product (sublingual buprenorphine), when used alone (i.e., without naloxone), is marketed as Subutex®. Currently being studied is the possibility of using ultra-low dose naltrexone in combination with oxycodone (Oxytrex®) to suppress opioid tolerance. Peripherally acting mu receptor antagonists such as methylnaltrexone and alvimopan are being studied for their potential to treat opioid-induced bowel dysfunction and postoperative ileus (Benyamin et al., 2008).

Tramadol

Tramadol is a special analgesic that is an atypical opioid, a 4-phenyl-piperidine analogue of codeine, with central GABA, catecholamine, and serotonergic activities combined with partial mu agonist activity. Although its primary use is as an analgesic, tramadol has also been shown to be effective in treating opioid withdrawal.

Opioid Metabolism

Opioid metabolites may be connected to numerous opioid side effects and effects themselves. Most people assume that the liver is where most metabolism takes place. Genetics, age, gender, and environment—including food, illness, and concurrent medication use—all affect the basal rate of metabolism. Renal metabolism is not well demonstrated, despite the kidney being a significant excretory organ. The P450 (CYP) system or glucuronidation are the two main methods used to metabolize opioids. The mu opioid peptide (MOP) receptor is encoded by the human OPRM1 gene, and there is evidence that polymorphism in this gene may also be a factor in the large range of opioid sensitivity. After reviewing the state of research on opioid receptor genes, Ikeda et al. came to the conclusion that variations in the OPRM1 gene are likely to impact opioid analgesia, tolerance, and dependence; further research on mice suggests that this gene may also be involved in the abuse of alcohol and other drugs that are not opioids (Helander et al., 2017).

In medicine, drug interactions can be extremely confusing. Over the past ten years, the average number of papers cited in PubMed with the term "drug interaction" in the title has been 60 per year. The heme-containing, microsomal drug-metabolizing CYP450 enzymes are a super-family of enzymes that play a crucial role in the biosynthesis and breakdown of chemicals, toxins, endogenous compounds, and pharmaceuticals. There are currently over 2,700 distinct members of the CYP450 superfamily and 57 human cytochrome P450 enzymes known to exist. The most common isoenzyme involved in drug metabolism, CYP3A4, is responsible for about half of the metabolism of marketed drugs. Individual differences in CYP3A4 levels can range up to thirty times, which causes a significant amount of variability in blood levels. Seven CYP isozymes (3A4, 3A5, 1A2, 2C9, 2C19, 2D6, and 2E1) are responsible for the metabolism of over 90% of the most clinically significant drugs. The enzymes consist of approximately 10% CYP1A2, CYP2C8, and CYP2C9, 5% each CYP2D6 and CYP2E1, and 1% CYP2C19. In certain populations, CYP2D6 is completely absent; for instance, 6–10% of Caucasians are deficient in this enzyme, whereas other people have high levels of it, which causes their medication to be metabolized quickly. A recent Danish study demonstrated the high potential for drug interactions. A total of two hundred medical and surgical patients who were released from the hospital were visited and surveyed to find out what medications they kept at home and how often they took them (Helander et al., 2017). To ascertain the significance of the potential interactions, this data was cross-referenced with hospital records and a drug-interaction database. Patients ranged in age from 1 to 24 years old, with an average age of 75 years. The median number of drugs used was 8. Prescription drugs accounted for 93% of drug usage among patients, followed by over-the-counter drugs (91%), herbal drugs, and dietary supplements (63%). In all, 476 possible drug interactions involving 63 % of the patients were found. Only 21 (4.4%) of these interactions were categorized as relative contraindications, and none of them represented absolute prohibitions against using the interacting medications together.

7.1.7 Pharmacology of Specific Opioids

Morphine

A Schedule II drug, morphine is used to treat moderately to severely painful conditions. German pharmacist Freidrich Wilhelm Adam Serturner isolated this medication in 1804, naming it "morphium" after the god of sleep. The invention of the hypodermic needle increased the amount of this medication used to manage pain. One hundred thousand soldiers experienced "soldier's disease," or addiction to morphine, following the American Civil War. The classic mu receptor opiate is morphine, which is a derivative of phenanthrene.

Merely 40 to 50 % of the dose taken orally eventually makes its way to the central nervous system; this happens in 30 minutes for morphine with immediate release and 90 minutes for any form with extended release. The drug's low lipid solubility, protein binding, quick conjugation with glucuronic acid, and ionization at a physiological pH are the causes of its poor penetration. The blood-brain barrier can be crossed more easily by the non-alkalized form of morphine, and blood alkalinization raises the proportion of non-ionized morphine. It is noteworthy that respiratory acidosis raises morphine concentrations in the brain due to enhanced cerebral blood flow brought on by elevated carbon dioxide tension and easier non-ionized form delivery to the blood-brain barrier. Morphine has an elimination half-life of about 120 minutes (Dorn et al., 2014).

The two main metabolic pathways for morphine are glucuronidation and demethylation. The former produces morphine-6 glucuronide (M6G) and morphine-3 glucuronide (M3G) in a ratio of 6:1, while the latter converts about 5% of the drug into normorphine. Both hepatic and extrahepatic sites experience glutaronidation almost immediately after morphine enters the serum, and there may be some intrahepatic recycling taking place. When M3G concentrations are high enough, it may cause hyperalgesia; M6G is thought to be in charge of some of the extra analgesic effects of morphine. CYP450 is responsible for phase one of this metabolism, while UGT2B7 is responsible for phase two. Normorphine is produced by CYP3A4 and CYP2C8-mediated demethylation. According to Ferrari et al., only 8 out of 12 patients receiving morphine produced normorphine. In small quantities, morphine can also be metabolized to produce the drugs hydromorphone and codeine. Sixty-six percent of morphine users do not exhibit aberrant drug behavior; this is typically the case at doses greater than 100 mg/day.

Although studies have shown that drugs that inhibit the UGT2B7 pathway may change the amount of M3G and M6G available, drug-drug interactions (DDIs) with morphine are thought to be uncommon. The most effective medications that block this pathway are benzodiazepines, tricyclic and heterocyclic antidepressants, tamoxifen, diclofenac, naloxone, and carbamazepine. Even so, these changes might not have any clinical significance. According to other research, ranitidine and rifampin may change the way morphine is metabolized (Dorn et al., 2014).

It is said that morphine is an opioid with a comparatively long half-life. Its side effect profile is linked to direct respiratory depression mediated by the nucleus accumbens in the brain stem, which causes a decreased response to the arterial carbon dioxide tension and shifts the response curve to the right, and histamine release, which can cause bronchospasm and hypotension. Remember that morphine will be delivered to the brain compartment at a higher rate in respiratory acidosis, increasing respiratory compromise.

Additionally, morphine has the potential to lower sympathetic nervous system tone, which could lead to peripheral vein hypotony, venous pooling, and orthostatic hypotension. The effects of morphine on the digestive tract include constipation due to decreased intestinal motility, spasm of the sphincter of Oddi, and spasm of the biliary smooth muscle. Urinary retention is caused by similar effects on the genitourinary system, which include spasms of the bladder trigone. By directly stimulating the chemoreceptor trigger zone in the fourth ventricle's floor, morphine may cause nausea and vomiting. Because morphine releases histamine, it can cause cutaneous changes, such as peripheral vasodilatation and urticaria, which is a flushing of the skin. For people with sulfa allergies, the parenteral forms of morphine contain sulfites that could result in anaphylactic shock or potentially fatal allergic reactions.

Codeine

The first of the weak opioid analgesics, codeine had a weak affinity for μ opioid receptors and was first isolated in 1832. When combined with other analgesics, codeine is classified as a Schedule III drug rather than a Schedule II substance in its pure form. Its half-life is 2.5–3 hours, and its analgesic potency is roughly 50% that of morphine. It is thought that codeine converts to morphine through metabolism, which produces the analgesic effect. The metabolite codeine-6 glucuronide appears to be active based on certain evidence. Codeine is prone to DDIs because it is metabolized by CYP2D6. This includes the inducers rifampin and dexamethasone as well as the inhibitors bupropion, celecoxib, cimetidine, and cocaine. Since the CYP450 enzymes exhibit significant variability, codeine may not be a useful medication for all populations, given its pro-drug nature. With a three-hour half-life, over 80% of the dosage is eliminated in a few hours. Like other opiate agonists, codeine has a similar side effect profile. Due to potential competing effects on the chemoreceptor trigger zone, a low dose of codeine paradoxically causes more emesis than a higher dose. Over 65 mg of codeine is not well tolerated in doses (Dorn et al., 2014).

The FDA recently released a Public Health Advisory about a very uncommon but dangerous side effect in nursing babies whose moms use codeine. These babies appear to be ultra-rapid codeine metabolizers, which causes higher and faster levels of morphine to be metabolized in the breast milk and potentially fatal neonatal respiratory depression. The doctor should use the least amount of medication that works best for the shortest amount of time when prescribing codeine-containing drugs to nursing mothers.

Dihydrocodeine

Dihydrocodeine, as the name suggests, has a structure very similar to that of codeine. The only distinction is that instead of a double bond connecting carbons 7 and 8, there is just one. Its analgesic qualities are typically regarded as complementing those of codeine. Like codeine, dihydromorphine (a minor metabolite, less than 5%) is produced by 2D6 demethylation at the 3-carbon site, while 3A4 activity produces nor-dihydrocodeine. The primary cause of the analgesic effects of dihydrocodeine is unknown; it could be the parent drug, its metabolites, or a combination of them.

Hydrocodone

The most widely used opioid, hydrocodone, is indicated for both symptomatic relief of nonproductive cough and moderate-to-moderately severe pain. Although hydrocodone is only available for pain management as a Schedule III combination product with non-opioid analgesics like ibuprofen and acetaminophen, it would be classified as a Schedule II substance in its pure form. After oral administration, hydrocodone has a high bioavailability and a half-life of 2.5 to 4 hours. With a keto (=O) group at carbon 6 instead of a hydroxyl (–OH) group, and a single bond at carbons 7 and 8, hydrocodone shares structural similarities with codeine. When the 2D6 enzyme demethylates hydrocodone at the 3-carbon position, it forms hydromorphone, which has much stronger μ binding than hydrocodone, although hydrocodone still exhibits weak binding capacity for the μ receptor. It has been suggested that hydrocodone is a prodrug, similar to codeine and dihydrocodeine. Put differently, individuals with CYP2D6 deficiency or those taking CYP2D6 inhibitors might not generate these analgesic metabolites and might experience less analgesia than normal. Regretfully, there are few studies that could support the claim that hydrocodone is a prodrug, and neither human nor pain model studies have been conducted with pain patients (Misailidi et al., 2018).

Oxycodone

A member of the phenanthrene class of opioids, oxycodone is available as a Schedule II drug, either alone or in combination with aspirin or Tylenol. The κ receptor is one of the several opiate receptors that oxycodone activates. With the exception of the addition of a hydroxyl group at carbon #14, oxycodone and hydrocodone are comparable. When taken orally, oxycodone has a high bioavailability and a half-life of 2.5 to 3 hours. It is extensively conjugated in the liver and degraded by oxidation to produce a range of metabolites that are primarily excreted in urine. Oxycodone is metabolized by 2D6 to oxymorphone and by glucuronidation to noroxycodone, which has less than 1% of the analgesic potency of oxycodone. Although oxymorphone, an active metabolite of oxycodone, may have some effect on analgesia, the majority of the analgesic effect is produced by the parent compound, oxycodone. Oxycodone is an analgesic and not a pro-drug. DDIs with 2D6 inhibitors are possible because oxycodone's clearance is dependent on the 2D6 pathway.

Oxymorphone

While oxymorphone exhibits a strong affinity for the μ receptor and minimal interaction with the κ and δ receptors, oxycodone exhibits activity at multiple receptors. About ten times as potent as morphine, oxymorphone is unaffected by CY2D6 or CY3A4. After oral dosing, there was significant individual variability in the excretion of both free and conjugated oxymorphone by six human subjects. It is now accessible in formulations for both sustained release and immediate release.

Hydromorphone

A hydrogenated ketone of morphine, hydromorphone is a Schedule II semi-synthetic opioid agonist. Similar to morphine, it mainly affects delta receptors to a lesser extent and μ opioid receptors in particular. With estimates of a relative potency of 7:1 to 11:1 when compared to morphine, hydromorphone is much more potent than morphine. Its high water solubility also enables the creation of very concentrated formulations. It might be preferred over morphine in patients with renal failure because of the latter's potential for hazardous metabolite accumulation. The liver metabolizes hydromorphone in great detail; on the first pass, the liver excretes about 62% of the oral dosage. The duration of action for oral immediate release preparations is 4 hours, with an approximate start of action at 30 minutes. Parenterally, hydromorphone can also be injected subcutaneously, intramuscularly, or intravenously (Misailidi et al., 2018).

The main product of hydromorphone metabolism is hydromorphone-3-glucuronide (H3G). Like its corresponding M3G, H3G exhibits a variety of dose-dependent excited behaviors in animal models, including myoclonus, allodynia, and seizures. It also lacks any analgesic effect.

Methadone

Methadone is a Schedule II drug that is a synthetic μ opioid receptor agonist and an antagonist of the Nmethyl-D-aspartate (NMDA) receptor in addition to its opioid receptor activity. Methadone is a racemic mixture of two enantiomers; S-methadone is an NMDA antagonist and the R form is more potent, having a 10-fold higher affinity for opioid receptors, which accounts for almost all of its analgesic effect. Because of its innate NMDA antagonistic properties, it may be helpful in "opioid-resistant" and severe neuropathic pain conditions. Additionally, the S isomer prevents serotonin and norepinephrine from being reabsorbed, which is something to be aware of when taking SSRIs and TCAs. Despite the fact that it has historically been used to treat heroin addicts, its affordability, ease of dosage, and ability to relieve neuropathic pain have all contributed to a recent rise in its use. Unfortunately, there has been a sharp rise in the number of deaths linked to this medication due to a lack of knowledge about its metabolism, possible drug interactions, and lengthy half-life.

Because methadone is a distinct synthetic opioid and has no relation to conventional opioids, it can be helpful for patients who have "true" morphine allergies. This medication is simple, lipophilic, and has a good, albeit very variable, oral bioavailability (40–100%). It is also available as a liquid and can be crushed or dissolved to deliver down an NG tube. One benefit for patients with renal failure or insufficiency is that methadone is almost entirely eliminated through feces after being metabolized in the liver and intestines. Its high lipid solubility causes it to be redistributed to fat tissues, where it remains for a very long time before being eliminated—between 12 and 150 hours. It is also incredibly cheap and might induce less constipation than morphine.

Methadone metabolism is never constant. CYP2D6 preferentially metabolizes R-methadone, whereas CYP3A4 and CYP1A2 metabolize both enantiomers of methadone. CYP3A4 is the primary metabolizer of methadone, with CYP2D6 having a secondary role. It's possible that CYP1B2 is involved, and CYP2B6, a recently discovered enzyme, might be a significant metabolic intermediary. There can be a 30-fold variation in CYP3A4 expression, and CYP2D6 genetic polymorphism can range from slow to fast metabolism. When methadone therapy is started, the CYP3A4 enzyme can be stimulated for 5–7 days. This can result in low blood levels at first, but if the medication has been rapidly titrated upward, it can also cause unexpectedly high levels about a week later. Additionally, an intestinal CYP3A4 transport enzyme may be involved. These enzymes can also be induced or inhibited by a wide range of substances. The inconsistent observed half-life could be explained by variations in methadone's enzymatic metabolic conversion. Since methadone doesn't produce any active metabolites, it may be less neurotoxic, cause myoclonus, and cause hyperalgia than morphine. Its analgesic action (4–8 hours) is much shorter than its elimination half-life (up to 150 hours), and patient self-directed redosing and a long half-life may increase the risk of respiratory depression and death. It might be unique in that it does not produce profound euphoria (Armenian et al., 2018).

Furthermore, Torsades de Pointes, a potentially lethal arrhythmia brought on by an extension of the QT interval, can be brought on by methadone. That risk may be increased by congenital QT prolongation, high methadone levels (typically more than 60 mg daily), and conditions that worsen QT prolongation (like hypokalemia and hypomagnesemia).

The interaction between methadone and other opioids is not fully cross-tolerated. The lengthy half-life of methadone may be overlooked when titrating dosage to analgesic effect, even when prescribed in small doses and used correctly by people skilled with opioids. Methadone dosages that are 10% of the estimated equianalgesic doses of conventional opioids generally result in better relief.

Known CYP3A4 inhibitor venlafaxine may show additional interactions.

Fentanyl

Strong opioid agonist fentanyl is a Schedule II drug that can be obtained in parenteral, transdermal, and transbuccal forms. The most ancient synthetic piperidine opioid agonist, fentanyl, mainly interacts with mu receptors. It binds to plasma proteins strongly, is highly lipophilic, and has about 80 times the potency of morphine.

The liver extensively metabolizes fentanyl. A portion of the medication swallowed when taken as a lozenge for oral trans-mucosal absorption is metabolized first-pass in the liver and possibly the small intestine. It is broken down into norfentanyl and hydroxyfentanyl.

CYP3A4 breaks down fentanyl into inert and nontoxic metabolites. On the other hand, CYP3A4 inhibitors might raise the blood levels of fentanyl. After application, the transdermal formulation takes 6–12 hours to start working, and it usually takes 3–6 days to reach a steady state. A subcutaneous reservoir is left behind after removing a patch, and it could take up to 24 hours for the drug to clear (Socías and Wood, 2017).

Meperidine

Meperidine, a Schedule II drug, has an oral-to-parental ratio of 4:1 and is a relatively weak opioid μ agonist, only 10% as effective as morphine. It also possesses strong anticholinergic and local anesthetic qualities. Meperidine has a half-life of roughly three hours. The liver breaks it down into normeperidine, which has a half-life of 15 to 30 hours and strong neurotoxic effects. Monoamine oxidase inhibitors (MAOIs) patients should not take meperidine; when combined with MAOIs, meperidine can cause severe respiratory depression, hyperpyrexia, excitation of the central nervous system, delirium, and seizures.

Meperidine is converted to normeperidine through glucuronidation. Normeperidine has T1/2 of 8–12 hours, meaning that substantial amounts can build up in just two days. Naloxone cannot reverse normeperidine's negative effects. At first, this is typified by mild affective changes (e.g., anxiety), which are sometimes followed by seizures, multifocal myoclonus, and tremors. Although it can happen after repeated administration in patients with normal renal function, CNS hyperexcitability is more common in patients with renal disease.

Levorphanol

Levorphanol is the optical isomer of dextromethorphan and a synthetic analogue of morphine. It lasts longer than hydromorphone and has the same potency. It is an NMDA antagonist as well as a mu, kappa, and delta agonist. After metabolism, a 3-glucuronide with unclear function is produced.

Lorafenol, like methadone, has garnered attention as a potential treatment for refractory pain recently. Similar to methadone, there is a variable equivalent for dosage; the conversion factor has been reported to be 12:1 for morphine doses under 100 mg and to be 25:1 for doses exceeding 600 mg. Regrettably, levorphanol shows potential for interaction at the glucuronidation enzyme sites; interactions with NSAIDs, valproic acid, lorazepam, and rifampin are possible, but they have not been confirmed. It was mentioned that aminophylline, amobarbital, heparin, methicillin, pentobarbital, phenobarbital, phenytoin, secobarbital, and thiopental were "pharmaceutically incompatible" with it.

Buprenorphine

The use of buprenorphine (Buprenex®) has been authorized in the U. S. since December of 1981. In Europe, there is a 72-hour transdermal product that releases buprenorphine continuously at 35, 52, or 70 mcg/hr (though not in the U.S.) in order to address chronic pain. In 2002, the Subutex® oral or sublingual form received approval. Suboxone®, which contains naloxone, is also an option. There is very little oral and nearly no sublingual absorption of the naloxone component. Its addition aims to counteract any potential effects of buprenorphine administered via IV or IM. It has a great sublingual bioavailability due to its high lipid solubility. The effects of sublingual administration start to take effect quickly (30–60 minutes), peaking between 90 and 100 minutes later. For maintenance therapy, it is taken once daily. P450 3A4 is the primary metabolite of buprenorphine. The induction or inhibition of the 3A4 system can result in a wide range of DDIs. Buprenorphine dosages for opioid addiction typically range from 4 to 32 mg per day. Common side effects of buprenorphine include drowsiness, headaches, nausea, vomiting, and respiratory depression. In patients who have developed physical dependence after receiving repeated doses of a morphine-like agonist, it may hasten withdrawal symptoms. The only thing that can counteract the respiratory depressant effects of buprenorphine is comparatively high doses of naloxone (Moy et al., 2020).

Propoxyphene

Propoxyphene is a Schedule IV drug that is used as a mild opioid agonist for mild to moderate pain. When propoxyphene is combined with other medications that can make drowsiness worse, the central nervous system effects of propoxyphene—dizziness, sedation, weakness and falls, mild visual disturbances, agitation, paradoxical excitement, and insomnia—can lead to drug-related deaths. Following two studies in 1991 and 1995, the Government Accountability Office (GAO) recommended against the use of propoxyphene in elderly patients due to the availability of safer and more effective alternatives to analgesics. Propoxyphene is a synthetic analgesic with an opioid dose equipotency akin to codeine and structural similarities to methadone. With a half-life of 6 to 12 hours, the analgesic action is limited to its d-stereoisomer (dextropropoxyphene), and the duration of effective analgesia is 3 to 5 hours. It is not metabolized by CYP2D6 in the liver but rather by norpropoxyphene, which has a lengthy half-life of 30 to 60 hours, is thought to be harmful to the heart. Furthermore, an overdose of propoxyphene itself may result in naloxone-reversible seizures. Propoxyphene is a weak and noncompetitive antagonist of the NMDA receptor in addition to being an agonist of the ε receptor. Additionally, because it is a CYP3A4 inhibitor, it may raise blood levels of ritonavir, carbamazepine, and methadone.

Propoxyphene, which is not a prodrug, would have more effect than hydrocodone (which must be metabolized by CYP2D6 to its more active form), as well as its NMDA antagonist activity. Clinically, some people report better relief with propoxyphene than hydrocodone; this could be indicative of a CYP2D6 deficiency.

Tramadol

Tramadol, an atypical opioid and codeine's 4-phenyl-piperidine analog, is a special kind of analgesic. O-demethyl tramadol, the M1 derivative generated by CYP2D6, binds to the μ receptor up to six times more strongly than the original compound. Tramadol is a racemic mixture of two enantiomers, the main one of which inhibits norepinephrine reuptake, and the other is a selective ε agonist that inhibits serotonin reuptake. The daily maximum dose is 400 mg. Seizures and CNS excitation result from toxic dosages (Moy et al., 2020).

Drugs not on the federal schedule include tramadol; state regulations may differ. Following oral dosages, tramadol is quickly and widely absorbed, matching codeine's analgesic potency. Although its primary use is as an analgesic, tramadol has also been shown to be effective in treating opioid withdrawal.

7.1.8 Drug Interactions

When two or more drugs are administered together, they can change a drug's dosage or mode of action. This is known as a drug interaction. Table 7.5 illustrates how multiple hepatic drug interactions can affect the levels of opioid drugs.

- There have been isolated reports of interactions between opioid and H2 blockers (cimetidine and ranitidine) causing breathing difficulties, confusion, and muscle twitching.
- A patient taking Tamoxifen (a CY2D6 substrate) was noted to get poor relief with oxycodone (which is metabolized by CY2D6) but excellent relief with morphine.

There are several drug interactions with methadone. Methadone metabolism is induced by phenytoin, carbamazepine, rifampin, erythromycin, barbiturates, and several anti-retrovirals. This lowers blood levels methadone and increases the risk of withdrawal. Methadone levels may rise in response to SSRIs, tricyclic antidepressants, and azole antifungals. TCA levels may also rise while on methadone. Withdrawal symptoms that take a week or longer are typically caused by CYP induction, whereas overmedication that occurs within a few days is typically caused by P450 (CYP) inhibition. In certain situations, methadone may also result in cardiac arrhythmias, such as prolonged QTc intervals and/or Torsade de Pointes. This risk can be raised by taking methadone along with a CYP3A4 inhibitor, such as ciprofloxin or even grapefruit. (However, this seems to be primarily theoretical and not clinically relevant in the case of grapefruit juice). A significant (50–90%) drop in the computed equipotent dose is advised when transitioning from another opioid to methadone.

Table 7.5: Drug interactions of opioids.

Tricyclic antidepressants	Inhibit morphine glucuronidation leading to ⇑ blood levels --- Nortriptyline inhibits non-competitively --- Amitriptyline and clomipramine inhibit competitively
Methadone and morphine	⇓ metabolism of TCAs, leading to toxicity
Quinine	⇓ conversion of codeine to morphine leading to ⇓ analgesia
Metoclopramide	Earlier peak plasma levels with controlled-released opioids
Meperidine	MAO inhibitors trigger hyperpyrexia
Propoxyphene	⇑ carbamazepine, doxepin, metoprolol, propranolol levels ⇓ excretion of benzodiazepines, leading to accumulation and overdose
Erythromycin	⇑ opioid effects
Venlafaxine	⇑ methadone levels
Rifampin Phenytoin Carbamazine	⇓ methadone levels
Phenytoin Phenobarbital	⇓ meperidine levels
CY2D6 inhibitors	⇑ tramadol levels ⇓ analgesia from hydrocodone/codeine
CY2D6 substrates	⇑ tramadol levels because of competition for metabolism
CYP3A4 inhibitors	⇑ methadone levels
CYP3A4 inducers	⇓ methadone levels

Source: Andrea M. Trescot, Sukdeb Datta, Marion Lee, and Hans Hansen. Opioid Pharmacology. Pain Physician 2008: Opioid Special Issue: 11: S133-S153. ISSN 1533-3159. https://www.painphysicianjournal.com/current/pdf?article=OTg3&journal=42

Drug Conversions

Although many opioid conversion charts have been created, none of them are trustworthy or account for the wide variations in effectiveness and drug metabolism among patients and prescriptions. The bioavailability of brand-name and generic drugs may differ significantly, and genetic polymorphism and drug interactions may have an impact on how well drugs are metabolized. Importantly, even "equipotent" dosages of drugs can result in drastically different levels of analgesia and adverse effects. Generally speaking, in order to transition between drugs, the doctor has to figure out an approximate equivalent 24-hour dose, divide it by the recommended dosage, and then "under-dose," titrating the medication until it takes effect.

The apparent potency of methadone in relation to other opioids is dependent on the patient's current exposure to other opioids, which is a significant characteristic. The current dosage of the opioid to be converted determines the conversion factor (Table 7.6).

Table 7.6: Oral morphine to oral methadone conversion.

Oral morphine dose	Morphine: methadone ratio
<100 mg	3:1
101 -300 mg	5:1
301-600 mg	10:1
601-800 mg	12:1
801-1000 mg	15:1
> 1000 mg	20:1

Source: Andrea M. Trescot, Sukdeb Datta, Marion Lee, and Hans Hansen. Opioid Pharmacology. Pain Physician 2008: Opioid Special Issue: 11: S133-S153. ISSN 1533-3159. https://www.painphysicianjournal.com/current/pdf?article=OTg3&journal=42

The ratio of oral morphine to intravenous (IV) morphine during chronic administration is 3:1. The potency of hydromorphone is 5-8 times that of morphine. The approximate equivalent of 25 mcg of transdermal fentanyl (TDF) is ten to twenty mg of IV morphine (and possibly up to ninety mg of oral morphine). Likewise, 12 mg of oral hydromorphone or 45 mg of oral oxycodone per day are approximately equal to 25 mcg of TDF. It has been stated that methadone and morphine are equipotent; however, it is now more obvious that administering methadone on a milligram-for-milligram basis will result in a potentially fatal overdose. A 3:1 ratio may be suitable for morphine dosages under 100 mg, while a 20 mg morphine to 1 mg methadone ratio may be suitable for higher morphine dosages. Maybe due to intestinal CYP3A4 metabolism, methadone seems to be much more potent when administered IV. It cannot be overstated that methadone dosage needs to be taken carefully and with knowledge because it has the potential to be fatal (Belzak and Halverson, 2018).

Pharmacokinetics

The plasma half-life values of opioids vary significantly (Table 7.7). Therefore, levorphanol and methadone are long half-life opioids that, on average, may require 70 to 120 hours to achieve a steady state, whereas morphine and hydromorphone are short half-life opioids that, upon repeated dosing, reach a steady state in 10 to 12 hours.

Table 7.7: Plasma half-life values for opioids and their active metabolites.

Drug	Plasma half-life (hours)
Short Half-Life Opioids	
Morphine	2 -3.5
Morphine 6 glucoronide	2
Hydromorphone	2-3
Oxycodone	2-3
Fentanyl	3-4
Codeine	3
Meperidine	3-4
Nalbuphine	5
Butorphanol	2.5 -3.5
Buprenorphine	3-5
Long Half-Life Opioids	
Methadone	24
Levorphanol	12-16
Propoxyphene	12
Norpropoxyphene	30-40
Normeperidine	14-21

Source: Andrea M. Trescot, Sukdeb Datta, Marion Lee, and Hans Hansen. Opioid Pharmacology. Pain Physician 2008: Opioid Special Issue: 11: S133-S153. ISSN 1533-3159. https://www.painphysicianjournal.com/current/pdf?article=OTg3&journal=42

The maximum (peak) effects of a dose change for a short-half-life opioid will manifest relatively quickly during dose titration, whereas the peak effects of a dose change for a long-half-life opioid will take longer to manifest. For instance, if a patient's initial methadone dosage is fixed and not adjusted as needed during the five to ten-day accumulation period, they may experience excessive sedation even though they report adequate pain relief after the initial dose.

The plasma half-lives of active metabolites, like normeperidine and norpropoxyphene, may be longer than those of their parent medications, propoxyphene and meperidine (Belzak and Halverson, 2018).

7.2 Synthetic Opioids and Their Analogs

Synthetic opioids are drugs created in a lab that function on the same brain receptors as their natural counterparts, such as e. g. morphine and codeine, in order to generate analgesic (pain-relieving) results. On the other hand, naturally occurring substances that are extracted from the seed pod of specific types of poppies are known as natural opioids. Methadone and fentanyl are two examples of synthetic opioids that have been authorized for medical use.

In the late 1970s and early 1980s, illicitly manufactured synthetic opioids that shared structural similarities with the Schedule II opioid analgesic fentanyl were abused and trafficked on the West Coast. Alphamethylfentanyl, 3-methylthiofentanyl, acetyl-alphamethylfentanyl, beta-hydroxy-3-methylfentanyl, alpha-methylthiofentanyl, thiofentanyl, betahydroxyfentanyl, para-fluorofentanyl, and 3-methylfentanyl were among the illicitly produced synthetic opioids that the DEA controlled in the 1980s.

The trafficking and abuse of various illicitly produced synthetic opioids, including several substances related to fentanyl, have resurfaced as of 2013. The following are a few examples of frequently encountered illegally manufactured synthetic opioids by law enforcement: acetyl fentanyl, butyryl fentanyl, furanyl fentanyl, furanyl fentanyl, 4-fluoroisobutyryl fentanyl, acryl fentanyl, and U-47700 (Belzak and Halverson, 2018).

7.2.1 Historical Emergence

In Mesopotamia, around 3400 BC, the Sumerians extracted opium from the plant's milky sap and called the bright red flowers of the plant "the joy plant." This is when the history of the opium poppy plant (*P. somniferum*) as an analgesic began. The plant's natural alkaloids and active components, however, were not thoroughly isolated and analyzed until the nineteenth century, which is when morphine (1805), codeine (1832), and thebaine (1835) were discovered. This was followed by the creation of more powerful and effective semi-synthetic opioid drugs, such as diamorphine (heroin) (1874), oxymorphone (1914), oxycodone (1916), and hydrocodone (1920), which were synthesized in laboratories from naturally occurring opium compounds. Heroin was originally discovered to have euphoric and uplifting effects; however, these effects were quickly sought after for non-medical purposes, raising concerns about dependence as early as the 20th century.

Legislation to Address Controlled Use

International law shifted in favor of tighter regulations after The Hague Opium Convention was ratified in 1912 and required signatories to restrict the production, distribution, and use of heroin and morphine to mainly medicinal and scientific purposes. Along with the adoption of the Limitation Convention in 1931, the Geneva Convention of 1925 imposed additional restrictions on the production and international trade of heroin, and a notable decline in both production and consumption was noted. Opioids (and their precursors), such as heroin, methadone, morphine, and opium, were classified as "substances with addictive properties, presenting a serious risk of abuse" and were subject to stringent international controls under the 1961 Single Convention on Narcotic Drugs and successive conventions in 1971 and 1988. The profitability of the then-controlled opioids prompted covert organizations to act in defiance of these international regulations, which resulted in the growth of an illicit global drug market.

Creation of Synthetic Opioids

Throughout the 20th century, pharmaceutical companies continued to develop synthetic opioids, which are defined as "opium compounds that are synthesized in the laboratory without the use of naturally occurring opium compounds" for use in human and veterinary medicine. This effort resulted in the discovery of meperidine in 1939, which has a different chemical structure than morphine but similar pharmacological properties, and the synthesis of methadone in 1946. Fentanyl was created in 1959 and quickly rose to prominence as a major analgesic and anesthetic drug because of its greater potency—50–100 times greater than that of morphine and heroin—faster absorption and shorter half-life. These characteristics, however, also attracted non-medical users, and fentanyl and its analogs quickly found their way onto the regulated market. As a result, they have been placed under UN Single Convention control in 1961 (scheduled under Schedule I, and Schedule IV for those without any medical use). In the past ten years or so, novel synthetic opioids (e.g., Carfentanil and ocfentanil), as well as non-pharmaceutical products, have been linked to the global opioid crisis and the rise in accidental overdoses, poisonings, and drug-related fatalities that has resulted from it. Synthetic opioids are a major and complex challenge to global public health because of their increasing prevalence on the market for controlled drugs, their ease of transportation in relatively small amounts (like via the postal service), and their associated morbidity and mortality (Brook et al., 2017).

Mortality Rates

Fentanyl and other synthetic opioids produced illegally in North America have greatly increased the rate at which the "opioid overdose crisis" is becoming worse. According to reports, there has been a "triple wave" of opioid-related deaths in the US: a rise in mortality from prescription opioids in the late 1990s, a sharp rise in deaths from heroin starting in 2010, and then from 2014 on, deaths from fentanyl and other synthetic opioids. These are not separate waves; rather, they overlap and each one adds to the total number of deaths within the wave. According to data from the Centers for Disease Control and Prevention (CDC), there were 100,306 drug overdose deaths in the US in the 12 months leading up to April 2021. The majority of these deaths (75,673; 75.4%) were caused by synthetic opioids. In the 12 months leading up to March 2021, 7224 opioid-related deaths were reported in Canada, a 95% increase. The vast majority of these deaths involved fentanyl or other synthetic opioids. Around the same time, the UK's Advisory Council on the Misuse of Drugs (ACMD) released a report on synthetic opioids. In it, they noted that over the previous ten years, the number of drug-related deaths had increased steadily and that deaths involving novel synthetic opioids were probably underreported because there were insufficient detailed forensic analyses available. Nonetheless, compared to North America, the percentage of deaths linked to fentanyl and novel synthetic opioids is said to be substantially lower in the United Kingdom. For instance, according to death registration data for 2020, there were 60 deaths linked to fentanyl, fentanyl analogs, or new synthetic opioids, compared to 1337 deaths linked to heroin and morphine.

International Response

In 2018, the United Nations Office on Drugs and Crime (UNODC) launched an integrated strategy in response to a growing global public health crisis. This strategy aimed to assist nations in tackling the global issue of synthetic opioids and included coordinating the international response, reducing supply through modifications to substance control laws, and promoting effective prevention and treatment options for substance use disorders. Other policymakers, organizations, and researchers have suggested, in addition to traditional preventive and treatment approaches, the following strategies in markets at high risk of exposure to new opioids: expanding the number of supervised drug consumption facilities, expanding the coverage of an expanded range of opioid agonist therapies; and introducing community-based "drug checking," which would quickly provide information on substances that are circulating in a local market (Brook et al., 2017).

Appearance of New Synthetic Opioids

The number of newly discovered synthetic opioids produced illegally climbed dramatically from one in 2009 to 55 in 2018, according to a 2020 UNODC report. Furthermore, they stated that the percentage of synthetic opioids in NPS increased from 2 % to 8 %, a fourfold increase between 2015 and 2019. Similar results were reported by the European Monitoring Centre for Drugs and Drug Addiction (EMCDDA), which states that since 2009, 57 new synthetic opioids have been found in Europe for the first time, with eight of those cases occurring in 2019. Unlike previous years, only two of these were derivatives of fentanyl; the other six were all chemically different from fentanyl, even though their potential for toxicity was similar, and they were referred to as non-fentanyl opioids. The ACMD in the UK came to the conclusion that synthetic opioids constituted a serious risk to public health and suggested that the monitoring and surveillance systems in place be modified in order to better determine the extent of the real threat to public health.

Emerging Markets

In addition to being marketed as separate items, synthetic opioids can also be found as fake opioid prescriptions and as adulterants in illicit supply lines of benzodiazepines, heroin, and other controlled substances. While some individuals will consciously search for these synthetic opioids, many others may inadvertently come into contact with substances with unknown pharmacology and toxicity because they are unaware of the ingredients in the products they have bought. While production and distribution are driven by financial gain, research indicates that the reasons behind their emergence may vary depending on the region. Analysis, for instance, indicates that the first wave of opioid deaths in the early 2000s in the United States may have been caused by restrictions on access to prescription opioids; in contrast, heroin shortages in certain European countries may have contributed to the growth in synthetic opioid consumption.

7.2.2 Mechanism of Action

Three opioid receptors—the mu, delta, and kappa opioid receptors—that are G-protein coupled, seven transmembrane domain inhibitory receptors make up the endogenous opioid system. In addition to their euphoric, sedative, and respiratory depressant effects, mu-opioid receptors are expressed throughout the peripheral and central nervous systems and are linked to the development of analgesia and dependence. They are also known to cause constipation. Agonism [combining a chemical substance (such as a drug) with a specific receptor on a cell thereby initiating the same reaction or activity typically produced by the binding of an endogenous substance] at both delta- and kappa-opioid receptors is also associated with analgesia, and additionally, agonism at kappa-opioid receptors is responsible for the dysphoric effects of opioids, which may also contribute partly to dependence formation. The human limbic system, hypothalamus, caudate nuclei, periaqueductal grey, dorsal horn of the spinal cord, and dorsal root ganglia are the areas where opioid receptor expression is most concentrated. These receptors are present on both pre- and post-synaptic membranes. Opioid receptors function at the spinal level to impede dorsal horn afferent nociceptive signaling. Peripheral opioid receptors are thought to be important in pain perception after injury based on observations of opioid receptor expression on peripheral sensory neurons and the efficacy of opioid analgesia administered peripherally (Brook et al., 2017).

Leu-enkephalin, met-enkephalin, dynorphin, and beta-endorphin are the four canonical endogenous opioid receptor ligands. All three opioid receptor subtypes are agonistic to these ligands, which have different affinities for them. For example, beta-endorphin acts as a full agonist on all three opioid receptors, while enkephalins have a higher affinity for delta opioid receptors than dynorphin does for kappa opioid receptors. Increased mu-opioid receptor stimulation leads to the G-protein complex's exchange of guanosine triphosphate (GTP) for guanosine diphosphate (GDP). This process inhibits the cells' adenylate cyclase, which lowers intracellular cyclic adenosine monophosphate (cAMP). The conductance of potassium and calcium ion channels is also inhibited by the activation of mu-opioid receptors. The release of various neurotransmitters, such as acetylcholine, noradrenaline, substance P, GABA, and dopamine, is subsequently reduced as a result of these events, which also cause neuronal membrane hyperpolarization and inhibition of tonic neural activity.

Synthetic opioids produce depressant effects like analgesia, sedation, and a lowering of consciousness level in addition to stimulating the limbic and midbrain dopaminergic circuitry, which is assumed to underlie the euphoric effect users seek. Nausea and vomiting may result from direct stimulation of the chemoreceptor trigger zone in the postrema area. Synthetic opioid toxicity is partially attributed to their lipophilicity and strong affinity for mu-opioid receptors, which can lead to the development of opioid toxicity at very low dosages (Wilson et al., 2020).

7.2.3 Mode of Use and Clinical Presentation

Synthetic opioids can be taken orally, by injection, by smoking, by swallowing, by nasal insufflation (snorting), by tablet (including lozenges), by transdermal patch, or by applying sublingually, vaginally, or rectally. One of the reported novel ways to consume these compounds is by vaping or the inhalation of electronic nicotine delivery devices. Chewing before swallowing can improve the absorption of synthetic opioids from transdermal patches that have been swallowed. Furthermore, since transdermal patches hold a significant amount of medication even after therapeutic use, it is possible to remove them for use via other routes, such as injection or nasal insufflation. The main desired effects of using synthetic opioids are analgesia, euphoria, and relaxation, similar to other natural and semi-synthetic opioid use. However, synthetic opioids produce significant inter-individual variability in dose/response, which can result in different toxic doses and clinical presentations. All of the body's major systems are impacted by synthetic opioids, which can cause cyanosis, hypoxia, bradycardia, nausea, vomiting, constipation, weight loss, chest pain, and hypoxia. The most frequent negative neurological consequence is a decrease in consciousness. Individuals who have ingested novel non-fentanyl compounds exhibit a variety of non-opioid adverse effects, such as skin rashes, paraesthesia, limb weakness, and disturbances in balance.

7.2.4 Compound-Specific Chemical Structure

Fentanyl, which was discovered in 1959, and its analogs sufentanil (1974), alfentanil (1976), and remifentanil (1987), which are used in medical therapy, are examples of synthetic opioids. The term "non-pharmaceutical fentanyls" refers to fentanyls such as acetylfentanyl (1962), carfentanil (1974), ocfentanil (1984), and furanylfentanyl (1986) that are not authorized for use in human medicine. Since 2010, new synthetic opioids, also known as non-fentanyl compounds, have entered the global drug market.

Table 7.8: Synthetic opioids.

Class	Drug name	Opioid receptor selectivity			Relative potency compared with morphine	Blood concentration found to be lethal (ng/ml)
		μ	κ	δ		
Fentanyl and pharmaceutical analogues	Fentanyl	+ + +			50–100	0.3–383
	Sufentanil	+ + +	+	+	1000–4000	27
	Alfentanil	+ + +			72	100–200
Illicit fentanyl analogues	Acetylfentanyl	+ + +			15.7	153–260
	Acrylfentanyl	+ + +			170	1.86 ± 3.08
	3-methyl-fentanyl	+ + +			48.5–569	0.3–1.9
	β-hydroxy-3-methyl-fentanyl	+ + +			6300	NA
	α-methyl-fentanyl	+ + +			56.9	3.1
	α-methyl-acetyl-fentanyl	+ + +			3.1	NA
	4-fluoro-fentanyl	+ + +			15.7	0.24 ± 0.21
	Butyr-fentanyl	+ + +			1.5–7	0.1–99
	Carfentanil	+ + +			10,000	0.1–4.9
	Isobutyrylfentanyl	+ + +			NA	NA
	Ocfentanil	+ + +			90	5.3–15.3
	Furanyl-fentanyl	+ + +			7	0.4–26
Non-fentanyl analogues	U-47000	+ + +			7.5	13.8–490
	AH-7921	+ + +	+		1–1.7	31–6600
	MT-45	+ + +	+	+	~1	8.3–1989

"+/++/+++" are markers of approximate increasing affinity for the relevant receptor subtype.

Source: Abu Shafi, Alex J. Berry, Harry Sumnall, David M. Wood, and Derek K. Tracy. Synthetic opioids: a review and clinical update. Therapeutic Advances in Psychopharmacology. Sage Journals. https://journals.sagepub.com/doi/10.1177/20451253221139616

These include MT-45 [1-cyclohexyl-4-(1,2-diphenylethyl) piperazine], AH-7921 [3,4-dichloro-N-{[1(dimethylamino) cyclohexyl]methyl} benzamide], and U-47700 [3,4-dichloro-N-[(1R,2R)-

2-(dimethy-lamino) cyclohexyl]-N-methylbenzamide]. Table 7.8 lists synthetic opioids along with their potency and receptor affinity for morphine. Now, we go over some of the more widely accessible synthetic opioids, discussing their pharmacological profiles and, where applicable, any unusual side effects that have been linked to their use.

Fentanyl and Its Analogues

Fentanyl is an opioid analgesic that is prescribed. In Belgium, fentanyl was initially created in the late 1950s. Fentanyl analogs analogs are made by modifying the chemical structure of fentanyl in certain places but otherwise, share a similar structure with the original drug. The amount of illegally produced fentanyl and its many analogs that law enforcement has come into contact with, as well as the abuse of these drugs and the deaths that result from it, have significantly increased in the past few years.

In addition to anesthesia, fentanyl, and its primary analogs, alfentanil, sufentanil, and remifentanil, are used in surgery to treat both acute and chronic pain and to induce sedation. Fentanyl is a derivative of 4-anilinopiperidine that is 2-phenylethyl-substituted and has a propionylamide moiety attached to the aniline-nitrogen. To create a wide range of fentanyl analogs, four structural features can be changed: (a) the piperidine ring; (b) the anilinophenyl ring; (c) the 2-phenylethyl substituent; and (d) a carboxamide moiety connected to the anilino-nitrogen.

Fentanyl

Fentanyl, a lipophilic phenylpiperidine synthetic opioid, selectively binds to the mu-receptor in the central nervous system [N-phenyl-N-[1-(2-phenylethyl) piperidin-4-yl] propanamide]. Because of its high lipophilicity, it can easily cross many membranes, including the blood-brain barrier, and spread throughout the body. Bioavailability is contingent upon the mode of delivery. Fentanyl has a low oral bioavailability, with an intranasal bioavailability of 89% and an oral bioavailability of 50%, respectively.

Sufentanil

Another phenylpiperidine synthetic opioid is sufentanil (N-[4-(methoxymethyl)-1-(2-thiophen-2-ylethyl)piperidin-4-yl]-N-phenylpropanamide]. It is distinct from fentanyl by having a methoxymethyl group added to the piperidine ring, which increases its potency and shortens its duration of action, and by substituting thiophene for the phenyl ring. It is five to fifteen times more potent than fentanyl and very selective for the mu-receptor site.

Alfentanil

Another phenylpiperidine synthetic opioid is alfentanil N-[1-[2-(4-ethyl-5-oxotetrazol-1-yl) ethyl]-4-(methoxymethyl)piperidin-4-yl]-N-phenylpropanamide. It was also produced by adding more substituents to the piperidine ring of fentanyl at the fourth position. In this instance, the methoxymethyl group was added along with the substitution of a tetrazolyl ring for the phenyl ring of the phenethyl. It is roughly thirty times more potent than morphine, despite not being as potent as fentanyl. It has the fastest analgesic onset and the time-to-peak effect when compared to fentanyl and sufentanil. It also has the shortest half-life of distribution and elimination, a small volume of distribution, increased binding to plasma proteins, and less lipid solubility (Belzak and Halverson, 2018).

Remifentanil

The compound known as remifentanil {methyl 1-(3-methoxy-3-oxopropyl)-4-[phenyl(propanoyl) amino]piperidine-4-carboxylate} was synthesized by substituting a carbomethoxy group for the phenyl ring located in the first position of the piperidine ring. Its ultra-short duration of action stems from its direct metabolism in the plasma by non-specific esterases, an active group of enzymes found in blood and tissues throughout the body, giving it an analgesic potency comparable to fentanyl.

Non-pharmaceutical Fentanyls

Strong synthetic opioids like ocfentanil and carfentanil have been linked to the global opioid overdose epidemic, especially in the US and certain European nations. Recently, overdose and fatalities in the US have also been linked to acetylfentanyl and furanylfentanyl.

Carfentanil

An extra methyl-carboxylate moiety is present at the 4-position of the piperidine ring in carfentanil [methyl 1-(2-phenylethyl)-4-(N-propanoylanilino)-piperidine-4-carboxylate], one of the N-4 substituted fentanyl analogues. Among the strongest opioids, it is only permitted for use in veterinary medicine as a general anesthetic or to tranquilize large animals, like elephants. Due to its extreme potency, it should not be used on humans. About 10,000 times the potency of morphine and 100 times the potency of fentanyl, respectively, are found in it. Carfentanil primarily affects the mu-opioid receptor subtype, although it is a very strong agonist at all opioid receptors. There have been hundreds of opioid overdoses, many of which are fatal, as a result of carfentanil being mislabeled as other drugs, including heroin, or used as a replacement to allegedly increase profitability. This opioid is currently the strongest available on the restricted market (Misailidi et al., 2018).

Ocfentanil

Ocfentanil [N-(2-fluorophenyl)-2-methoxy-N-[1-(2-phenylethyl)-piperidin-4-yl] acetamide has a fluorine atom on the ortho position of the aniline group and a methoxy group in place of a methyl group. It was discovered that ocfentanil had about 200 times the potency of morphine and 2.5 times the potency of fentanyl. After 2010, occfentanil was found on the market for controlled substances, despite never having been intended for use in pharmaceuticals.

Acetylfentanyl

The acetyl amide analog of fentanyl is called acetylfentanyl [N-Phenyl-N-[1-(2-phenylethyl)-4-piperidinyl] acetamide], where the N-propionyl moiety is replaced with an acetyl moiety. It is about 15 times more potent than morphine, but it is three times less potent than fentanyl. It shares some characteristics with heroin, such as color, consistency, and pharmacologic activity. There have been reports of novel ways to consume acetylfentanyl, including its combination with alcohol and use in electronic cigarettes made of propylene glycol.

Furanylfentanyl

With a furanyl ring in place of the methyl group next to the carbonyl bridge, furanylfentanyl [N-(1-(2-phenylethyl)-4-piperidinyl)-N-phenyl-furan-2-carboxamide] has a potency similar to fentanyl. In a study conducted between 2013 and 2017, 417 deaths involving fentanyl and analogs were reported in five counties in New York; the number of cases increased from 10 in 2013 to 184 in 2017, with fentanyl being one of the most frequently used drugs.

Non-fentanyl Opioids

Since 2010, a new class of synthetic opioids has entered the recreational drug market. These opioids differ structurally from fentanyl. Their chemical structures fall into the classes of compounds known as piperazine (MT-45), acetamide (U-50488, U-51754), or benzamide (U-47700, U-48800, or AH-7921).

U-47700

U-47700 [3,4-dichloro-N-[(1R,2R)-2-(dimethylamino)yclohexyl]-N-methylbenzamide] is a structural isomer of AH-7921. Slang terms for it include "fake morphine" or "U4". It is also occasionally referred to as "pink" because the powder that makes up the ingredient is colored pink due to impurities during production. It has been linked to recent intoxication cases and fatalities in the United States. It is 7:5 times more potent than morphine and has an affinity for the mu-opioid receptor.

U-50488

A kappa-opioid receptor agonist, U-50488 [trans-3,4-dichloro-N-methyl-N-[2-(1-pyrrolidinyl) cyclohexyl]-benzeneacetamide], has been shown to have some respiratory antagonist effects on mu-opioid receptors. Research conducted on animals has demonstrated that U-50488 induces dysphoria and diuresis as opposed to constipation or respiratory depression. Although the toxicological profile of U-50488 is still being investigated, its structural resemblance to U-47700 raises the possibility that it could be extremely dangerous.

MT-45

With a structure different from other therapeutic opioids, MT-45 [1-cyclohexyl-4-(1,2-diphenylethyl)piperazine] exhibits selective agonism of mu-opioid receptors, significantly lower affinities for delta and kappa opioid receptors, and potency comparable to morphine. Hair depigmentation and loss, dermatitis, folliculitis, disordered keratinization, and bilateral secondary cataracts necessitating surgery are among the side effects that have been reported. There have been fatal intoxication reports linked to MT-45 in Europe. Between November 2013 and July 2014, it was linked to 28 analytically confirmed deaths in Sweden.

7.2.5 Management of Acute Toxicity and Overdose

Clinical Features

Due to their strong affinity for mu-opioid receptors, fentanyl, and its analogsanalogs cause significant morbidity and mortality as well as respiratory and central nervous system depression. Miosis, also known as "pinpoint pupils," respiratory depression, and a lowered state of consciousness or coma are typical signs of an overdose. This is referred to as the "triad of opioid overdose." This can result in respiratory arrest and even death in cases of severe opioid toxicity. Aspiration risk can be elevated when vomiting occurs in the presence of diminished unconsciousness and/or protective airway reflexes. Consequently, intubation may be required for airway protection if there is a loss of protective airway reflexes and/or a significant central nervous system depression that does not improve with antidote therapy. Some of these synthetic opioids have longer half-lives than natural opioids, which may contribute to the reported prolonged admissions to intensive care for ongoing management. Changes in muscle tone, chest wall rigidity, "seizure-like" activity, confusion, affective changes, suppression of cough, orthostatic hypotension, urinary urgency or retention, folliculitis and dermatitis with hair loss, dry eyes, elevated liver enzymes, and delayed bilateral hearing loss are other side effects associated with synthetic opioids that have been reported. There have been reports of nasal burn or drip following inhalation and a bitter taste following oral ingestion; these effects are frequently observed with a variety of NPS, including non-opioid NPS (Misailidi et al., 2018).

Clinical Management

Respiratory depression and possibly death occur from a prolonged effect on the brainstem and cortical centers that control breathing rate during an overdose. As in any emergency, the primary goals of management should be to preserve breathing and circulation while safeguarding the airway. Naloxone reverses the effects of opioids quickly, both centrally and peripherally. It is a competitive mu-opioid receptor antagonist. The intramuscular, intranasal, intraosseous, subcutaneous, endotracheal, inhalational, and sublingual routes can all be used to administer naloxone. When possible, it should be administered intravenously as this lowers the risk of side effects like acute withdrawal and enables dose titration to the desired clinical response. Although there is a higher risk of side effects and acute withdrawal due to the unpredictable absorption of naloxone, intramuscular injection would be appropriate in the pre-hospital setting or where intravenous access is not possible. In order to lower the risk of needlestick injuries associated with intramuscular injection, there has been a growing interest in the use of intranasal naloxone in the pre-hospital setting. It is important to remember, though, that synthetic opioids' high potency, quick start of action, and lengthy half-life present unique difficulties for naloxone reversal. According to reports, administering larger or more frequent repeated doses of naloxone than is generally advised may be necessary to treat a synthetic opioid overdose.

7.2.6 Dependence and Withdrawal Syndromes

A variety of symptoms are associated with opioid dependence, such as decreased self-control over substance use, the prominence of substance use in a person's life, and physiological symptoms like tolerance and withdrawal. The best way to describe it is as a chronic, relapsing condition that often takes years or decades to fully heal between active use and periods of abstinence and relapse. Reduction of tolerance following a period of abstinence, like incarceration, raises the risk of overdose death. The evidence that is currently available indicates that non-fentanyl opioids are linked to the highest risk of all synthetic opioids and that repeated use of fentanyl and their analogs cause tolerance and dependence more quickly than with natural or semi-synthetic opioids. Similar to both natural and semi-synthetic opioids, typical withdrawal symptoms from these drugs include anxiety, sweating, diarrhea, cramping in the abdomen, bone pain, and shivers that resemble "goose flesh skin.". Withdrawal from synthetic opioids has been linked to psychotic symptoms and restless legs syndrome.

Structured drug treatment interventions (e.g., opioid agonist therapies, psychosocial interventions) are effective in treating opioid use disorders, and pharmacotherapies (e.g., methadone, buprenorphine) reduce the risk of all-cause and drug poisoning mortality. Hence, creating opportunities for those who may be exposed to new opioids to access drug treatment is an essential component of a comprehensive strategic response to the emergence of these compounds.

7.2.7 Laboratory Testing

Analytical techniques are crucial for determining synthetic opioids; the focus should be on identifying the parent drug and its metabolites, and the results should be correlated with intoxication symptoms and clinical outcomes. One significant issue is the steady influx of new synthetic opioids onto the market for controlled substances. Due to the low doses of the highly potent drugs, the concentrations expected in the biological samples are in the low ng to pg/ml or ng to pg/g range, requiring extremely sensitive methods of analysis. The majority of these new substances are not detected by routine screening and confirmation methods. Because the results do not alter the outcome and are not available in a timely manner, routine screening is not done in clinical practice (Misailidi et al., 2018).

Due to their increased sensitivity and specificity, current reliable methods for identifying synthetic opioids include liquid chromatography coupled to tandem mass spectrometry (LC-MS/MS) and gas chromatography coupled with mass spectrometry (GC-MS), which enable both qualitative and quantitative analyses in various biological matrices. In the past, GC-MS has been the preferred analyzer in toxicology and the gold standard test for detecting and quantifying drugs. The sample preparation may necessitate multiple post-extraction derivatization steps following the micro-extraction of the sample. Additionally, the detection of non-volatile or polar molecules may be limited, particularly when considering the excretion of hydrophilic metabolites in urine. For the analysis of synthetic opioids, LC-MS/MS is preferred because it can analyze polar molecules with fewer sample preparation steps and lower detection limits.

For the purpose of identifying synthetic opioids, both GC-MS and LC-MS/MS need current reference libraries and must contend with the ongoing emergence of new structural derivatives. The development of high-resolution (LC-HRMS) techniques with both targeted and untargeted workflows for synthetic opioid identification has been made possible by recent developments in mass spectrometry. Although most forensic labs do not have easy access to high-resolution mass spectrometry (time-of-flight, Orbitrap), it has the potential to be advantageous in identifying unknown compounds in the absence of a reference standard.

7.3 Public Health Crisis and Impact of Opioid Abuse

The abuse of heroin, prescription opioid analgesics, and illicitly produced fentanyl and its analogs is causing overdoses and overdose deaths in the United States, an unprecedented public health crisis. The misuse of prescription opioid analgesics has become an epidemic threat to public health over the last 20 years, affecting large areas of the US. The National Survey on Drug Use and Health (NSDUH) estimates that in 2015, 2.1 million individuals aged 12 or older "misused" opioid analgesics for the first time, and an estimated 12.5 (4.7%) million people "misused" pain relievers in the previous year. In 2015, there were about 2 million adults over the age of 12 who had "pain reliever use disorder."

Since the early 2000s, there has been a significant increase in overdose deaths in the United States related to prescription opioid analgesics, surpassing those from cocaine and heroin combined. Recent data from the CDC reveals that deaths from synthetic opioids like fentanyl and tramadol, excluding methadone, have also surpassed those from natural and semisynthetic opioids as well as methadone combined. Additionally, the CDC reports that illegally made fentanyl, its analogs, and heroin are the primary contributors to the alarming rise in opioid overdose deaths in recent years. The more recent data from the CDC suggests that fentanyl and its analogs might be developing into a distinct class of abuse that doesn't combine with other illegal opioids. The President of the United States declared the opioid crisis a national public health emergency on October 26, 2017, in response to the extraordinary, dramatic, and ongoing rise in overdoses and overdose deaths related to opioids.

7.3.1 Public Health Impact of Abuse of Fentanyl and Its Analogues Relative to Prescription Opioid Analgesics

Pharmacological Considerations

The two primary pharmacological effects of opioid painkillers (e.g., morphine, hydrocodone, oxycodone, etc.) are largely responsible for their detrimental effects on public health: (1) opioid analgesics, a highly addictive class of drugs, activate the brain's reward pathways to produce intense euphoria; and (2) when taken in high doses, opioid analgesics consistently depress the brain's respiratory center. The most common cause of death from overdoses on these drugs is respiratory depression, which results in total respiratory failure. An individual's opioid tolerance is a significant additional risk factor for overdose. Individuals with low or nonexistent tolerance are more vulnerable to fatal overdoses from opioid analgesics.

Furthermore, the depressant effects of opioid analgesics, including fentanyl and its analogs, may be enhanced by the concurrent use of other central nervous system depressant medications, such as other opioids, sedatives or hypnotics, general anesthetics, phenothiazines (antipsychotics), tranquilizers, skeletal muscle relaxants, sedating antihistamines, or alcohol-containing beverages. A lethal fentanyl overdose can also occur from the concurrent use of medications that block fentanyl metabolism and the cessation of medications that promote fentanyl metabolism (Socías and Wood, 2017).

Public Health Impact of Abuse of Prescription Opioid Analgesics and Pharmaceutical Fentanyl

A significant change in the way prescription opioid analgesics are used clinically to treat pain has occurred in the United States since the 1990s. This increase has been both gradual and noticeable. The total number of opioid analgesic prescriptions written each year increased gradually and peaked in 2010 or 2011. When all opioid analgesics were combined, 303 million prescriptions were written in 2011. Prescriptions for opioid analgesics increased concurrently with a gradual and noticeable rise in diversion (forensic drug exhibits), emergency department visits, inpatient hospital admissions, admissions for addiction treatment, and deaths linked to these opioid analgesics (Table 7.9). As an illustration, the National Forensic Laboratory System (NFLIS) annual reports from the DEA for the years 2000 and 2010 listed 7,680 and 137,670 forensic drug exhibits for all prescription opioid analgesics, respectively. With the exception of methadone, 17,545 inpatient hospitalizations for prescription opioid analgesics occurred in 2006. 366,181 emergency department visits in 2011 were connected to the non-medical use of opioid analgesics or narcotic painkillers. In 2010, 16,651 deaths were linked to opioid analgesics, according to the CDC (Socías and Wood, 2017).

Increases in prescriptions, forensic drug exhibits, and emergency room visits involving fentanyl and deaths involving synthetic opioids excluding methadone (e.g., such as tramadol, fentanyl, etc.) also increased in tandem with the overall rise in prescription opioid analgesics. In 2000 and 2010, the NFLIS annual reports referenced 23 and 579 fentanyl-related forensic drug exhibits, respectively. The CDC reports that from 730 in 1999 to 3,007 in 2010, deaths associated with synthetic opioids—apart from methadone—rose. Deaths from synthetic opioids, other than methadone, increased significantly between 2013 and 2016. Illegal fentanyl production is primarily responsible for the recent rise in opioid-related drug-related deaths, with illicit fentanyl analog production playing a smaller role.

The DEA is not currently aware of any diversion or abuse of pharmaceutical products containing fentanyl analogs, such as alfentanil, remifentanil, sufentanil, carfentanil, and thiafentanil that have been approved by the FDA for medical purposes. However, there has been recent evidence of carfentanil on the illicit market. Law enforcement has determined that the carfentanil discovered thus far is of illicit origin and is produced in clandestine labs.

Table 7.9: Increases in annual prescriptions (or kilograms) and adverse health impact (emergency department admissions, inpatient hospitalizations, addiction treatment admissions, and deaths) related to prescription opioid analgesics as compared to fentanyl or synthetic opioids

Drugs	Increase in opioid prescriptions from 1998 to 2011 (Increase in kilograms sold from 1999 to 2010)	Increase in Emergency Department visits from 2004 to 2011	Increase in impatient hospitalizations from 1999 to 2006	Increase in admissions for addiction treatment from 1999 to 2009	Increase in deaths from 1999 to 2010
All Prescription Opioid analgesics	2.0-fold (4.0-fold)	2.5-fold	2.6-fold	6-fold	4.1-fold
Fentanyl (or) Synthetic opioids	4.4-fold	2.0-fold			4.1-fold

Source: https://www.ussc.gov/sites/default/files/pdf/amendment-process/public-hearings-and-meetings/20171205/Tella.pdf

Public Health Impact of Abuse of Illicitly Manufactured Fentanyl and Its Analogues

Evidence from law enforcement and public health indicates that the current opioid public health crisis has primarily been caused in recent years by fentanyl and its analogs produced illegally. The total number of annual prescriptions for opioid analgesics showed a slight decline after peaking around 2010–2011, particularly from 2014 through 2016. Fentanyl prescriptions also followed a similar pattern, peaking in 2008 and then declining slightly between 2014 and 2016. The number of fentanyl-related encounters with law enforcement has sharply increased in recent years, in contrast to the decrease in fentanyl prescriptions (Table 7.10). Fentanyl-containing forensic drug exhibits increased from 978 in 2013 to 36,134 in 2016, according to the NFLIS database (database queried on October 30, 2017). As of October 30, 2017, there were 21,872 fentanyl reports from January through June 2017 on NFLIS and 6,808 corresponding data for fentanyl analogs. In line with the rise in fentanyl-related encounters with law enforcement, deaths associated with synthetic opioids, other than methadone (e.g., tramadol, fentanyl, etc.) have also significantly increased recently (Table 7.10). Evidence suggests that fentanyl produced illegally is the main cause of deaths related to this class of opioid drugs.

According to the CDC, drug overdose deaths involving synthetic opioids (e.g., fentanyl and tramadol, etc.), excluding methadone, increased from 3,105 in 2013 to 9,580 in 2015. Drug overdose deaths involving synthetic opioids, excluding methadone, for the 12-month period ending in January 2017 (20,145 deaths) approximately doubled from the corresponding data for the period ending in January 2016 (9,945 deaths), according to provisional data released in August 2017 by the CDC, National Center for Health Statistics. A daily average of fifty-five Americans are thought to pass away from synthetic opioid overdoses, excluding methadone. Excluding methadone, the number of deaths linked to synthetic opioids outnumbered those linked to natural and semisynthetic opioids as well as methadone combined. Many recently released studies concluded that the majority of these synthetic opioids (apart from methadone) related deaths were not caused by pharmaceutical fentanyl, but rather by illegally produced fentanyl and, to a lesser extent, illicitly manufactured fentanyl analogs. While deaths from prescription opioid analgesics have stabilized, overdose deaths from illicitly manufactured fentanyl and its analogs have increased recently (Socías and Wood, 2017).

Table 7.10: Changes in annual prescriptions and increases in forensic drug exhibits for fentanyl and deaths related to synthetic opioids excluding methadone

Change in fentanyl prescriptions from 2013 to 2016	**Change in forensic drug exhibits for fentanyl from 2013 to 2016**	**Change in deaths related to synthetic opioids excluding methadone, from 2013 to 2016**	**Change in deaths related to synthetic opioids excluding methadone, from 1999 to 2016**
13.8% decline	37-fold increase	6.5-fold increase	27.6-fold increase

Source: https://www.ussc.gov/sites/default/files/pdf/amendment-process/public-hearings-and-meetings/20171205/Tella.pdf

According to the CDC data, deaths caused by synthetic opioids, not including methadone (such as fentanyl, tramadol, etc.), skyrocketed from 730 in 1999 to 20,145 in 2016, marking a 27.6-fold increase.

There is a population that uses heroin, fentanyl, and other prescription opioid analgesics that is also likely to use fentanyl analogs. As is the case with heroin and prescription opioid analgesics, someone who takes a fentanyl analog runs the risk of becoming addicted to drugs, overdosing, and passing away. The identity, purity, and quantity of illegally produced fentanyl and its analogs are unknown and inconsistent, resulting in serious health risks for the user. This is because the drugs are sourced from unregulated sources. Users may unknowingly consume unknown amounts of fentanyl and/or its analogs in products marketed as heroin or in counterfeit prescription pills, which increases the harm associated with the abuse of these substances. According to recent CDC data, injection is the most often used method of administration for fentanyl and its analogs in fatalities. The high potencies of fentanyl and its analogs, along with this mode of administration, raise the possibility of overdoses and overdose deaths related to these substances.

A Closer Look

Dangers of Synthetic Opioids

Since the early 2010s, synthetic opioids have significantly contributed to overall opioid-related overdose mortalities. For reference, of the 68,630 opioid-related deaths recorded in 2020, 56,516 involved synthetic opioids (primarily fentanyl and its analogs). This rise in synthetic-opioid-related use in recent years has been accompanied by a corresponding decrease in the use of other illicit opioids, such as heroin. Some potential reasons why synthetic opioid use has become so ubiquitous have been postulated to include lower production costs, stronger or longer-lasting highs, and increasingly efficient synthesis by manufacturers. As noted by the US Drug Enforcement Agency, a relatively common factor in synthetic opioid overdoses is their utilization as cheap adulterants in preparations of other illicit drugs. This is not to say that there are no users who intentionally seek out synthetic opioids. Still, the role of synthetic opioids as additives unknown to the user is nevertheless thought to play a significant role. Fentanyl and other synthetic opioids have been detected as components in mixtures of cocaine, methamphetamine, heroin, and counterfeit pills. The increased danger of overdose from synthetic opioids versus substances such as heroin is simply related to their greatly increased potency and efficacy, as well as increased availability in the drug supply. What may be a "typical" dose of an opioid like heroin is certainly lethal without rapid intervention when a synthetic opioid like fentanyl or carfentanil is substituted in its place. Furthermore, a heroin overdose can take 20–30 min before it leads to a fatality. Fentanyl, on the other hand, can precipitate a profoundly dangerous and life-threatening respiratory arrest within 2–5 min.

Presentation

The signs and symptoms of overdose from synthetic opioids are essentially the same as those seen from overdose secondary to natural and semisynthetic opioids. Through various pharmacological mechanisms, synthetic opioids potently act on the CNS to produce various effects, ranging from euphoria and analgesia to respiratory depression, coma, and death. Respiratory arrest followed by death is the most serious outcome of an overdose. However, even nonfatal overdoses can produce variably debilitating results, with life-altering effects such as permanent parkinsonism or psychosis secondary to hypoxic brain injury. The treatment of opioid overdose revolves chiefly around restoring a patient's ability to breathe spontaneously. As is standard in treating opioid overdoses in general, the MOR antagonist naloxone is the first-line medication for reversal in the case of synthetic opioid overdose. Given the increased potency of synthetic opioids, it has been hypothesized that increased dosages of naloxone are necessary to reverse their effects. Additionally, given the wide therapeutic window of naloxone, and with the increasing prevalence of these substances in circulation, suggestions have been made to simply increase the standard doses of naloxone administered by the first responders who initially arrive on the scene to an opioid overdose.

Summary

- Opioids are a group of analgesic agents commonly used in clinical practice. There are three classical opioid receptors (DOP, KOP, and MOP), while the novel NOP receptor is considered to be a non-opioid branch of the opioid receptor family.
- Buprenorphine is classified as a partial agonist. It has a high affinity but low efficacy at the mu receptor, where it yields a partial effect upon binding, yet possesses kappa receptor antagonist activity, making it useful as an analgesic, and in opioid abuse deterrence, detoxification, and maintenance therapies. Buprenorphine has a poor bioavailability with extensive first-pass effect by the liver.
- The opioid receptor antagonists naloxone and naltrexone are competitive antagonists at the mu, kappa, and delta receptors, with a high affinity for the mu receptor but lacking any mu receptor efficacy. Naloxone and naltrexone act centrally and peripherally but have differing pharmacokinetic profiles favoring different therapeutic uses.
- A unique analgesic, tramadol is an atypical opioid, a 4-phenyl-piperidine analog of codeine, with partial mu agonist activity in addition to central GABA, catecholamine, and serotonergic activities. Tramadol is used primarily as an analgesic but has demonstrated usefulness in treating opioid withdrawal.
- Morphine is metabolized by demethylation and glucuronidation; glucuronidation is the predominant mode of metabolism, producing morphine-6 glucuronide (M6G) and morphine-3 glucuronide (M3G) in a ratio of 6:1, while approximately 5% of the drug is demethylated into normorphine.
- Hydrocodone is indicated for moderate-to-moderately severe pain as well as symptomatic relief of nonproductive cough, and it is the most commonly used opioid.
- Hydromorphone is metabolized primarily to hydromorphone-3-glucuronide (H3G), which, similar to the corresponding M3G, is not only devoid of analgesic activity but also evokes a range of dose-dependent excited behaviors, including allodynia, myoclonus, and seizures in animal models.
- Methadone is a unique synthetic opioid, unrelated to standard opioids (leading to its usefulness in patients with "true" morphine allergies). It is a basic and lipophilic drug with an excellent (though highly variable) oral bioavailability (from 40% to 100%). It can be crushed or dissolved to deliver down an NG tube and is also available in a liquid.
- Levorphanol is a synthetic morphine analog, the optical isomer of dextromethorphan. It is as potent as hydromorphone but longer lasting. It is a mu, kappa, and delta agonist, as well as being an NMDA antagonist. It is metabolized to a 3-glucuronide of unknown activity.
- Synthetic opioids are substances that are synthesized in a laboratory and that act on the same targets in the brain as natural opioids (e.g., morphine and codeine) to produce analgesic (pain relief) effects. In contrast, natural opioids are naturally occurring substances extracted from the seed pod of certain varieties of poppy plants. Some synthetic opioids, such as fentanyl and methadone, have been approved for medical use.

- Carfentanil and ocfentanil are two potent synthetic opioids that have been implicated in the international opioid overdose crisis, particularly in the United States and some European countries. Acetylfentanyl and furanylfentanyl have also recently been associated with cases of overdose and death in the United States.

References

1. Armenian P, Vo KT, Barr-Walker J, et al. Fentanyl, fentanyl analogues and novel synthetic opioids: a comprehensive review. Neuropharmacology 2018; 134: 121–132.
2. Belzak L, Halverson J. The opioid crisis in Canada: a national perspective. Health Promot Chronic Dis Prev Can 2018; 38: 224–233.
3. Benyamin R, Trescot AM, Datta S, et al. Opioid complications and side effects. Pain Phys 2008; 11: S105–20.
4. Brook K, Bennett J, Desai SP. The chemical history of morphine: an 8000-year journey, from resin to de-novo synthesis. J Anesth Hist 2017; 3: 50–55.
5. Dorn S, Lembo A, Cremonini F. Opioid-induced bowel dysfunction: epidemiology, pathophysiology, diagnosis, and initial therapeutic approach. Am J Gastroenterol Suppl 2014; 2: 31.
6. Ghelardini C, Mannelli LD, Bianchi E. The pharmacological basis of opioids. Clin Case Min Bone Metab 2015; 12: 219.
7. Helander A, Bradley M, Hasselblad A, et al. Acute skin and hair symptoms followed by severe, delayed eye complications in subjects using the synthetic opioid MT-45. Br J Dermatol 2017; 176: 1021–1027.
8. Manchikanti L, Sanapati J, Benyamin RM, et al. Reframing the prevention strategies of the opioid crisis: focusing on prescription opioids, fentanyl, and heroin epidemic. Pain Phys 2018; 21: 309–326.
9. Misailidi N, Papoutsis I, Nikolaou P, et al. Furanylfentanyl: another fentanyl analogue, another hazard for public health. Forensic Toxicol 2018; 36: 1.
10. Moy JK, Hartung JE, Duque MG, et al. Distribution of functional opioid receptors in human dorsal root ganglion neurons. Pain 2020; 161: 1636–1649.
11. Pardo B, Taylor J, Caulkins J, et al. The dawn of a new synthetic opioid era: the need for innovative interventions. Addiction 2020; 16: 1304–1312.
12. Prekupec MP, Mansky PA, Baumann MH. Misuse of novel synthetic opioids: a deadly new trend. J Addict Med 2017; 11: 256–265.
13. Socías ME, Wood E. Epidemic of deaths from fentanyl overdose. BMJ 2017; 358: j4355. DOI: 10.1136/bmj.j4355.
14. Suzuki J, El-Haddad S. A review: fentanyl and non-pharmaceutical fentanyls. Drug Alcohol Depend 2017; 171: 107–116.
15. Wilson N, Kariisa M, Seth P, et al. Drug and opioid-involved overdose deaths: United States, 2017–2018. Morb Mort Weekly Rep 2020; 69: 290–297.

Chapter

DESIGNER STEROIDS AND PERFORMANCE-ENHANCING DRUGS

8

Contents

Introduction

Designer steroids are artificial steroids made by slightly altering the chemical makeup of anabolic steroids that already exist. With these changes, their androgenic (masculinizing) effects should be minimized while their anabolic effects are maximized. This could make them more potent or harder to find in drug tests. Designer steroids have historically been used by bodybuilders and athletes to obtain an advantage over their rivals or to evade detection in doping tests.

Nevertheless, there are a lot of risks associated with using designer steroids. As a result of their frequent covert creation and lack of thorough safety or effectiveness testing, they may have severe and unexpected side effects. Hormonal imbalances, liver damage, cardiovascular issues, and psychological effects are a few examples of these side effects.

Athletes looking to avoid sanctions run the risk of using designer steroids because numerous sports organizations and anti-doping agencies regularly add them to their lists of prohibited substances.

It's crucial to remember that most sports organizations forbid the use of performance-enhancing substances, including designer steroids, and that athletes who are found using them risk severe penalties. Furthermore, using these substances to enhance one's physical appearance or athletic performance is risky due to the health risks involved (Jones et al., 2018).

Orientation and Directional Terms

Term	Definition	Illustration
Tamoxifen	Tamoxifen is a selective estrogen receptor modulator used to prevent breast cancer in women and men. It is also being studied for other types of cancer. It has been used for Albright syndrome. Tamoxifen is typically taken daily by mouth for five years for breast cancer.	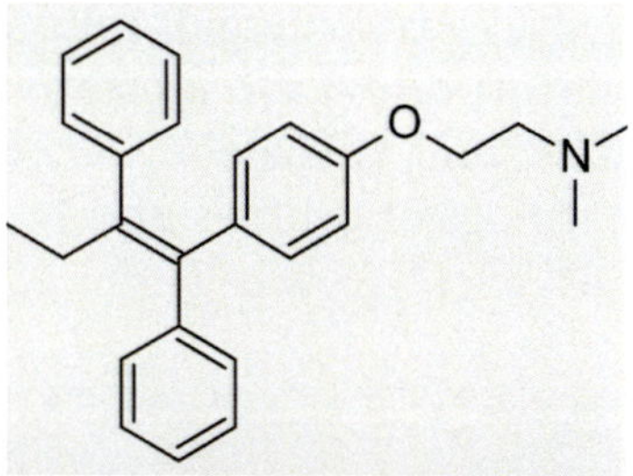
Mineralocorticoid	Mineralocorticoids are a class of corticosteroids, which in turn are a class of steroid hormones. Mineralocorticoids are produced in the adrenal cortex and influence salt and water balances (electrolyte balance and fluid balance). The primary mineralocorticoid is aldosterone.	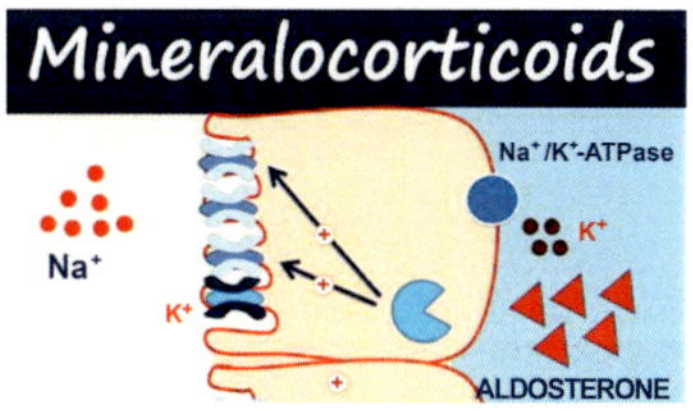
Heat shock proteins (HSP)	HSPs are a family of proteins that are produced by cells in response to exposure to stressful conditions, including exposure to heat, cold, UV light, infection, exercise, starvation; fasting and hypoxia. HSPs are classified by their molecular weight.	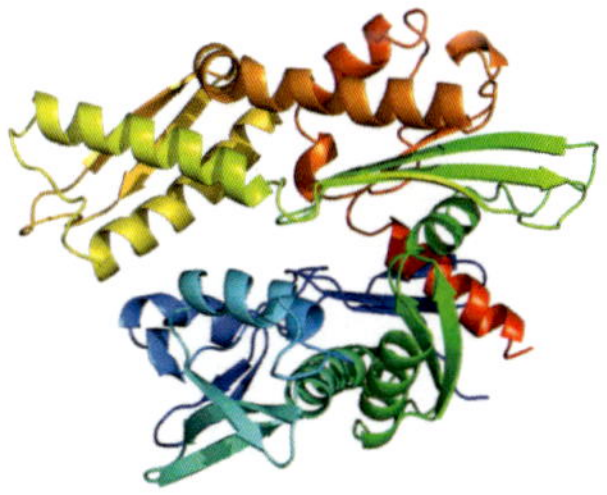
Dihydrotestosterone	Dihydrotestosterone is an endogenous androgen sex steroid and hormone primarily involved in the growth and repair of the prostate and the penis, as well as the production of sebum and body hair composition.	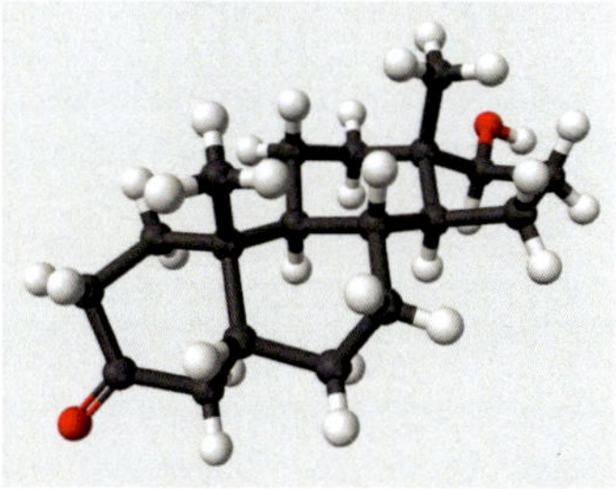
Methylclostebol	Methylclostebol is a synthetic, orally active anabolic-androgenic steroid (AAS) and designer steroid that has been sold on the Internet as a "dietary supplement", but it has never been studied for medical use. It is the 17α-alkylated variant of clostebol (4-chlorotestosterone).	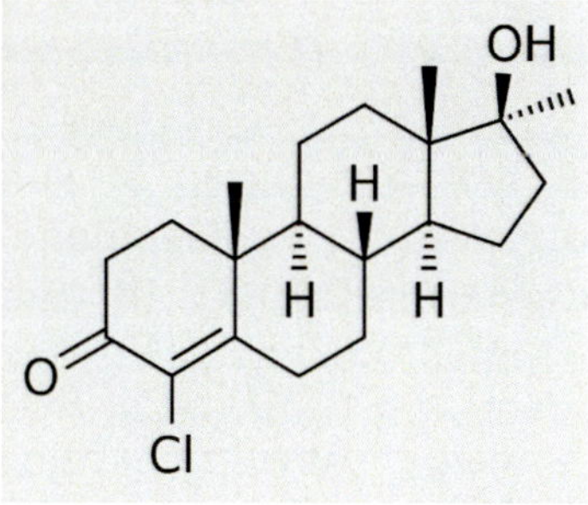

8.1 Steroid Hormones

Steroid hormones are lipophilic compounds that are derived from cholesterol. They are classified as corticosteroids (glucocorticoids and mineralocorticoids) and sex steroids (androgens, estrogens, and gestagens) according to their pharmacological profiles and receptor-binding affinities.

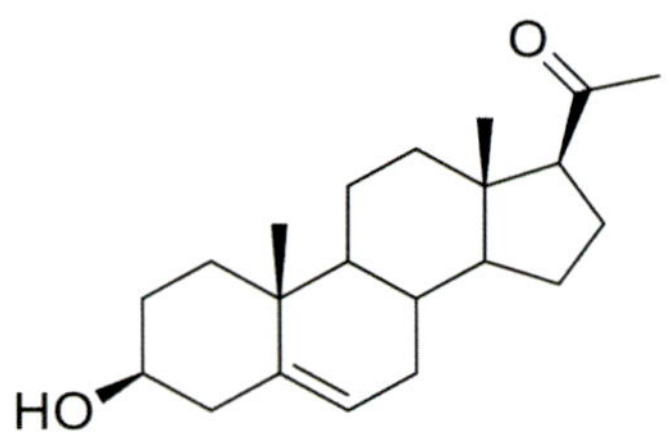

(I)

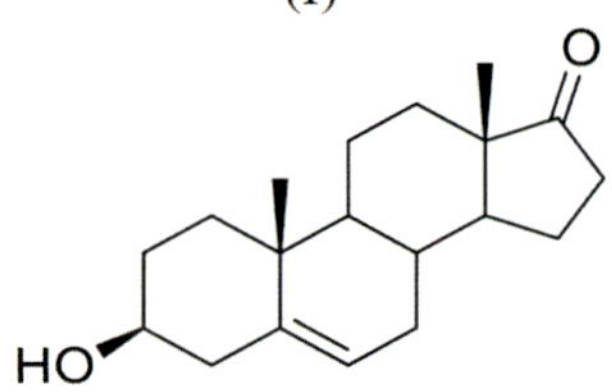

(II)

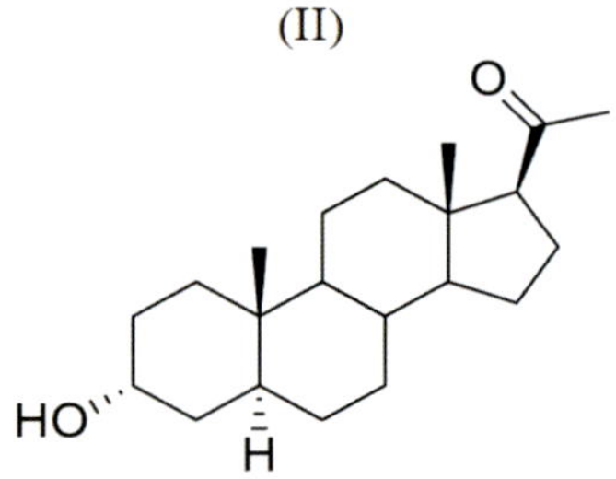

(III)

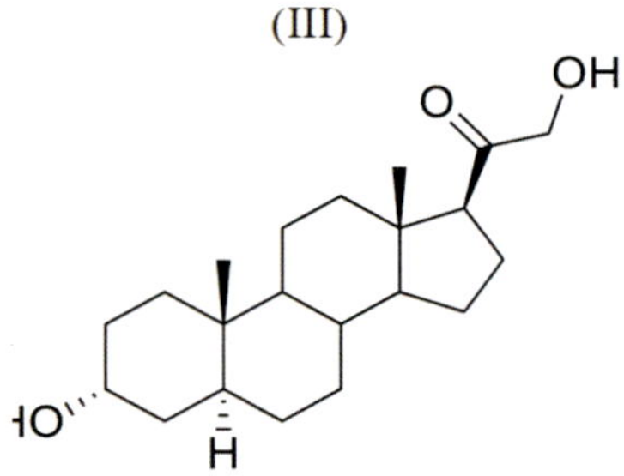

(IV)

Figure 8.1. Structures of some important neurosteroids: (I) Pregnenolone, (II) dehydro-epiandrosterone (DHEA), (III) Allopregnanolone, (IV) Tetrahydrodeoxycorticosterone.

Source: https://www.ncbi.nlm.nih.gov/pmc/articles/PMC4462045/figure/F2/

Pregnenolone is the primary pregnane that remains after the cytochrome P450 enzyme CYPscc cleaves the cholesterol side chain. The general precursor of androgens, estrogens, and corticosteroids is prostenoid hormone (pregnenolone). The adrenal gland is the primary site of corticosteroid synthesis. Mineral and water transport (mineralcorticoids), energy metabolism, and the immune system's reaction to stress (glucocorticoids) are all regulated by corticosteroids. The androgens and estrogens are produced when the molecule loses its C_{20}/C_{21} bonds. The development of female sex traits, menstrual cycle regulation, and pregnancy maintenance are all aided by the female sex steroids, estrogens, and gestagens. They also have an impact on how male spermatogenesis and sperm maturation are regulated. Androgens are the source of estrogens. Estrone and estradiol are produced from androstenedione and testosterone, respectively, by the enzyme complex aromatase, CYP19. Apart from their previously mentioned roles, steroids have a significant impact on the brain. These include neuroactive steroids, which are exclusively synthesized within the central nervous system, and peripheral steroids, which are involved in brain functioning (Jones et al., 2018).

8.1.1 Androgens

There has been a thorough review of the pharmacology of androgens and the androgen receptor. Male sex hormones known as androgens stimulate anabolic and androgenic effects. Other endogenous androgens such as androstenedione, dehydro-epiandrosterone (DHEA) and its sulfate (DHEAS), and androstenediol, in addition to testosterone and its 5α-hydrogenated form, the more active metabolite 5α-dihydrostestosterone (5α-DHT), also play important roles in humans. The testis's Leydig cells are where men produce the majority of their testosterone. Women's ovaries generate testosterone and androstenedione. The hypothalamic-pituitary-gonadal (HPG) axis controls androgen biosynthesis in the testa and ovaries. When gonadotropin-releasing hormone (GnRH) is released by the hypothalamus, the anterior pituitary stimulates the release of luteinizing hormone (LH), which in turn causes the production of testosterone. Reduced pituitary sensitivity to GnRH and reduced hypothalamic release of GnRH are the two mechanisms by which testosterone produces negative feedback. Adrenocorticotropic hormone (ACTH) controls the adrenal cortex in both sexes, where the production of the weaker androgens occurs. The main proteins to which testosterone is bound in the bloodstream are albumin and sex hormone binding globulin (SHBG). After being transported to its intended tissues, free testosterone primarily diffuses into the cells where it binds to the androgen receptor (AR), gets reduced to 5α-DHT by 5α-reductase, or gets aromatized to estradiol by aromatase (Lusetti et al., 2018).

8.1.2 Androgen Receptor-Mediated Action

Androgens primarily work through the androgen receptor, which is part of the nuclear receptor superfamily. The receptor is found in the cytosol, supported by heat shock proteins and other chaperones. When an androgen binds to the receptor, it causes the complex to break apart, allowing the receptor to interact with coregulators. This interaction enables the androgen receptor to move into the cell nucleus and form a homodimer. Once dimerized, the receptor complex attaches to specific promoter regions of target genes called androgen response elements (AREs) and acts as a ligand-dependent transcription factor. While it is possible for the androgen receptor to form heterodimers with estrogen receptor α or orphan nuclear receptors, this is less common and leads to the activation of different target genes. The action of the androgen receptor can be influenced by allosteric modulation, phosphorylation, and coregulators. Coregulators play a significant role in regulating the androgen receptor and other steroid hormone receptors, with recent studies highlighting their importance as coactivators or corepressors. Variations in coregulator expression in tissues targeted by androgens help explain the diverse effects of these hormones (Dahmani et al., 2018).

8.1.3 Non-Classical Actions

Steroid hormones have been shown to act through non-genomic pathways in addition to the traditional, genomic mechanism of action. It is well known that estrogens can cause fast steroid hormone actions by interfering with the intracellular trans-membrane orphan G-protein coupled receptor (GPCR) GPR30. Recently, the effects of rapid estrogen action on human behavior have been reviewed. Additionally, progesterone and androgens can interact through non-genomic pathways. It was discovered that non-classical testosterone actions mediated their effects in a number of tissues, including the immune, cardiovascular, musculoskeletal, and reproductive systems. There is discussion of membrane-associated ARs that impact intracellular Ca^{2+} levels, signaling pathways via an SHBG receptor, androgen-tyrosine kinase interactions that modify coregulator function through phosphorylation. A group recently offered support to the theory that fast androgen signaling is carried out by a membrane-bound GPCR (Lusetti et al., 2018).

8.2 Designer Androgens

The endogenous androgens, testosterone and 5α-DHT, are the source of androgenic anabolic steroids. These compounds underwent chemical changes to increase their oral bioavailability, minimize their estrogenic side effects, improve their pharmacokinetics, and produce more selective anabolic effects. It was completely unsuccessful to distinguish between androgenic and anabolic activity. Some AAS, like nandrolone and stanozolol, have a relatively high anabolic-androgenic index, meaning that although their anabolic effects outweigh their androgenic effects, they are still inseparable. Oral administration is made possible by 17α-methylation's reduction of inactivation during first pass metabolism, but concurrently increased liver toxicity. It is still not possible to totally prevent estrogen-related side effects, but they can be lessened by methylating at C2, introducing a 1,2-double bond, or removing the C19-methyl group, which prevents the aromatase enzyme complex from aromatizing the A-ring. Additional changes include the addition of extra double bonds in rings A, B, and/or C, the halogenation, hydroxylation, or methylation at C-1, C-2, C-4, C-6, C-7, or C-11, as well as the attachment of an extra ring at C-2/C-3 (Lusetti et al., 2018).

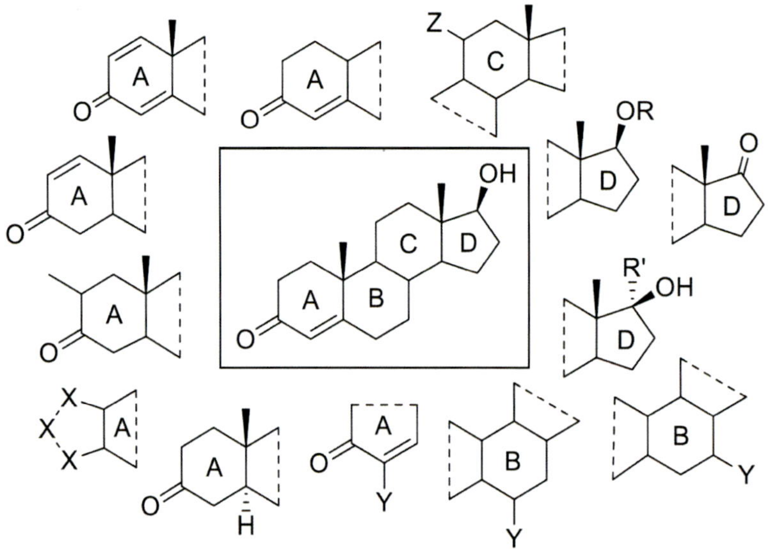

Figure 8.2. Modifications of the testosterone molecule to yield designer anabolics.

Source: https://www.ncbi.nlm.nih.gov/pmc/articles/PMC4462045/figure/F1/

8.3 Anabolic Steroid

The class of medications known as anabolic steroids, or anabolic-androgenic steroids (AAS), is structurally related to testosterone, the primary hormone involved in the male sex, and exerts its effects by binding to the androgen receptor. In addition to their many medical applications, anabolic steroids are used by athletes to improve their performance, strength, and muscle mass.

Excessive dosages or prolonged use of AAS can pose health risks. These side effects include high blood pressure, acne, liver damage (primarily from most oral AAS), left ventricular hypertrophy, and detrimental changes in cholesterol levels (increased low-density lipoprotein and decreased high-density lipoprotein). When athletes use steroids in addition to other drugs, these risks are exacerbated and their bodies are severely harmed. The effects of anabolic steroids on the heart can result in strokes and myocardial infarctions. AAS may also be the cause of conditions related to hormone imbalances, such as gynecomastia and reduced testicular size. AAS has the potential to irreversibly masculinize women and children.

AAS are controversial when used as performance-enhancing drugs in bodybuilding, sports, and racing because of their negative side effects and ability to give athletes an unfair advantage in physical contests. The majority of significant sporting organizations forbid their use, which is known as doping. Since the beginning of the Olympics in Ancient Greece, athletes have searched for drugs to improve their performance. In IOC-accredited laboratories, AAS have been the most frequently found doping agent for a long time. In many nations, anabolic steroids are categorized as Schedule III controlled substances. There is frequently a black market where users can purchase illegally obtained, covertly produced, or even counterfeit medications in nations where AAS are prohibited substances (Smit and de Ronde, 2018).

8.3.1 Uses

With differing degrees of success, doctors have employed AAS for a variety of purposes since the 1930s, when testosterone was discovered and synthesized. These fall into the broad categories of androgenic, anabolic, and other uses.

Medical

Anabolic

- Bone marrow stimulation: AAS constituted the cornerstone of treatment for hypoplastic anemias resulting from leukemia, renal failure, or aplastic anemia for many years.
- Growth stimulation: Pediatric endocrinologists can treat children with AAS who are experiencing growth failure. However, this is only a secondary treatment because synthetic growth hormone, which has fewer side effects, is readily available.
- Patients with chronic wasting diseases like cancer and AIDS have been administered AAS, which stimulates appetite and preserves and increases muscle mass.
- In older men, stimulation of lean body mass and prevention of bone loss are suggested by certain studies.
- On the other hand, low-dose testosterone supplementation in elderly men with low testosterone levels was found to have no beneficial effects on quality of life, insulin sensitivity, body composition, or physical performance in a 2006 placebo-controlled trial.
- Prevention or treatment of osteoporosis in postmenopausal women. This use of nandrolone decanoate is authorized. AAS saw very little use for this purpose despite being indicated for this indication because of their virilizing side effects.
- Aiding weight gain following surgery or physical trauma, during chronic infection, or in the context of unexplained weight loss.
- Counteracting the catabolic effect of long-term corticosteroid therapy.
- It is well known that oxyandrolone is a safe treatment for individuals recovering from severe burns, as it improves both short- and long-term outcomes.
- Treatment for alcoholic hepatitis, hypogonadism, inherited angioedema, and idiopathic short stature.
- Methyltestosterone is used to treat menopausal symptoms (particularly for osteoporosis, hot flashes, and to increase libido and energy),

postpartum breast pain and engorgement, and breast cancer in women. It is also used to treat delayed puberty, hypogonadism, cryptorchidism, and erectile dysfunction in males.

(Smit and de Ronde, 2018)

Androgenic

- For men with low testosterone levels, such as those with late-onset hypogonadism, androgen replacement therapy is beneficial in boosting libido in older men.
- Male puberty induction: Many boys who are worried about their severely delayed puberty are given androgens. In boys with delayed puberty, testosterone has been shown to increase height, weight, and fat-free mass. It is currently almost the only androgen used for this purpose.
- By causing masculine secondary sexual characteristics like a deepening of the voice, increased bone and muscle mass, masculine fat distribution, facial and body hair, and clitoral enlargement, as well as mental changes like a reduction in gender dysphoria and an increase in sex drive, masculinizing hormone therapy is beneficial for transgender men, other transmasculine people, and intersex people.

Enhancing Performance

Many who use steroids are not athletes. It is estimated that between one million and three million Americans, or 1% of the total population, have used AAS. Studies conducted in the US have revealed that the majority of AAS users are middle-class men, with a median age of approximately 25, who use the drugs primarily for cosmetic purposes and are not competitive bodybuilders or athletes.

According to a study by insurance company Blue Cross Blue Shield, the use of steroids and related drugs increased by 25% among boys aged 12 to 17 between 1999 and 2000. Of these, 20% claimed to take the drugs more for their appearance than for athletic purposes. According to a different study, less than 1% of college students used AAS for non-medical purposes. In a recent survey, 78.4% of steroid users identified as noncompetitive bodybuilders and non-athletes. Approximately 13% of users reported engaging in unsafe injection practices, like sharing or reusing needles or sharing multidose vials. However, a 2007 study discovered that sharing needles was incredibly rare among people using AAS for non-medical purposes—less than 1% of users reported doing so. According to a different 2007 study, 74 % of non-medical AAS users had post-secondary degrees, more had graduated from college, and fewer had not completed high school, compared to what is typically found in the general population. According to the same study, people who use AAS for non-medical reasons are more likely than the general population to be employed and have higher household incomes (Andrews et al., 2018).

AAS users typically take issue with the media's and politicians' portrayal of AAS as lethal. One study found that people who use AAS also have mistrust for their doctors and that 56% of the sample had not told their doctors they used AAS. Similar results were found in another study conducted in 2007. It showed that although 66% of people using AAS for non-medical purposes were willing to seek medical supervision for their steroid use, 58% did not trust their doctors, 92% thought the medical community did not know enough about AAS use for non-medical purposes, and 100% thought that the public exaggerated the risks associated with AAS use. A new study has also revealed that long-term users of AAS exhibited stronger support for more traditional male roles and were more likely to exhibit symptoms of muscular dysmorphia.

Men and women in a wide range of professional sports have utilized AAS to gain a competitive advantage or aid in injury recovery. Bodybuilding, weightlifting, track and field events such as shot put, cycling, baseball, wrestling, mixed martial arts, boxing, football, and cricket are among these sports. The regulations of the majority of sports' governing bodies forbid such use. Teenagers do use AAS, particularly those who play sports that are competitive. It has been suggested that the prevalence of use among high-school students in the U. S. could reach a maximum of 2 % (Mullen et al., 2020).

Dosages

The most frequently utilized AAS in medicine are metandienone (methandrostenolone), stanozolol, testosterone and its various esters (mostly testosterone undecanoate, testosterone enanthate, testosterone cypionate, and testosterone propionate), and nandrolone esters (usually nandrolone decanoate and nandrolone phenylpropionate). Methyltestosterone, oxandrolone, mesterolone, and oxymetholone, along with metenolone (methylandrostenolone) esters (particularly metenolone acetate and metenolone enanthate) and fluoxymesterone, have also been accessible and used frequently, albeit to a lesser degree. Dihydrotestosterone (DHT), which is also notable in its esters but is not commonly used in medicine, is also known as androstanolone or stanolone when used medicinally. In veterinary medicine, trenbolone acetate and belindone undecylenate are used. Designer steroids are AAS that are sold on the black market but have not been authorized for use in medicine. Renowned designer steroids comprise desoxymethyltestosterone, methasterone, trenbolone enanthate, 1-testosterone (dihydroboldenone), tetrahydrogestrinone, and methylstenbolone.

Oral pills, injectable steroids, topical creams and gels, and skin patches are the four common ways that AAS are administered. The most convenient method is oral administration. Oral testosterone is quickly absorbed, but only around one-sixth of it is available in active form before it is mostly converted to inactive metabolites. To make testosterone derivatives sufficiently active when taken orally, they are alkylated at the 17α position, for example. fluoxymesterone and methyltestosterone. Because of this alteration, the liver is less able to break down these substances before they enter the bloodstream.

Parenterally administered testosterone has a more irregular prolonged absorption time and exhibits higher muscle activity when administered in the form of enanthate, undecanoate, or cypionate ester. At the injection site, these derivatives hydrolyze to release free testosterone. The frequency of injections for medical purposes varies depending on the esters used but typically ranges from once every 12 weeks to twice a week. To keep the hormone levels in the system more consistent, a more frequent schedule might be preferable. In order to prevent abrupt fluctuations in the drug's concentration in the blood, injectable steroids are normally injected into the muscle rather than the vein. Furthermore, intravenous injection of estered testosterone carries the risk of causing a dangerous embolism (clot) in the bloodstream due to its dissolution in oil (Kanayama et al., 2018).

Another option for delivering a continuous dosage through the skin and into the bloodstream is to use transdermal patches, which are adhesive patches applied to the skin. There are also daily skin creams and gels that contain testosterone; however, these treatments are typically more expensive, and the absorption rate is inefficient (approximately 10%, depending on the individual). People who take frequent baths or engage in intense physical activity might not be the best candidates because the medication can wash off and take up to six hours to fully absorb. Since women and children are particularly sensitive to testosterone and can experience unintentional masculinization and negative health effects even from small doses, there is also a chance that an intimate partner or child will come into contact with the application site and unintentionally dose themselves. When administering AAS for non-medical purposes, injection is the most common method used.

The conventional methods of administering the medication have no different impact on its effectiveness. Studies show that despite variations in pharmacokinetic principles like first-pass metabolism, the anabolic qualities of AAS are generally comparable. On the other hand, excessive dosages of the oral forms of AAS may harm the liver.

8.3.2 Mechanism of Action

Men's sex organs grow and develop as a result of endogenous androgen, which also keeps secondary sex traits in place. Both synthetic and endogenous anabolic steroids, including testosterone and dihydrotestosterone, work by binding to and activating androgen receptors to mediate their effects. Anabolic steroids control the transcription of target genes in skeletal muscle, which in turn controls the build-up of DNA in skeletal muscle necessary for muscle growth.

Additionally, anabolic steroids increase the number and upregulate androgen receptors, which allows for higher training intensities and indirectly contributes to larger and stronger muscles. Through their varied effects on different neurotransmitters in the central nervous system, their antagonistic effects on glucocorticoids, and their stimulation of the growth hormone-insulin-like growth factor-1 axis, they also have a stimulatory effect on the brain.

An increased ratio of anabolic activity to androgenic activity is linked to nandrolone decanoate and nandrolone phenpropionate. The only goal of the slow-acting anabolic steroid nandrolone decanoate is to increase muscle mass. It works by encouraging muscle retention of nitrogen, which results in larger muscles. It also relieves joint pain by boosting collagen synthesis and improving bone mineralization. In addition, nandrolone phenpropionate stimulates hunger, promotes the growth of muscle, and increases red blood cell production (Hakansson et al., 2012).

Dromeostanolone, a synthetic anabolic steroid with anti-estrogenic qualities, is five times more potent than methyltestosterone, which bodybuilders use extensively to get ready for competitions. It improves the retention of potassium, phosphorus, and nitrogen, which raises protein anabolism and lowers amino acid catabolism, increasing muscle density and hardness.

8.3.3 Adverse Effects of Anabolic-Androgenic Steroids

The negative effects of AAS are caused by multiple mechanisms, all of which require further clarification. Many organs and systems, in both humans and animals, are affected by AAS-related side effects. This could be because endogenous steroids are not properly synthesized, transformed, or degraded and because AR is widely distributed throughout the body. AASs bind to a particular type of androgen receptor, and at supraphysiological doses, they may cause secondary effects once the receptors are saturated. It is necessary to distinguish between side effects linked to AAS use (i.e., when used under medical supervision) and abuse (i.e., when multiple drugs are taken at high doses or when these substances are used for purposes other than medicine). Athletes who take more than just anabolic steroids may also use alcohol, cocaine, opiates, marijuana, and gamma-hydroxybutyrate, some of which have negative interactions with AASs. It is challenging to assign the observed effects to a single drug due to the polydrug assumption. The effects of AAS are also influenced by sex, dosage, and administration time. The majority of the effects in this regard become apparent after prolonged use.

Brain and Behavior

AASs' neurotoxic effects are linked to G-protein coupled receptors as well as membrane AR receptors. Additionally, a number of studies demonstrated how apoptosis influences brain damage assessment. In fact, it has been shown that high levels of methandienone and 17βmethyltestosterone have a deleterious effect on neuron cell cultures that express AR. These effects include the inhibition of neurite network maintenance, which ultimately results in cell death via apoptosis and the cleavage of protective chaperone proteins, like Hsp90. According to a recent study, brain damage caused by AAS may be characterized by mechanisms involving miRNA dysregulation. Three groups were examined in this study: "AAS" users, "Cocaine" abusers, and "Aging" individuals. In this context, the "AAS" group exhibited significantly higher levels of miR-34 and miR-132 (Alsiö et al., 2009).

A recent study suggested that rats treated with long-term nandrolone administration had areas of their brains where apoptosis was present. This is because oxidative stress and NF-Kb signaling have been linked to promote brain injury in particular regions of the brain, including the striatum, frontal cortex, and hippocampal regions. Furthermore, it was discovered that by activating apoptotic and pre-apoptotic cells, daily injections of stanozol in male adult rats for 28 days resulted in histopathologic alterations in the hippocampus. Furthermore, an additional study showed that the positive effects of exercise on hippocampal cell proliferation and apoptotic signaling are counteracted by supraphysiological doses of AASs. By stabilizing the mitochondrial membrane, endurance exercise enhances the redox system balance and lessens the apoptotic effects of ND in neural cells.

Abuse of AAS may also have an adverse effect on cognitive function. When compared to nonexposed subjects, weightlifters exposed to AASs exhibited reduced cognitive functions, including motor and executive performance. A recent study that examined AAS users using neuroimaging found that AAS users had thinner cortex, smaller putamen volume, and smaller overall gray matter in widespread regions when compared to weightlifters who did not use AAS. Additionally, a different imaging study revealed significantly higher volumes in the right amygdala, significantly lower volumes in the right amygdala, and lower levels of scyllo-inositol and dACCgln/glu in comparison to non-users. Recent research demonstrating a cognitive dysfunction resulting from long-term high AAS exposure was conducted on weightlifters, both AAS users and nonusers, using neuropsychological tests. In this sense, long-term users, adolescents, and young adults are particularly susceptible to neurodegeneration and dementia as a result of oxidative stress and apoptosis brought on by AAS abuse (Alsiö et al., 2009).

Particularly in those who are predisposed, AASs in supraphysiological concentrations affect a number of central nervous system functions, including memory, aggression, anxiety, and depression. By influencing the production, breakdown, and metabolism of neurotransmitters, the underlying mechanisms impact neurotransmission. Furthermore, a study conducted on animals revealed that prolonged use of ND causes memory loss and anxiolytic behavior. High doses of AASs administered over time have been linked to anxiety-like behavior by augmenting the GABAergic inhibitory effects from the central amygdala onto the bed nucleus of stria terminalis through the corticotrophin release factor. Furthermore, long-term AAS treatment modifies the expression of neurotransmitters involved in the regulation of aggression. Last but not least, AASs may phosphorylate the NMDA receptor to boost excitatory neurotransmission, which would escalate aggression. In this sense, aggressiveness and violent behavior brought on by AAS consumption may be influenced by the orbitofrontal cortex. In fact, the absence of inhibitory control may result from the reduction of the orbitofrontal cortex seen in these situations. Individuals who use AASs are more likely to abuse drugs or alcohol. To elucidate the mechanisms and the biological and social processes involved in the neuropsychiatric effects of AAS abuse, more extensive research is required (Sessa et al., 2018).

Cardiovascular System

Even with increased morbidity and mortality, the effects of AAS abuse on the heart and metabolism remain unknown. Because the heart has a higher metabolic activity than other body tissues and organs and is more sensitive to oxidative stress, cardiac injury is the most common side effect of exogenous steroid administration. Tonic cardiac autonomic regulation dysfunction is caused by the chronic high-dose administration of AASs. In fact, an experiment showed that rats given AASs had reduced heart rate variability, diminished high-frequency power, and impaired parasympathetic cardiac modulation. Moreover, in AAS abusers, the inflammatory process might contribute to the development of cardiac injury. Indeed, in a mouse model, anabolic steroid-treated mice showed a greater cytokine response than the control group, indicating that TNF-α plays a part in determining myocardial injury. Furthermore, it was shown that treated animals lost the adaptive response of exercise-induced amelioration of antioxidant activity after receiving anabolic steroids. When AAS is used at supraphysiological doses, abnormal plasma lipoproteins are linked to it. A human study with hypogonadal men receiving testosterone replacement therapy revealed lower plasma levels of HDL (high-density lipoprotein) cholesterol. Additional research highlights the promotion of atherogenesis of these substances by observing hyperomociysteinaemia and elevated low-density lipoprotein (LDL) cholesterol levels following long-term AAS administration. There was a noticeable rise in sympathetic activity following the administration of AAS. Furthermore, high AAS concentrations stimulate the renin-angiotensin-aldosterone system by activating ARs, cell membrane receptors, and secondary transmitters. This results in increased heart muscle synthesis, left ventricular hypertrophy, and hypertension. Compared to non-users, AAS users exhibit myocardial mechanical dysfunction, a higher left ventricular mass index, thicker left ventricular walls, and more concentric left geometry. Extended training in conjunction with AAS delivery diminishes the relaxation characteristics of the left ventricle. In this sense, the positive effects of exercise on left ventricular function are linked to the loss of these effects when anabolic steroids are used. Reports of arrhythmic events occurred after long-term AAS administration (Sessa et al., 2018). The most common occurrence is atrial fibrillation, although literature has also reported on ventricular arrhythmias and sudden cardiac death. Research on both humans and animals indicated a link between the administration of testosterone and a decrease in cardiac repolarization. Furthermore, an important factor in cardiac morphologic and electric disturbances is the cardiac hypertrophy brought on by AASs. An increased volume of atherosclerotic plaque is a characteristic of AAS users. Furthermore, 3.0% of AAS users experienced a myocardial infarction as a result of atherosclerotic disease. The real me.

According to a recent study, Doppler myocardial imaging can help identify subclinical left ventricular dysfunction in athletes who abuse performance-enhancing substances. In these situations, new imaging modalities like magnetic resonance might provide basic details about cardiac tissue. To consider AAS abuse in differential diagnosis and perform primary and secondary prevention in their patients, clinicians need to understand the mechanisms underlying cardiotoxicity, the pathological and clinical consequences, as well as the diagnostic tools to highlight cardiac damage in AAS abusers.

Liver

One of the most common adverse effects of AAS abuse is hepatotoxicity. It was proposed that oxidative stress in hepatic cells was connected to AAS-induced hepatotoxicity. When the AR receptor is activated, there is a rise in mitochondrial b-oxidation, which leads to an increase in reactive oxygen species. Furthermore, anti-oxidant compounds guard against hepatotoxicity caused by AASs. It has also been shown that the degree of liver damage is positively correlated with androgenic potency and metabolic resistance (Hakansson et al., 2012).

Genetic factors play a role in AS-induced hepatotoxicity, which is linked to the infiltration of inflammatory cells like neutrophils, eosinophils, and lymphocytes in liver tissue. Because oxidative stress activates androgen receptors, which cause hepatic cell mitochondria to degenerate, it may play a part in the liver damage resulting from AAS abuse. A recent study assessed the effects of five weeks of ND administration on rats' livers. The findings showed elevated liver necrosis marker plasma levels as well as increased collagen deposition in the liver parenchyma, portal space, and centrilobular vein. An increase in Kuppfer cell activity and quantity may be the mechanism underlying collagen deposition. In this sense, the activation of Kuppfer cells results in the production of numerous inflammatory cytokines associated with the process of liver fibrosis, including TGF-b1, NF-Kb, and IL-1b (Hakansson et al., 2012).

Peliosis and cholestasis are two of the most frequent liver effects that occur after supraphysiological doses of AASs. Histologically speaking, peliosis is defined by the presence of numerous small, blood-filled cystic spaces dispersed throughout the liver parenchyma. The process at play might be the induction of hepatocyte hyperplasia, which is in charge of the development of nodules and tumors, as well as the mechanical blockage of hepatic veins. Furthermore, research on animals has shown that a decrease in the animal's capacity for transportation can lead to an accumulation of bile. Necrosis and inflammation, however, are not features of AAS-associated cholestasis. In AAS-induced hepatotoxicity, inflammation and necrosis may trigger a regenerative signal. The literature has reported a relationship between androgen steroid therapy and hepatocellular adenoma, and it appears that the potency and dosage of AAS administration affect the risk of androgen-associated liver tumors. In order to implement preventive measures, more research is necessary to elucidate the relationship between the administration of AASs and hepatocellular proliferation.

Urinary System

Numerous studies have shown that long-term androgen exposure directly damages the kidneys, particularly the glomerular cells, leading to the buildup of mesangial matrix, depletion of podocytes, and structural changes. In this sense, AR expression is a characteristic of kidney tissues. In the kidney, AR activation causes cell proliferation and hypertrophy. According to a recent report, exposure to ND may induce hypertrophy in the kidneys of mice, specifically in the proximal and distal convoluted tubules. Moreover, following prolonged ND exposure, kidney fibrosis may be initiated by both direct ND action to AR and testosterone activity.

It has been demonstrated that long-term ND administration in mice results in dose-dependent oxidative kidney stress and damage. Increased lipid peroxidation and decreased antioxidant enzyme activity, including glutathione reductase and glutathione peroxidase, were observed in the kidneys of mice treated with ND. A recent study on mouse kidneys receiving long-term ND treatment revealed dose-related oxidative stress. The authors noticed a decrease in antioxidant enzymes along with an increase in pro-inflammatory and pro-apoptotic markers like TNF, IL-1B, and Hsp90. These changes may result in secondary focal segmental glomerulosclerosis.

Morphological alterations were noted in mice receiving ND. After three months of androgen intramuscular injection, a number of histopathological changes were observed, including kidney samples containing eosinophilic cell cytoplasm, a sign of chronicity, and vascular congestion, as well as glomerular atrophy and fragmentation, tubular wall rupture, vacuolar degeneration of the epithelium lining the proximal convoluted tubules and blood hemorrhage between the tubules, basal lamina thickening in distal convoluted tubules and tubes with only the basal lamina, numerous hyaline cylinders, and some areas of necrosis. Urinary system damage is largely influenced by oxidative stress, apoptosis, and inflammation, just like in other tissues and organs. This knowledge is essential for both preventative and therapeutic approaches.

Muscoloskeletal System

The administration of AAS seems to impact muscle mass. In fact, testosterone stimulates the differentiation of pluripotent mesenchymal cells into a myogenic lineage, lowers the expression of myostatin, and increases the production of IGF-1 by binding to AR. These processes result in increased muscle mass, strength, and capacity for exercise by increasing protein synthesis, decreasing protein breakdown, forming new myotubes, and increasing the number of myonuclei.

High AAS concentrations can also result in major skeletal muscle injuries. AASs at supraphysiological doses have been shown in an experiment to cause a reduction in matrix metalloproteinase-2 (MMP-2) activity in the muscles of jumping rat agonists. It was proposed that the mechanism underlying skeletal exercise adaptation may involve the vascular endothelial growth factor (VEGF). Rats that received ND treatment had lower levels of VEGF expression, which may be connected to a dysfunction in MMP-2 activity as MMPs control the amount of VEGF extracellular stores. Moreover, poor remodeling and vascularization resulting from AASs may contribute to skeletal damage, which could be caused by decreased VEGF expression. However, tendon damage may also be related to AASs. Physical activity can alter the organization and morphology of collagen fibers. AAS abuse results in increased muscle mass, strength, and a decreased ability to respond, particularly during exercise, therefore, it also raises the risk of tendon rupture. In rat tendons, it was shown that ND enhanced tendon remodeling even in the face of MMP-2 activity declines. AAS-related MMP dysregulation still requires further clarification, though. One of the most common reasons why young people and athletes abuse AASs is for aesthetic reasons, such as to gain more muscle mass and strength. Public health initiatives and information campaigns are required to raise youth awareness of the musculoskeletal side effects of AAS misuse (Anawalt, 2019).

Reproductive System

Androgens are essential for the development of the male reproductive system. Both puberty and male sexual function require them. When AAS is administered, the hypothalamic-pituitary axis experiences a negative feedback loop that modifies the release of both FSH and LH, ultimately leading to infertility. A recent study using Leydig cell cultures treated with ND revealed that these cells' interference with STARR and CYP17A1 expression impaired their ability to produce testosterone.

Previous research revealed that morning erection frequency, sexual thoughts, and satisfaction were all higher among both current and former AAS users. However, a number of adverse effects, including anorgasmia, premature ejaculation, and erectile dysfunction, were noted. However, new research lends credence to the idea that prolonged and high-frequency use of AASs can cause sexual dysfunction when stopped. Young men with hypogonadism frequently used AAS in the past, and this factor needs to be taken into account when doing a clinical evaluation of hypogonadism.

Hematologic Consequences

Since AASs can increase erythropoietin (EPO) secretion, they were used to treat anemias prior to the development of recombinant human EPO. Erythrocytosis and an increase in hematocrit are two more adverse effects of AAS. Abuse of AAS is harmful to cardiovascular health and is frequently linked to an increased risk of thrombosis. But case reports have been the association's main source of information. An elevated risk of cardiovascular disease is associated with elevated LDL and decreased HDL. Following intramuscular testosterone enanthate (200 mg every 3 or 4 weeks for 24 weeks), mild but significant increases in mean red blood cell, hematocrit, hemoglobin, and white blood cell concentrations were reported in 33 men in a study. The type and dosage of the anabolic steroid determine how AASs affect plasma concentration and the activity of coagulation factors. Regarding this, it has been shown that endothelial cells' release of plasminogen activator inhibitor type 1 is inhibited by physiological testosterone, while tissue plasminogen activator and tissue factor pathway inhibitor are stimulated. The existing literature has not provided enough clarity on the relationship between AAS abuse and thrombosis, with only a few reports addressing actual thrombotic outcomes. According to a recent report, there may be a connection between immunodeficiency and AAS abuse that is related to corticosteroid activity mimicking. Furthermore, this report recommended that when an uncommon death occurs in immunocompromised patients, AAS abuse should be looked into (Anawalt, 2019).

Anabolic steroids (AASs) and Cancer

AASs and testosterone share a similar biochemical mechanism. AASs bind to specific DNA sequences to change the expression of genes. The toxicity, mutagenicity, genotoxicity, and carcinogenicity of sexual hormones are caused by a combination of genetic and epigenetic factors, according to a recent review on the effects of androgen on cellular functions. The genotoxicity associated with AAS is still unknown, though. Three epigenetic molecular processes—DNA methylation, histone modifications, and chromatin condensation—lead to genetic transcription control. DNA methylation prevents transcriptional expression activation by blocking the binding of transcriptional factors to their target sequences, which includes both promoters and introns. Transcriptional expression is likewise controlled by chromatin condensation. Synthetic testosterone derivatives have the ability to be metabolized into 17β-estradiol, a steroid that has been linked to cancer and mutagenesis in adipose, cerebral, and testicular tissues. Moreover, 17 beta-estradiol and its metabolites are thought to stimulate cell division. AASs also exhibit an oxidative role during catabolism, producing more reactive oxygen species (ROS), which are extremely unstable, readily lose hydrogen atoms, form covalent bonds with DNA bases or sequences, and have the potential to cause genetic harm.

There is a suggestion that the number of stem cell divisions that occur in a given tissue during its lifetime is strictly positively correlated with the incidence of cancer in that tissue. This leads to the hypothesis that long-term nandrolone administration may represent a preconditioning that, in addition to multiple hits, may increase the risk of carcinogenesis onset, particularly in tissues with a high concentration of stem cells like the liver. This is because chronic nandrolone administration may favor the persistence and viability of stem cells in various tissues.

The adverse effects on the body's natural production of anabolic steroids may influence hormonal fluctuations and regulation and may be the root cause of some carcinogenic processes. Additionally, through a variety of process pathways, widely distributed and readily accessible AASs like stanozolol and nandrolone may contribute to the etiology of cancers like Leydig cell tumors. It has been shown that there is a link between the abuse of AASs and cancer, so it is imperative to prevent its abuse and run awareness campaigns among young athletes and in gyms. To achieve an early diagnosis in this case, monitoring long-term abusers is necessary (Tokish et al., 2004).

8.3.4 Monitoring

Measurements of early morning testosterone levels on two different days are necessary to confirm the diagnosis of hypogonadism prior to starting testosterone treatment. Before starting treatment, a patient must have a lipid profile, hepatic function tests, hemoglobin, hematocrit, prostate-specific antigen, and a prostate exam if they are over 40.

Clinicians should get the patient's lipid profile, hematocrit, hemoglobin, and hepatic function tests (every year, after three to six months of anabolic steroid treatment). It's important to watch out for any signs of virilization in women receiving testosterone treatment for breast cancer. Three to six months after starting therapy and then annually, especially for cardiac adverse events, patients taking testosterone should have their response to treatment and side effects observed.

Every three to six months, men over 40 who have a baseline prostate-specific antigen (PSA) level greater than 0.6 ng/mL should have their PSA levels checked as well as a prostate examination. Men who have a palpable prostate nodule or a prostate-specific antigen level greater than 4 ng/mL, as well as patients who are at high risk of prostate cancer and have a level greater than 3 ng/mL, should not receive treatment.

Testosterone levels for both testosterone enanthate and testosterone cypionate should be checked halfway between shots, and changes to dosage and frequency should be made to maintain a concentration of testosterone between 400 and 700 ng/dL. When a patient is using a topical testosterone solution, their serum testosterone level should be measured two to eight hours after application, fourteen days after beginning therapy, or after dose titration (Tokish et al., 2004).

When patients using nasal testosterone gel begin therapy, their total serum testosterone levels should be checked on a regular basis. If the total testosterone level rises above 1050 ng/dL, the patient's treatment should be stopped. Serum testosterone levels should be checked at least 14 days after therapy begins, in the morning, before transdermal testosterone is applied, at the conclusion of the testosterone pellet dosage interval, and 4 to 12 weeks after treatment begins, prior to the morning dose in patients taking testosterone orally.

8.4 Currently Popular Designer Steroids

8.4.1 Dimethazin

Due to its strong anabolic properties, "DMZ" was initially investigated in Italy in the 1960s. It was used to treat a number of conditions, such as gynecologic cancer, osteoporosis, fibrocystic dysplasia, tuberculosis, and childhood cachexia. Dimethazine was shown to have a stronger myotropic effect in animal experiments compared to methyltestosterone, oxymetholone (Anadrol), and testosterone propionate. In 2008, dimethazine was listed as an ingredient in dietary supplements for the first time. One supplement manufacturer was fined $125,000 by the FDA in 2009 for selling drugs that were not authorized, including dimethazine. A press release from the FDA in 2013 alerted consumers to the presence of dimethazine and the controlled AAS methasteron (Superdol) in a vitamin B dietary supplement. Despite these measures, dimethazine is still listed on the labels of 17 currently marketed products and is known as 2a,17a-dimethyl-5a-androstan-17b-ol-3-one-azine when it comes to dietary supplements.

8.4.2 Methylclostebol

Clostebol (4-chloro-17b-hydroxyandrost-4-en-3-one) is the chlorinated derivative of testosterone (17b-hydroxyandrost-4- en-3-one).

A Schedule III controlled substance, clostebol is applied topically to treat dermatological and ophthalmologic conditions. Chemical analysis revealed that methylclostebol, a 17-alpha-alkylated form of clostebol, was present in a nutritional supplement in considerable amounts. We discovered that four "dietary supplements" that are presently on the market list methylclostebol as an ingredient. The labeled ingredient (4-chloro-17amethyl-androst-4-en-17b-ol-3-one), which is present in many designer steroids products, is written in an archaic and confusing nomenclature and is more accurately described as 4-chloro-17a-methyltestosterone (methylclostebol). Like clostebol, methylclostebol is a 4-chlorinated derivative of testosterone and is not a substrate for 5-alpha reductase or aromatase. Therefore, it stands to reason that this compound would be less likely to cause virilization and gynecomastia. German athletes used methylclostebol as an ergogenic in the 1960s and 1970s, probably because of its non-virilizing side effect profile, but this oral androgen has never been investigated for medical use. Oral methylclostebol was shown to be considerably less androgenic and about half as anabolic as testosterone in animal tests conducted in vivo.

8.4.3 Mentabolan

When 7-alpha-alkylated nandrolone derivatives were created in the 1960s, it was discovered that they had more androgenic potential. 7-alpha-methyl-19-nortestosterone (MENT) was one such substance. In studies funded by the Population Council, MENT, commonly known as Trestolone, is presently being assessed as an experimental male contraceptive. A related substance known as 7a-methyl-19-nor-androstenedione, also known as metabolan or trestione, has recently gained popularity as a designer steroid. Our systematic product search revealed it to be listed as an ingredient in two products. Trestione is just the "dione" form of trestolone, much like androstenedione is to testosterone, so the name's resemblance to MENT (Trestolone) is justified. According to preliminary research, mentabolan, and trestolone are more androgenic than other 19-nor androgens like nandrolone (Deca Durabolin). More so than nandrolone but less so than trestolone or testosterone, oral metabolan administration effectively suppressed gonadotropins while increasing the weight of the ventral prostate, seminal vesicles, and levator ani.

8.4.4 Methoxygonadiene

Some of the first synthetic oral contraceptives were developed as a result of a series of patents filed by organic chemist Herchel Smith and associates in the 1960s and 1970s. Methoxygonadiene (18-methyl-19-nortestosterone) was one of these early experimental compounds. Our systematic search turned up this compound, which goes by the chemical name 13b-ethyl3-methoxy-gona-2,5(10)-dien-17-one, as a labeled ingredient in ten different products. Methoxygonadiene, a progestin that belongs to the levonorgestrel family, is a strong anabolic that can be obtained by injection. Its anabolic: androgenic ratio is roughly 54:27 vs. propionate testosterone and 90: 625 vs. 19-norethisterone. On the other hand, there is no data on methoxygonadiene's oral activity in humans (Kicman, 2008).

8.4.5 Methylepitiostanol

Known by most as "epistane," this substance is the 17-alpha-alkylated form of the androgen epitiostanol, which was created in Japan to treat breast cancer. Epitiostanol, which is regarded as a steroidal antiestrogen and an androgen, has the ability to induce ASIH because it inhibits the hypothalamic-pituitary-gonadal (HPG) axis. Because it is a 17-alpha-alykylated androgen, hepatotoxicity may occur. Chemical analysis of nutritional supplements has revealed the presence of methlyepithiostanol. It is believed that in some product containers, methlyepithiostanol may break down into the restricted AAS desoxymethyltestosterone (Madol). Methylepitiostanol (2a,3a-epithio-17amethyl-5a-androstan-17b-ol) is listed as an ingredient on the labels of more than thirty products that are currently on the market.

8.4.6 Methylstenbolone

Known by most as "Ultradrol," this substance was recently found in a dietary supplement and seems to be a well-liked new generation designer steroid. The 17-alpha alkylated oral form of the regulated AAS stenbolone is called methylstenbolone. Oral methylstenbolone is reported to be 124% androgenic and 660 % more myotrophic than oral methyltestosterone in early animal studies. Although methylstenebolone has never been investigated for medical purposes, it has the potential to cause ASIH and infertility because it is an androgen with activity at the HPG axis. At least twenty different, legitimately sold products with the ingredient methylstenbolone (2,17a-dimethyl-17bhydroxy-5a-androst-1-en-3-one) listed on the label were found using our Internet search.

8.5 Ergogenic Use of Anabolic Steroids

Anabolic steroids (AAS) have been around since they were discovered and have been used extensively as anti-aging, sports performance-enhancing, physical appearance-enhancing, and self-medication for injury recovery. It is debatable and sometimes illegal to use anabolic steroids for goals other than curing medical ailments. Prominent athletic associations have taken action to outlaw the use of anabolic steroids. Users have a variety of health-related concerns. Many nations have laws that prohibit and punish the trading and possession of AAS.

For thousands of years, cultures all over the world have utilized performance-enhancing drugs in traditional medicine to increase strength and vitality. Gonadal hormones were used before they were recognized and separated. Testicle extract was first used medicinally in the late 19th century when the research was still being done on its effects on strength. During a scientific meeting in 1889, Charles-Édouard Brown-Séquard, a 72-year-old Mauritian neurologist, reported that he had received several positive effects from injecting himself with an extract of dog and guinea pig testicles. But nearly all experts—including some of Brown-Sequard's contemporaries—agreed that Brown-Sequard was the one who caused these beneficial effects. Replicating Brown-Séquard's approach, a 2002 study found that the amount of testosterone obtained was insufficient to produce any meaningful clinical effect (Cheung et al., 2018).

In 1935, testosterone was isolated for the first time and subsequently synthesized chemically. It is the most potent anabolic-androgenic steroid produced by Leydig cells in the testes. Shortly after, synthetic testosterone derivatives were developed. By the end of the next decade, a variety of medical conditions had been treated with varying degrees of success using testosterone and its derivatives. However, athletes didn't start learning that anabolic steroids could help them gain more muscle mass until the 1950s. Sports physician John Ziegler claims that testosterone was used by Russian weightlifters at the 1954 weightlifting championships in Vienna, which was the first instance of anabolic steroid use in an international athletic competition.

The use of anabolic steroids was mostly limited to professional sports throughout the 1960s and 1970s. Training regimens in the former Soviet Union even required certain athletes to use anabolic steroids. Sports physicians like Ziegler and medical textbooks continued to widely declare that anabolic steroids were useless for helping athletes gain muscle in the United States. These medical professionals did concede that anabolic steroids could be helpful for severely disabled patients (Armstrong et al., 2018).

Dianabol, a popular anabolic steroid at the time, had a package insert that said, "Anabolic steroids do not enhance athletic ability." Notwithstanding these cautions, anabolic steroid use started in competitive bodybuilding, track and field competitions (e.g., shot put) and other sports where muscle strength or training recovery speed was a determining factor in performance.

8.5.1 Prevalence and User Profiles

General population

Because most studies rely on self-reporting, it is challenging to estimate the percentage of the population that has used anabolic steroids. Research conducted in the United States has indicated that the majority of anabolic steroid users are middle-class heterosexual men who are not competitive bodybuilders or athletes, with a median age of approximately 25. They mention using the medications for aesthetic goals. According to another study, less than 1% of college students used anabolic steroids for non-medical purposes. In a 2006 survey, noncompetitive bodybuilders and non-athletes made up 78.4% of steroid users. Reusing, sharing, and sharing multi-dose vials are among the unsafe injection practices that about 13 % of respondents reported doing. However, a 2007 study found that sharing of needles was very rare—less than 1 %—among those using anabolic steroids for purposes other than medical purposes. According to a different 2007 study, 74 % of non-medical anabolic steroid users had completed secondary college, more had graduated from college, and fewer had not completed high school as would be expected in the general population (Sessa et al., 2018). According to the same study, people who use anabolic steroids for non-medical reasons have greater employment rates and higher household incomes than people in general. Users of anabolic steroids do more research on the drugs they take than users of other controlled substances do. However, friends, non-medical handbooks, and fitness magazines are the main sources of information that steroid users consult, and these sources may contain false or dubious information. A 1998 study found that 2 % of American middle school students (ages 9 to 13) reported using steroids, with 2 % of female students and 2 % of male students reporting use. According to a 1988 study, 6.6 % of students in the 12th grade—or those who are 17 or 18 years old—use or have used steroids.

The media and political discourse frequently depict anabolic steroids as lethal, which demoralizes users of these drugs. One study found that people who use anabolic steroids also have mistrust for their doctors, and that 56% of the sample had not told their doctors they used anabolic steroids. Another study conducted in 2007 revealed that although 66% of people using anabolic steroids for non-medical purposes were willing to seek medical supervision for their steroid use, 58% did not trust their doctors, 92% thought the medical community knew too little about the use of anabolic steroids for non-medical purposes, and 100% thought that people's perceptions of the negative effects of anabolic steroids were exaggerated. Long-term users of anabolic steroids had higher rates of muscle dysmorphia symptoms and stronger support for more stereotypically masculine roles, according to a 2006 study (Patanè et al., 2020).

Sports

Professional athletes in track and field, weightlifting, bodybuilding, shot put, cycling, baseball, wrestling, mixed martial arts, boxing, and football have all used anabolic steroids. Many of the professional and amateur associations that oversee these sports forbid such use.

Adolescents do use anabolic steroids, particularly those who play competitive sports. It has been suggested that the prevalence of use among high-school students in the U. S. could reach a maximum of 2 %. Students who participated in sports generally used steroids more frequently than students who did not, and male students used anabolic steroids more frequently than female students (Pope et al., 2014).

8.5.2 Ergogenic Effects

Drugs known as "performance-enhancing drugs" (PEDs) are used to increase sports performance. They function through various mechanisms, such as boosting oxygen delivery, boosting muscle mass, sharpening focus and alertness, and lowering fatigue. The following are some typical ergogenic effects of drugs used to enhance performance:

Increased Muscle Mass

Probably the most well-known PEDs for gaining muscle mass are anabolic steroids. They function by stimulating the synthesis of proteins, which causes muscle hypertrophy (growth).

Improved Endurance

A hormone called EPO promotes the formation of

red blood cells, which supply oxygen to muscles. EPO can improve oxygen delivery and increase endurance by raising red blood cell counts.

Enhanced Strength and Power

Athletes can lift greater weights or use more force during explosive movements thanks to the effects of androgenic-anabolic steroids like testosterone, which can also increase muscle strength and power.

Faster Recovery

Certain PEDs, such as human growth hormone (HGH), encourage tissue regeneration and repair, which can hasten the healing process. This allows athletes to train harder and more frequently.

Improved Focus and Alertness

Athletes and caffeine are examples of stimulants that can improve focus, alertness, and reaction time—all of which are beneficial in sports that demand a high degree of concentration.

Reduced Fatigue

Athletes can maintain high-intensity efforts for extended periods of time by using stimulants and medications such as beta blockers, which can lessen perceived exertion and delay fatigue.

Increased Confidence and Aggression

Certain PEDs can have psychological side effects, like boosting aggression and confidence, which can give athletes a competitive advantage in some sports.

It is crucial to remember that although performance-enhancing drugs (PEDs) have the potential to improve performance in the short term, they also come with a number of health risks and can have major long-term effects, such as liver damage, cardiovascular problems, hormonal imbalances, and psychological dependence. PED use is also prohibited by law and unethical in the majority of sports organizations.

8.6 Gene Doping

Gene doping is the hypothetical, non-therapeutic use of gene therapy by athletes for purposes other than illness treatment in order to enhance their performance in those sports where such uses of genetic modification technology are prohibited. There is no proof that gene doping has ever been used to improve athletic performance in any sporting event as of April 2015. Gene doping is the use of gene transfer to alter the expression of a particular human gene and the biosynthesis of its protein; this can be achieved by injecting the gene carrier directly into the subject or by isolating the subject's cells, transfecting them, and then giving the subject's cells back.

Athletes' historical interest in gene doping and their concerns about its dangers and detection methods have developed in tandem with the field of gene therapy. This was particularly the case after research on a transgenic mouse that overexpressed insulin-like growth factor 1 was published in 1998 and showed the mouse to be significantly more robust than normal mice even in old age (El Osta et al., 2016; Roman et al., 2018).

8.6.1 Agents used in Gene Doping

Many genes are promising candidates for use as gene doping agents. They consist of endorphin, enkephalin, alpha-actinin-3, VEGF, fibroblast growth factor, myostatin, insulin-like growth factor 1, human growth hormone, and EPO.

Gene doping carries risks that are similar to those associated with gene therapy: a strong immune response to the native protein that could result in a genetic disease-like condition, a severe inflammatory response, cancer, and death. In each scenario, these risks would be taken in the hopes of making a quick profit rather than curing a serious illness.

Alpha-actinin-3

Only present in human skeletal muscle, alpha-actinin-3 has been shown in multiple genetic studies to exhibit a distinct polymorphism in elite athletes when compared to the general population. There are two forms of this gene: one causes the gene to produce more protein and is associated with increased power in sprinters; the other causes the gene to produce less protein and is associated with endurance athletes. A DNA construct that interfered with expression, such as a small interfering RNA or polymorphism, for endurance athletes, could be used to create gene doping agents.

Myostatin

The protein myostatin is in charge of preventing the development and differentiation of muscles. Muscle mass and strength increase when the myostatin gene is deleted, or its expression is restricted in another way. Schwarzenegger mice—knockout mice devoid of the gene—have served as proof of this. Humans with faulty genes at birth can also be used as "knockout models"; a German boy born with a myostatin gene mutation in both copies had developed muscles. After birth, the boy's advanced muscle growth persisted, and by the time he was 4 years old, he could lift 3 kg of weight. In a 2009 study, researchers used gene therapy to give non-human primates' quadriceps follistatin, which caused the animals' local muscles to grow in a manner akin to that of mice (Cheung and Grossmann, 2018).

Erythropoietin

A glycoprotein called EPO functions as a hormone to regulate the production of red blood cells. For many years, athletes have used EPO protein injections as a performance-enhancing drug (blood doping). An athlete's endurance is improved when the extra EPO produces more red blood cells in the bloodstream, which raises the amount of oxygen available to the muscle. According to recent research, it might be able to boost an animal's endogenous EPO production by introducing an additional EPO gene. It has been demonstrated that successfully introducing EPO genes into mice and monkeys can raise hematocrit levels by up to 80% in those species. However, some animals experienced severe anemia as a result of the autoimmune responses triggered by endogenous and transgene-derived EPO.

Insulin-like growth factor 1

One protein that aids in the growth hormone's mediation is called insulin-like growth factor 1. Mice given IGF-1 have shown increased muscle growth and faster regeneration of their muscles and nerves. If athletes took this, their bodies would produce too much IGF-1, which could lead to cancer and heart disease.

Others

Gene doping may also aim to alter the levels of proteins that influence psychology; for instance, endorphins and enkephalins influence pain perception, BDNF influences stress response, and increased monamine synthesis may elevate athletes' moods. Gene therapy with a replication-deficient herpes simplex virus, which targets nerves, has been used to administer preproenkephalin to mice. The results were good enough to support a Phase I clinical trial in individuals with terminal cancer who experience uncontrollable pain. It would be difficult to implement that strategy for athletes because the pain deadening would probably be irreversible.

Although VEGF has been investigated as a possible gene doping agent and tested in clinical trials to improve blood flow, long-term follow-up of trial participants has yielded negative results. Regarding the fibroblast growth factor, the same holds true. Increased gluconeogenesis in athletes would result in more energy being available and a decrease in the accumulation of lactic acid. Glucagon-like peptide-1 has been shown to increase the amount of glucose in the liver and has been given via gene therapy to the livers of mice models of diabetes (Creagh et al., 2018).

8.6.2 Detection

The primary regulatory body investigating the problem of gene doping detection is the World Anti-Doping Agency (WADA). The organization is researching both direct and indirect testing methods. Indirect methods involve analyzing the athlete to look for physical changes or structural differences between endogenous and recombinant proteins, whereas direct methods typically require the discovery of recombinant proteins or gene insertion vectors. As it becomes increasingly difficult to distinguish between anomalies that are clearly indicative of gene doping and those that are just peculiar but natural biological features, indirect methods are by their very nature more subjective. For instance, Olympic cross-country skier Eero Mäntyranta's body produced unusually high levels of red blood cells due to a mutation. Determining whether Mäntyranta's red blood cell levels were a result of an artificial or inherent genetic advantage would be extremely challenging (Melo Junior et al., 2018).

First generation of gene doping detecting methods

The idea for gene doping detection originated in 2004 when WADA added gene doping to its list of prohibited practices and began looking into a novel technique for identifying transgenes that have been inserted.

Transgene sequences were the target of polymerase chain reaction (PCR) tests, which were used in the first generation of gene doping detection methods. A blood sample containing both endogenous and transgene DNA can be used to obtain it, as a small amount of the transgene will seep into the bloodstream. Since the transgene will most likely use cDNA obtained from RNA that has had its intones removed by RNA splicing, leaving only exon-exon junctions that include only the coding sequences and some important sequences like promoters since the viral victors has a limited capacity, it can be easily distinguished from endogenous DNA because it lacks introns. Since these exon-exon junctions are a distinct sequence absent from gDNA, PCR can target them as such.

Real time polymerase chain reaction

In the field of molecular biology, PCR has numerous uses, one of which is DNA analysis. PCR is primarily used to exponentially amplify and double DNA sequences.

When it comes to gene doping detection, if the sequence began to amplify and produce an exponential graph, the test is considered positive and shows that the gene was present in the sample taken from that individual. However, the test is considered negative and the targeted DNA sequence was absent from that individual's sample if the sequence did not amplify and a linear graph was generated.

Next generation sequencing (NGS)

It was necessary to create a new technique in order to address the shortcomings of the first-generation detection methods. This new method must be highly accurate in order to detect manipulations in DNA sequences that PCR methods may miss.

Using NGS, which can target exon-exon junctions in transgenes and compare the results with reference gene sequences, was the solution. NGS can also determine the nucleotide orders of the entire genome. This approach has created new scientific opportunities that were previously unattainable, such as whole genome sequencing, and it is becoming increasingly affordable over time. It is also quick and accurate.

Two-dimensional chromatography laid the foundation for DNA sequencing in the 1970s, and the technology continued to advance until the human genome project was completed in 2001. The project cost roughly three billion dollars, and it took 15 years to sequence the entire genome. But thanks to advancements in sequencing technology, whole genome sequencing (WGS) can now be completed in a single day for about $1,000. Furthermore, a brand-new sequencing technique that will only cost $100 for WGS is being developed (Joseph and Parr, 2015; Melo Junior et al., 2018).

8.7 Detection of Doping Agents by Lc–Ms and Lc–Ms-Ms

When liquid chromatography–mass spectrometry (LC–MS) was first introduced into the doping analysis field, it was mainly used to detect compounds that were challenging to detect using other methods. The identification of the highly polar and thermally labile diuretics was the first use of LC-MS in antidoping analysis. Additional investigation also showed that LC-MS can produce good results for nonpolar doping agents. For instance, no other analytical method can match the sensitivity, selectivity, and specificity of corticosteroids. Over the past ten years, LC-MS screening applications for practically all classes of doping agents have been made available following research on the detection of all doping agent groups. Advancements in MS technology concerning polarity switching, scan speed, and sensitivity enable the simultaneous detection of various doping agent classes. Low physiological levels in plasma and urine make it challenging to detect peptide hormones using LC-MS. It is generally expected that LC-MS will be used more often in antidoping analysis.

These compounds can be analyzed by LC-MS without the need for a derivatization step, and attempts to interface mass spectrometry and liquid chromatography were made in large quantities in the 1980s. Commercial LC-MS equipment became available in doping control labs at the start of the 1990s, and research mainly concentrated on compounds for which GC-MS detection was challenging or impossible. A preliminary method for the LC-MS analysis of diuretics demonstrated encouraging outcomes in 1991. Even with these positive outcomes, routine application was hampered by technical issues. Over the next few years, both the cost of purchase and the quality of LC-MS instrumentation declined. By the end of the 1990s, routine LC-MS detection techniques were therefore available in many doping control laboratories. Consequently, routine techniques for detecting various classes of doping agents were created. In 2005, these early LC-MS techniques were examined (Moretti et al., 2018).

8.7.1 Compounds Prohibited in and Out of Competition

Anabolic steroids

Athletes use synthetic anabolic steroids, which are derivatives of the male hormone testosterone, to gain more strength. Even though they have been outlawed since 1976, approved laboratories continue to find steroids to be the most common doping agent. GC-MS is typically used to detect anabolic steroids in human urine following hydrolysis and derivatization.

The ability to identify anabolic steroids directly without derivatization was made possible by LC-MS. Regrettably, limited ionization occurs when employing traditional atmospheric pressure interfaces electrospray ionization (ESI) and atmospheric chemical ionization (APCI) for LC-MS analysis of these analytes. Because of this issue, the number of steroids that were initially included in LC-MS screening methods was restricted to those for which GC-MS detection provided difficulties. A screening method for 28 doping agents has included three steroids: gestrinone, tetrahydrogestrinone [THG], and 39OH-stanozolol. The limits of detection for 39OH-stanozolol, THG and gestrinone, respectively, were 2 ng/mL and 5 ng/mL. In our laboratory, comparable limits of detection (LODs) were achieved for the screening of 17α-trenbolone and these three anabolic steroids. Furthermore, it was mentioned that LC-MS is applicable for identifying various stanozolol metabolites (Moretti et al., 2018; Tokish et al., 2004).

The ESI of anabolic steroids has been studied recently in our lab. The results show that some anabolic steroids, such as $[M+NH_4]^+$, $[M+H+CH3OH]^+$, or $[M+H+CH_3CN-H_2O]^+$, can be better ionized after the formation of adducts with mobile phase components. Conversely, anabolic steroids with a conjugated keto function or nitrogen can be easily ionized as $[M+H]^+$. A thorough screening procedure for the identification of 34 anabolic steroids was subsequently developed using the results of these ionization experiments.

The identification of novel and unidentified designer steroids is one of the primary difficulties facing LC-MS doping analysis. Various methods have been explained. Thevis and associates devised a technique utilizing precursor ion scan, wherein multiple ions that are commonly present when steroids share a common structure are identified. This method has proven effective for analytics with a predetermined structure. Additionally, LC-MS has demonstrated its ability to identify new steroids, such as the novel metandienone long-term metabolite, or endogenous interferences that may impede the identification of exogenous anabolic steroids.

Peptide hormones and related substances

Following the introduction of LC-MS in the 1990s, doping laboratories concentrated on applying this method to the identification of small molecules (nonpeptide substances). These LC-MS techniques are currently highly optimized, and doping labs are looking into the detection of peptide hormones in blood or urine using LC-MS.

The main issue with peptide hormone detection is sensitivity. Because peptide hormones are typically administered at low dosages, blood and urine concentrations of these hormones are generally low (low nanograms or picograms per milliliter). Generally, immunological methods are used to detect them, but doping control laboratories are developing LC-MS methods to confirm the presence of peptides because scientific evidence obtained with MS is preferred (Basaria, 2010).

Certain types of diabetes mellitus are treated medicinally with insulin. Athletes are interested in insulin because it facilitates the uptake of glucose and amino acids by cells. Athletes with diabetes may be eligible for a 'therapeutic use exemption'. The range of endogenous insulin concentrations is 0–3.2 ng/mL. Thevis and colleagues reported the first doping-related LC–MS application in 2005, despite the fact that insulins have been off the list since 1999. Following an immunoaffinity clean-up, the fivefold protonated molecules $[M+5H]^{5+}$ were the focus of reversed-phase LC–ESI–MS–MS detection of the synthetic analogues Humalog, Novolog, and Lantus in plasma. A detection limit of 0.5 ng/mL should be adequate for antidoping control. An artificial version of human ACTH is called tetracosactide. Cortisol is released more when ACTH is present. This cortisol-releasing hormone is also forbidden since corticosteroids are on the list of prohibited substances. Thevis and associates have recently described the detection of synacthen. Solid-phase extraction and immunoaffinity chromatography were used to purify the plasma samples. Reversed-phase LC was used to separate the compounds. Selected reaction monitoring was done using ESI-MS-MS detection. The developed procedure allowed for an LOD of 100 fmol/mL (300 pg/mL) and required 2 mL of plasma (Basaria, 2010).

Artificial oxygen carriers are oxygen compounds based on hemoglobin. They can be utilized to improve oxygen transport in endurance sports. Hemopure is a significant compound in this group. Hemoglobin from cows is the source of hemopure. The amino acid sequence of human and bovine hemoglobins differs by 15%. Following tryptic digestion, bovine-specific fragments were found and chosen as target compounds for LC–ESI–MS–MS detection. Unlike other peptide compounds, the concentrations in blood are relatively high (1 mg/mL), so immunochromatographic purification was not necessary.

Beta2-agonists

Among the bronchodilator medications are beta2-agonists (β2 agonists), such as salbutamol (albuterol), clenbuterol, fenoterol, formoterol, and salmeterol. Because of the potential for anabolic side effects at high concentrations, the use of beta2-agonists is forbidden outside of competition. Additionally, because of their stimulating effect at higher levels than recommended therapeutically, beta2-agonists are prohibited in competition. Athletes are eligible to receive a therapeutic use exemption for certain beta2-agonists used in metered-dose inhalers because they are commonly used to treat exercise-induced asthma.

This class of substances is often extracted and analyzed in conjunction with other doping substance classes. The LC–ESI–MS–MS screening method for anabolic steroids and corticosteroids in the laboratory includes beta2-agonists. When inhaled beta2-agonists are abused frequently, the sensitivity of LC-MS for this class of substances leads to a large number of adverse analytical findings.

Agents with antiestrogenic activity

This group of drugs is separated into three categories: antiestrogenic drugs (like clomiphene and cyclofenil), selective estrogen receptor modulators (SERMs) (like raloxifene, tamoxifen, and toremifene), and aromatase inhibitors (like anastrozole, letrozole, and exemestane).

The majority of these drugs are used in cancer treatment. For example, the most commonly prescribed medication for treating breast cancer is tamoxifen. In sports, antiestrogenic agents can be used to prolong the anabolic activity of anabolic steroids administered by inhibiting the aromatase pathway or to treat the negative side effects of anabolic steroid abuse, such as gynecomastia and reduced testosterone production. An LC–ESI–MS–MS screening method for 28 doping agents, including five antiestrogenic drugs, is described by Mazzarino and colleagues. The process of preparing the sample involved liquid-liquid extraction at pH 9.2. Positive ionization mode was used for detection, and LODs ranged from 5 to 30 ng/mL. A different approach outlines the identification of fifteen antiestrogenic compounds. The sample was prepared by liquid-liquid extraction at pH 9.2, following hydrolysis. In 13 minutes, the LC-ESI-MS-MS analysis was completed. With the exception of formestane (300 ng/mL) and aminoglutethimide (100 ng/mL), all LODs were less than 10 ng/mL. This approach only included parent drugs, whereas Mareck and el.al. recommend screening for multiple antiestrogen metabolites. In a different paper, the detection of six antiestrogenic compounds via solid-phase extraction and enzymatic hydrolysis is described using LC-ESI-time-of-flight (TOF) MS. The LODs for every substance were 100 ng/mL (Pope et al., 2014).

In our lab, we looked into the metabolism and excretion of 6-OXO, a dietary supplement that is advertised online as an aromatase inhibitor. The active ingredient in this supplement is androst-4-ene-3,6,17-trione. The metabolites of androst-4-ene-3,6,17-trione are androst-4-ene-6α-ol-3,17-dione and androst-4-ene-6α,17β-diol-3-one. For the purpose of quantifying androst-4-ene-3,6,17-trione and its metabolites in urine, an LC–APCI ion-trap MS method was created and verified. After enzymatic hydrolysis, the sample is cleaned up by performing a liquid-liquid extraction using diethyl ether at pH 9.2. Using this technique, it was possible to identify androst-4-ene-6α-ol-3,17-dione as a minor metabolite and androst-4-ene-6α,17β-diol-3-one as a major urinary metabolite.

Diuretics and other masking agents

Treatment for fluid retention involves the use of diuretics. They don't improve performance in sports, but by diluting the urine, they can cover up drug use. Diuretics are also used in sports like boxing, judo, and wrestling where weight limits are enforced to help athletes lose weight quickly before competition. Diuretics are polar substances with a broad range of physico-chemical characteristics and significant structural variations. Variations in ionization are noted as a result of these variations in molecular structure. In negative ionization, thiazide diuretics form a significant group of diuretics and a large amount of deprotonated molecular ions. Amiloride, triamterene, and canrenone—a diuretic with a steroid skeleton—are only found in positive ionization. Because of this, it takes both polarities to identify them all. To detect these compounds in a single run, scan-to-scan polarity switching is required because they can coelute. Initially, two consecutive runs were required because scan-to-scan polarity switching was not possible due to instrument limitations. By the end of the 1990s, positively and negatively charged diuretics could be identified in a single chromatographic run thanks to the availability of LC-MS instruments that allowed for quick and accurate polarity switching. Consequently, a number of doping laboratories have created screening techniques that use scan-to-scan polarity-switching to identify diuretics (Pope et al., 2014).

In our laboratory, LC-MS screening for diuretics was first implemented in 2001. The method included probenecid and eighteen diuretics. It was easy to add new compounds to this screening method without changing the MS-method because full-scan MS in both polarities was applied throughout the entire chromatographic run. This approach is currently expanded to include carboxy-finasteride, some stimulants, 21 beta-blockers, and 26 diuretics. The compound carboxy-finasteride is the target for identifying finasteride abuse, as it is a 5a-reductase inhibitor. This compound, which is used in diuretics, has acidic properties and is easily extracted at pH 5.2 (Rahnema et al., 2015).

8.7.2 Compounds Prohibited in Competition

Stimulants

Amphetamines are the most well-known stimulants. Amphetamines can extend the tolerance to anaerobic metabolism in endurance sports that demand high levels of anaerobic exercise. In most cases, stimulants are forbidden in any amount. Nonetheless, a threshold is set for some compounds similar to ephedrine.

Traditionally, GC with nitrogen-phosphorus detection or GC-MS with moderate to good sensitivity have been used to analyze this class of substances. Because of this, the routine use of LC-MS for this class of drugs is still restricted to stimulants that are challenging for GC to detect. These drugs include strychnine, mesocarb-hydroxysulphate (a mesocarb metabolite), ritalinic acid (a methylphenidate metabolite), modafinil, adrafinil, and modafinil-acid (a metabolite for adrafinil and modafinil). These compounds are used in a full-scan ion-trap mass spectrometry screening procedure for diuretics in the laboratory (Rahnema et al., 2015).

The ion at m/z 296 is associated with the sodium adduct of modafinil, while the ion at m/z 167 is associated with a benzyltropylium that results from the neutral loss of modafinil's sulfonyl-side chain. In positive ionization, no sodium-adduct was seen for modafinil acid, but a benzyltropylium was visible as well. Together with a phenyl-benzyl anion, the [M–H]–could be found in negative ionization. Additionally, this phenyl-benzyl anion has an m/z of 167. At any temperature in the heated capillary, the spontaneous fragmentation of modafinil and modafinil-acid into this kathion or anion, stabilized by the aromatic rings, could not be prevented. Ritalinc is an additional stimulant that is a part of our LC–MS screening protocol for diuretics. Ritalinic acid is a methylphenidate metabolite that remains in urine considerably longer than the original drug. By using full-scan MS^2 monitoring of a single product ion at m/z 84, retinic acid is screened for. To ensure accuracy, extra diagnostic ions are produced in MS^3. The quantification of ephedrine and cathine (threshold levels 10 and 5 μg/mL, respectively) is another use for LC-MS. The only steps involved in sample preparation are filtering the urine and then injecting it into the LC-MS system.

We have looked into the complete detection of 27 stimulants in our lab. Diethyl ether was used in a liquid–liquid extraction process at pH 14, and the extracts were then analyzed using an ion-trap device using APCI in positive ionization mode. There was a 15-minute run time total. Every compound underwent an MS2 or MS3 analysis. With the exception of chlorphentermine (detection limit: 250 ng/mL), all compounds had LODs less than 25 ng/mL. LODs of 1 ng/mL were found for a number of substances (Tokish et al., 2004).

Narcotics

Athletes can use opioids to treat moderate to severe pain in order to continue playing even though they are truly injured.

While a number of screening techniques have been published for other fields, LC–ESI-TOFMS has only recently described routine LC–MS screening of drugs for antidoping purposes. Using this method, drugs were found following solid-phase cleanup and enzymatic hydrolysis.

In our lab, we looked into the LC-ESI-MS-MS method of drug detection. A low percentage of organic modifier was added at the beginning of the chromatography process on a C18 column in order to enhance the retention of morphine and hydromorphone. Buprenorphine and methadone are examples of hydrophobic compounds that require high percentages of organic modifier to be eluted. Nalorphine was utilized as the internal standard. Diethyl ether and methylene chloride (CH_2Cl_2) were the two extraction solvents that were tested. LODs for diethyl ether varied from 0 to 20 ng/mL, while those for methylene chloride varied from 0 to 10 ng/mL.

The only drug with a threshold level of 1 μg/mL is morphine. For its quantification, a direct injection of the urine into the LC-MS system following filtration has been described using the LC-ESI-MS-MS method. This eliminates the requirement for hydrolysis and extraction in GC-MS analysis for the detection of morphine and morphine-glucuronides (Kanayama et al., 2010).

Glucocorticosteroids

Corticosteroids are highly effective anti-inflammatory drugs that are used to treat inflammatory conditions. Prior to the development of LC-MS, GC-MS was used for their detection. Selectivity was adequate, but because most corticosteroids have low volatility, a lengthy derivatization step was required. Corticosteroids proved to be the perfect compounds for LC–MS, according to research conducted in the latter part of the 1990s. They are detectable in both polarities using ESI and APCI. Protonated molecular ions are able to identify corticosteroids in the positive ionization mode. Since corticosteroids lack protons that exhibit an acidic gas-phase behavior, no [M–H]–can be seen in the negative mode. Rather, they combine to form highly abundant adducts with formic or acetic acid, which are commonly added to mobile phases. Due to their inability to form these adducts in the negative mode, endogenous anabolic steroids and endogenous corticosteroids can be distinguished from one another using this fact. Since the only differences between corticosteroids and anabolic steroids are the presence of C_{21} and C_{22}, it is likely that the hydroxyfunctions at C_{20} and C_{22}, as well as the keto at C_{21} contribute to the formation of adducts during negative ionization (Fortunato et al., 2006).

Negative ionization was favored in our initial corticosteroid LC–MS–MS screening method. The LODs for this technique varied from 0.5 to 5 ng/mL. As of right now, the LC–MS–MS screening method for anabolic steroids includes glucocorticosteroids.

A Closer Look

Recreational Use of Selective Androgen Receptor Modulators

As a vital intermediary between patients and healthcare professionals, pharmacists have to be aware that people aren't always completely honest about the drugs they use. One such supplement would be selective androgen receptor modulators (SARMs), which are gaining popularity as performance-enhancing agents because of their ability to increase lean muscle mass, burn fat, improve endurance, and speed up recovery. Those who are physically demanding in their jobs, fitness enthusiasts, and bodybuilders are among the people who use or may use products containing SARMs recreationally. In 2008, the World Anti-Doping Agency prohibited the use of SARMs in sports. The FDA warned the public in 2017 that SARMs were being used in bodybuilding supplements and that doing so increased the risk of liver damage, heart attack, and stroke. The trade group representing the dietary supplement industry, the Council for Responsible Nutrition, released voluntary guidelines encouraging the exclusion of SARMs from dietary supplements in response to the FDA's public warning on the drug. Military personnel, medical professionals, and DOD civilians have also been alerted by the Department of Defense's (DOD) "Operation Supplement Safety" that SARMs may artificially lower endogenous testosterone and have negative effects on cholesterol and liver function.

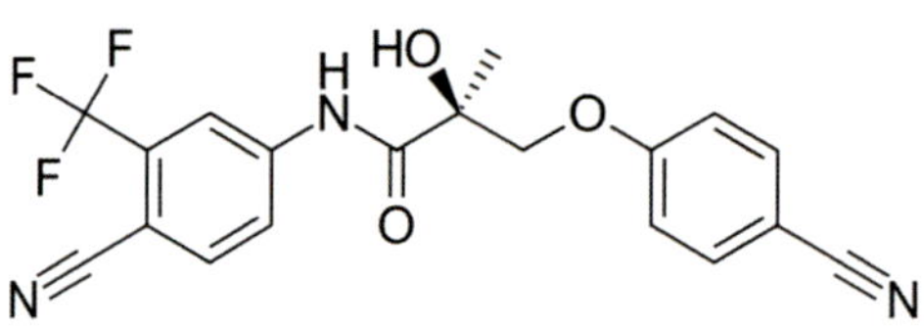

A recent study compared the contents of dietary supplements and products sold online as SARMs to their product labels in order to ascertain the chemical identities and amounts of each ingredient. Just 52% of the 44 products that were tested and marketed as SARMs actually contained one or more SARMs. Another unapproved medication was present in 39% of the products. Of the products, 25% contained ingredients not mentioned on the label, and 9% had no active compound detected at all. In just 41% of the products, the amount of active ingredient matched the amount listed on the label; in 59% of the products, the amount of compounds listed on the label significantly differed from that found through analysis. These results raise serious safety concerns about these products and show an alarming lack of regulatory oversight. At the moment, Ostarine (MK-2866), Ligandrol (LGD-4033), Testolone (RAD-140), and Andarine (GTx-007, S-4) are the most widely used SARMs available. Despite SARMs' increasing popularity and supposed safety in the bodybuilding and fitness industries, there haven't been many clinical studies done to better understand their pharmacokinetic profiles, spot possible side effects, or figure out how drugs interact with one another. As a result, it is still mostly unknown how they will affect the body in the long run. Clinical research has not produced much clinical experience with SARMs; instead, it comes from illicit use. In addition, SARMs are used in the fitness community at higher dosages and longer durations than those that have been clinically tested. When used chronically, especially at high doses, the interactions of SARMs with other substances (such as alcohol and other drugs) are still unknown.

As of right now, SARMs that are sold only as research chemicals can be legally purchased and sold online. On the other hand, those that are labelled as dietary supplements and/or packaged in capsules for human consumption are prohibited from being sold or purchased. In addition, they are not allowed to be sold to the general public as dietary supplements or have any kind of benefit statement made for them.

Nonsteroidal SARMs: Alternative to Androgenic-Anabolic Steroids

SARMs are performance-enhancing drugs that were found in the late 1990s. They promote anabolism, or the growth and development of muscle, and they also make it easier to recover from exercise. SARMs are synthetic ligands that bind to androgen receptors; they are not anabolic steroids. They can act as antagonists, partial agonists, or full agonists depending on their chemical makeup. Every SARM-AR complex has a distinct conformation, and the expression of AR varies across different tissues (such as the brain, skin, liver, prostate, skeletal muscle, and bone). Therefore, SARMs selectively target tissues to promote anabolic activity by interacting with coregulators, transcription factors, and signaling cascade proteins. Compared to anabolic-androgenic steroids, nonsteroidal SARMs are a preferred option due to fewer limitations. They have high oral bioavailability and lower androgenic activity since they are not converted to DHT by 5 alpha-reductase or estrogen by aromatase. These characteristics make nonsteroidal SARMs advantageous over steroidal options, showing promise in male contraception and treating various conditions such as osteoporosis, prostate cancer, sexual dysfunction, Alzheimer's disease, and muscle-related disorders.

Recreational users are now using the different anabolic profiles of different SARMs to selectively achieve results in terms of bulking and cutting, partly due to the belief that SARMs are safer than anabolic steroids. Cutting refers to a fat-loss phase that combines adherence to a strict weight-loss diet with aerobic exercise and less-intense weight training, whereas bulking refers to a muscle-gaining phase that combines a weight-gain diet and intense weight training. Because anecdotal evidence suggests that different SARMs produce different effects when it comes to bulking versus cutting, bodybuilders and other fitness enthusiasts frequently stack (or combine) SARMs.

Ostarine/Enobosarm/GTx-024/MK-2866/S-22

Developed in the late 1990s by Gtx, Inc., osteosarerine is an oral bioavailable nonsteroidal SARM used mainly to treat osteoporosis and muscle atrophy. The SARM with the best clinical characterization is ostarine. Its potential for treating skeletal muscle deficits associated with stress urinary incontinence, breast cancer, non-small-cell lung cancer, and cancer-related cachexia has been investigated in the few published clinical trials. Up to now, clinical trials have consistently shown a significant increase in total lean body mass, even in cancer patients. In certain research, there was no change in the overall body weight but a corresponding decrease in total fat mass. The most frequent low-grade side effects were back pain, fatigue, headaches, and nausea. Additional effects that were noted included a brief increase in alanine transaminase (ALT), as well as decreases in blood glucose, insulin, high density lipoprotein (HDL), and insulin resistance. As soon as the treatment was stopped, all of these changed parameters went back to normal. These are ten times the clinically studied doses. Lowered testosterone levels may result from taking ostarine at these high doses for this prolonged period of time, according to anecdotal evidence. Reduced sex drive, erectile dysfunction, infertility, muscle weakness, loss of bone density, weight gain with increased body fat, insomnia, and depression are among the side effects of low testosterone. Little evidence of clinically significant drug interactions has been found when ostarine (and its major metabolite) is studied in combination with probenecid, celecoxib, itraconazole, and rosuvastatin. One SARM-promoting website states that stacking SARMs will result in greater and more distinct benefits. It is unknown if taking higher doses of several SARMs consistently increases the chance of negative drug-drug interactions.

Ligandrol/LGD-4033/VK5211

Another oral bioavailable SARM is ligandrol. The medication, created by Ligand Pharmaceuticals, has only been the subject of one clinical trial. 76 healthy men were randomly assigned to receive a placebo or 0 mg, 0 mg, 0 mg, or 1 mg of LGD-4033 daily for three weeks in this placebo-controlled study. There were no major adverse drug-related events, and the medication was well tolerated. At any dose, there were no changes in hemoglobin, prostate-specific antigen, aspartate aminotransferase (AST), ALT, or QT intervals. Follicle-stimulating hormone and free testosterone were markedly suppressed at the 1.0 mg dose, while luteinizing hormone remained unchanged. Following the cessation of treatment, hormone levels returned to baseline. There were no statistically significant changes in fat or appendicular skeletal muscle mass, but lean body mass increased dose-dependently. Although not statistically significant, strength, power, and stair-climbing speed and power trended in the direction of a dose-dependent improvement. At any dose, the levels of total and low-density lipoprotein cholesterol did not differ substantially from the baseline. HDL rose at the 0.3 and 1.0 mg doses, but when the medication was stopped, it went back to normal. At all doses, triglyceride levels fell from the baseline. The most frequent adverse effects were dry mouth and headache. A 24-year-old man in good health showed symptoms of hepatocellular liver injury in a recent case report. These signs appeared one week after stopping the drugs. The man did not take regular medications, had a history of binge drinking, and did not have a history of liver disease. This hepatotoxicity is concerning since it falls into the category of liver damage brought on by androgenic anabolic steroids.

Testolone/RAD-140

One SARM that is mainly used to treat breast cancer and muscle atrophy is testosterone. Developed by Health Radius, Inc. According to reports, testosterone is still undergoing first-stage clinical trials; results are anticipated later this year. Therefore, not much is known at this time about its safety. On the other hand, a recent case report details a 49-year-old man who took the medication and suffered significant liver damage (dose not reported). Indicators of mixed hepatocellular-cholestatic liver injury included elevated bilirubin, AST, ALT, and creatinine levels. Inflammation was also seen in liver histology. However, a year after his initial presentation, every liver test had returned to normal. It was anecdotally suggested by SARMs users that Testolone be taken at 5 mg to 30 mg daily for 8 to 16 weeks in order to gain lean muscle mass and strength in the gym. More anecdotal evidence of adverse effects, such as fatigue and insomnia, exists.

Andarine/GTx-007/S-4

There haven't been any human clinical studies on andarine to date. It is promoted as a muscle-boosting supplement that causes weight loss and encourages muscle growth and repair in the fitness community and on numerous internet forums. But because it is thought to be somewhat weaker than other well-known SARMs, it is frequently stacked with other SARMs. Andarine taken alone at a dose of 25 mg daily is said to enhance mood and overall health; however, increasing the dose to 50 mg daily only slightly increases fat burning, lean mass, and strength. It is advised to stack andarine (50 mg) with testolone (10 mg) every day for 8 to 12 weeks in order to bulk. For maximum potency, it is advised to combine Ligandrol (10 mg) with Andarine (50 mg) once a day for two to three weeks. 25 It is recommended that it be stacked with 20 mg of Cardarine (a non-SARM paroxisome proliferator-activated receptor-delta agonist) every day for 12 weeks in order to facilitate cutting. 25 Andarine (50 mg) should be taken daily for nine to twelve weeks in combination with both Ostarine (25 mg) and Cardarine (20 mg) in order to achieve body recomposition (i.e., fat loss and muscle gain at the same time). The two main adverse effects of andarine that have been documented are testosterone suppression and yellowing of the eyesight.

Summary

- Designer steroids refer to synthetic steroids created with slight chemical modifications from existing anabolic steroids. These modifications are intended to enhance their anabolic effects while minimizing their androgenic (masculinizing) effects, potentially making them more potent or less detectable in drug tests.
- Steroid hormones are lipophilic substances derived from cholesterol and are subgrouped based on their pharmacological profile and their receptor binding affinity as sex steroids (androgens, estrogens, gestagens) and corticosteroids (gluco-, and mineralocorticoids).
- Besides the classical, genomic mechanism of action, steroid hormones are reported to act via non-genomic pathways. It is known that estrogens can interfere with the orphan G-protein coupled receptor (GPCR) GPR30, an intracellular trans-membrane receptor, and cause rapid steroid hormone actions.
- Anabolic steroids, also known as anabolic-androgenic steroids (AAS), are a class of drugs that are structurally related to testosterone, the main male sex hormone, and produce effects by binding to the androgen receptor.
- Endogenous androgen is responsible for the growth and development of the sex organs in men and maintaining secondary sex characteristics.
- Endogenous anabolic steroids such as testosterone and dihydrotestosterone and synthetic anabolic steroids mediate their effects by binding to and activating androgen receptors.
- The neurotoxic action of AASs is associated with both membrane AR and G-protein coupled receptors. Furthermore, several studies highlighted the role of apoptosis in determining brain damage.
- Hepatotoxicity is one of the most frequent side effects of AAS abuse. AAS-induced hepatotoxicity was hypothesized to be related to oxidative stress in hepatic cells.
- Before initiating treatment with testosterone, diagnosis of hypogonadism require confirmation by measuring early morning testosterone levels on two separate days.
- Anabolic steroids have been used by athletes in many professional sports, including track and field, weightlifting, bodybuilding, shot put, cycling, baseball, wrestling, mixed martial arts, boxing, and football.
- Performance-enhancing drugs are substances used to improve athletic performance. They work by various mechanisms, including increasing muscle mass, enhancing oxygen delivery, improving focus and alertness, and reducing fatigue.
- Gene doping is the hypothetical non-therapeutic use of gene therapy by athletes in order to improve their performance in those sporting events which prohibit such applications of genetic modification technology, and for reasons other than the treatment of disease.

References

1. Lusetti M, Licata M, Silingardi E, Bonsignore A, Palmiere C. Appearance/Image- and Performance-Enhancing Drug Users: A Forensic Approach. Am J Forensic Med Pathol. 2018 Dec;39(4):325-329.
2. Jones IA, Togashi R, Hatch GFR, Weber AE, Vangsness CT. Anabolic steroids and tendons: A review of their mechanical, structural, and biologic effects. J Orthop Res. 2018 Nov;36(11):2830-2841.
3. Armstrong JM, Avant RA, Charchenko CM, Westerman ME, Ziegelmann MJ, Miest TS, Trost LW. Impact of anabolic androgenic steroids on sexual function. Transl Androl Urol. 2018 Jun;7(3):483-489.
4. Melo Junior AF, Dalpiaz PLM, Sousa GJ, Oliveira PWC, Birocale AM, Andrade TU, Abreu GR, Bissoli NS. Nandrolone alter left ventricular contractility and promotes remodelling involving calcium-handling proteins and renin-angiotensin system in male SHR. Life Sci. 2018 Sep 01;208:239-245.
5. Moretti S, Lega F, Rigoni L, Saluti G, Giusepponi D, Gioiello A, Manuali E, Rossi R, Galarini R. Multiclass screening method to detect more than fifty banned substances in bovine bile and urine. Anal Chim Acta. 2018 Nov 22;1032:56-67.
6. Dahmani H, Louati K, Hajri A, Bahri S, Safta F. Development of an extraction method for anabolic androgenic steroids in dietary supplements and analysis by gas chromatography-mass spectrometry: Application for doping-control. Steroids. 2018 Oct;138:134-160.
7. Smit DL, de Ronde W. Outpatient clinic for users of anabolic androgenic steroids: an overview. Neth J Med. 2018 May;76(4):167.
8. Creagh S, Warden D, Latif MA, Paydar A. The New Classes of Synthetic Illicit Drugs Can Significantly Harm the Brain: A Neuro Imaging Perspective with Full Review of MRI Findings. Clin Radiol Imaging J. 2018;2(1).
9. Andrews MA, Magee CD, Combest TM, Allard RJ, Douglas KM. Physical Effects of Anabolic-androgenic Steroids in Healthy Exercising Adults: A Systematic Review and Meta-analysis. Curr Sports Med Rep. 2018 Jul;17(7):232-241.
10. Roman M., Roman D.L., Ostafe V., Ciorsac A., Isvoran A. Computational assessment of pharmacokinetics and biological effects of some anabolic and androgen steroids. Pharm. Res. 2018;35:41.
11. Patanè F.G., Liberto A., Maglitto A.N.M., Malandrino P., Esposito M., Amico F., Cocimano G., Li Rosi G., Condorelli D., Di Nunno N., et al. Nandrolone Decanoate: Use, Abuse and Side Effects. Medicina. 2020;56:606.
12. Mullen C., Whalley B.J., Schifano F., Baker J.S. Anabolic androgenic steroid abuse in the United Kingdom: An update. Br. J. Pharmacol. 2020;177:2180–2198.
13. Basaria S. Androgen abuse in athletes: Detection and consequences. J. Clin. Endocrinol. Metab. 2010;95:1533–1543.
14. El Osta R., Almont T., Diligent C., Hubert N., Eschwège P., Hubert J. Anabolic steroids abuse and male infertility. Basic Clin. Androl. 2016;26:2.

15. Joseph J.F., Parr M.K. Synthetic androgens as designer supplements. Curr. Neuropharmacol. 2015;13:89–100.

16. Hakansson A., Mickelsson K., Wallin C., Berglund M. Anabolic androgenic steroids in the general population: User characteristics and associations with substance use. Eur. Addict. Res. 2012;18:83–90.

17. Kanayama G., Kaufman M.J., Pope H.G., Jr. Public health impact of androgens. Curr. Opin. Endocrinol. Diabetes Obes. 2018;25:218.

18. Rahnema C.D., Crosnoe L.E., Kim E.D. Designer steroids-over-the-counter supplements and their androgenic component: Review of an increasing problem. Andrology. 2015;3:150–155.

19. Kanayama G., Hudson J.I., Pope H.G., Jr. Illicit anabolic–androgenic steroid use. Horm. Behav. 2010;58:111–121.

20. Anawalt B.D. Diagnosis and management of anabolic androgenic steroid use. J. Clin. Endocrinol. Metab. 2019;104:2490–2500. doi: 10.1210/jc.2018-01882.

21. Kicman A.T. Pharmacology of anabolic steroids. Br. J. Pharmacol. 2008;154:502–521. doi: 10.1038/bjp.2008.165.

22. Sessa F., Salerno M., Di Mizio G., Bertozzi G., Messina G., Tomaiuolo B., Pisanelli D., Maglietta F., Ricci P., Pomara C. Anabolic androgenic steroids: Searching new molecular biomarkers. Front. Pharmacol. 2018;9:1321.

23. Alsiö J., Birgner C., Björkblom L., Isaksson P., Bergström L., Schiöth H.B., Lindblom J. Impact of nandrolone decanoate on gene expression in endocrine systems related to the adverse effects of anabolic androgenic steroids. Basic Clin. Pharmacol. Toxicol. 2009;105:307–314. doi: 10.1111/j.1742-7843.2009.00439.x.

24. Cheung A.S., Grossmann M. Physiological basis behind ergogenic effects of anabolic androgens. Mol. Cell. Endocrinol. 2018;464:14–20. doi: 10.1016/j.mce.2017.01.047.

25. Fortunato R.S., Marassi M.P., Chaves E.A., Nascimento J.H., Rosenthal D., Carvalho D.P. Chronic administration of anabolic androgenic steroid alters murine thyroid function. Med. Sci. Sports Exerc. 2006;38:256–261. doi: 10.1249/01.mss.0000183357.19743.51.

26. Tokish J.M., Kocher M.S., Hawkins R.J. Ergogenic aids: a review of basic science, performance, side effects, and status in sports. Am. J. Sports Med. 2004;32(6):1543–1553. doi: 10.1177/0363546504268041.

27. Pope H.G., Jr, Kanayama G., Athey A., Ryan E., Hudson J.I., Baggish A. The lifetime prevalence of anabolic-androgenic steroid use and dependence in Americans. Current best estimates. Am J Addict. 2014;23(4):371–377. doi: 10.1111/j.1521-0391.2013.12118.x.

Chapter 9

SYNTHETIC CLUB DRUGS

Contents

Introduction

Teenagers and young adults most frequently use club drugs, which are a class of drugs that heighten sensory perceptions and lower inhibitions at bars, nightclubs, concerts, and parties. Consequences are difficult to ascertain because we do not fully understand the sources, compositions, and potential contaminants of many club drugs. Gamma hydroxybutyrate (GHB), rohypnol, ketamine, and 3,4-methylenedioxymethamphetamine (MDMA or ecstasy) are among the medications in this class.

Orientation and Directional Terms

Term	Definition	Illustration
Ecstasy	MDMA (3, 4-methylenedioxymethamphetamine), better known as ecstasy, is a synthetic, psychoactive drug that acts as both a stimulant and a hallucinogen. Users may call it XTC, X, E, Adam, Eve, clarity, hug, beans, love drug, lovers' speed, peace, uppers, or molly.	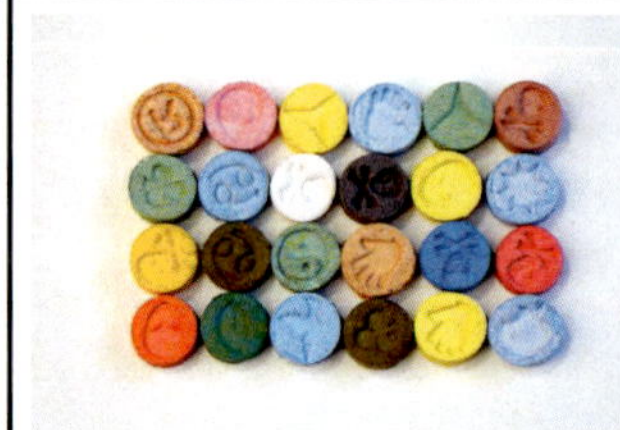
Rohypnol	Rohypnol (flunitrazepam) is a central nervous system depressant and is classified as a benzodiazepine. It is not approved for medical use in the United States, and its importation is banned.	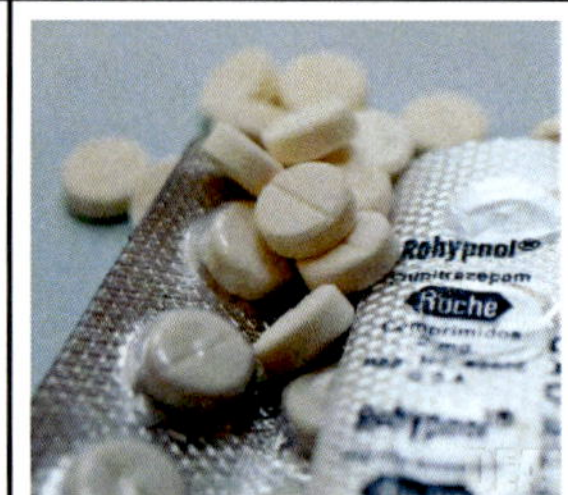
Gamma-hydroxybutyric acid (GHB)	Gamma-hydroxybutyric acid (GHB), also known as Xyrem®, is a central nervous system (CNS) depressant prescribed to treat narcolepsy (a sleep disorder). It exists naturally in the brain but at much lower concentrations than when GHB is taken recreationally.	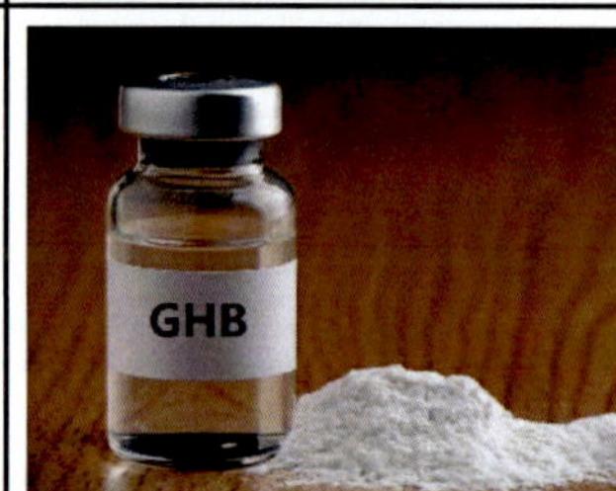
Ketamine	Ketamine is mostly used in veterinary practice as an animal tranquilizer. It causes detachment from pain and the environment. Ketamine is manufactured commercially as a powder or liquid. When sold illegally, it is usually a white crystalline powder.	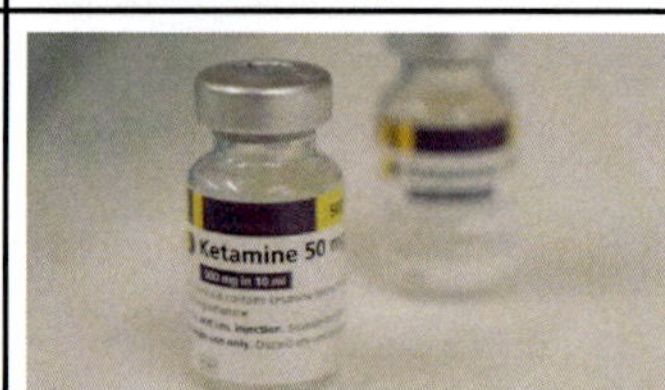
Ephedrine	Ephedrine is a stimulant similar to amphetamine and is found naturally in the Chinese herbal medicine "ma-huang" and in "Mormon's tea."	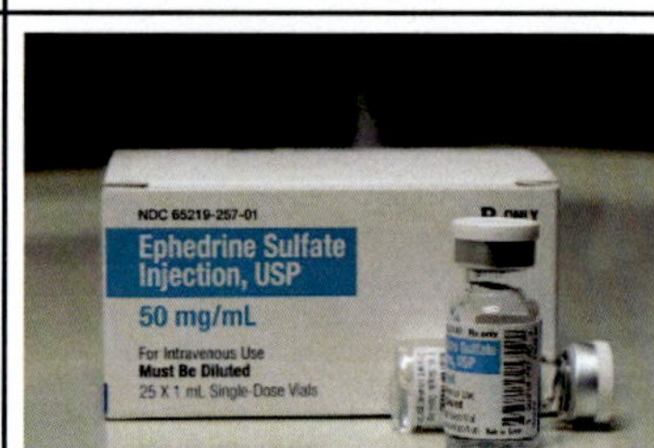

9.1 History

Club drugs, also known as rave drugs or party drugs, are a nebulously defined class of recreational drugs that have been linked to raves, electronic dance music (EDM) parties, nightclubs, and discothèques since the 1980s. Club drugs are classified in a "category of convenience" because they are consumed in certain places or the user travels to certain places while high, unlike many other categories, like opiates and benzodiazepines, which are based on pharmaceutical or chemical properties. Teenagers and young adults are typically the ones who use club drugs.

Club drugs range from entactogens such as MDMA ("ecstasy"), 2C-B ("nexus"), and inhalants (e.g., nitrous oxide and poppers) to stimulants (e.g., amphetamine and cocaine), depressants/sedatives (Quaaludes, GHB, Rohypnol) and psychedelic and hallucinogenic drugs (lysergic acid diethylamide or LSD and dimethyltryptamine or DMT). During the 1960s Mod subculture in the United States, dancers at all-night parties and dance events used some of these drugs for their stimulating properties whose members used amphetamine to stay up late. Substances of choice for clubbing in the 1970s disco scene included the stimulant cocaine and the depressant Quaaludes. Quaaludes were known as "disco biscuits" because they were so popular at discos. Methamphetamine and MDMA were sold and used in numerous clubs during the 1990s and 2000s. Each country and region has its own definition of "club drugs." Although it is not a common practice, some regions have allowed the sale of opiates like heroin and morphine in clubs. Narconon states that other synthetic drugs used in clubs or which are sold as "Ecstasy" include harmaline; piperazines (e.g., BZP and TFMPP); paramethoxyamphetamine/paramethoxymethamphetamine (PMA/PMMA); mephedrone (generally used outside the US) and MDPV.

Club drugs have different legal statuses depending on the drug and the area. Some drugs, like "poppers" (which are often sold as "leather polish" or "room deodorizer" to get around drug laws) and nitrous oxide (which is legal when used from a whipped cream can), are legal in some places. Other club drugs, like amphetamine, are typically prohibited unless the user has a prescription from a doctor. Certain club drugs, like MDMA and cocaine, are virtually always prohibited (Anthony et al., 2017).

Club drug use carries a number of risks. Like with all drugs, whether they are illegal like BZP or legal like alcohol, using them can raise your risk of getting hurt from falls or risky or dangerous behavior (e.g., unsafe sexual relations), as well as harm or death from drunk driving accidents if the user is a driver. Cocaine and amphetamines are two examples of club drugs that can become addictive after repeated use, making the user want more of the substance. Overdoses are more common with certain club drugs. Certain club drugs have negative health effects that can endanger the user; one such drug is MDMA, which can lead to dehydration when used in an all-night dance club.

9.2 Types

Every year, more synthetic club drugs are added to the list. These are some of the popular club drugs along with their street names.

9.2.1 Ecstasy

MDMA, also known as ecstasy, is a common club drug in nightclubs and the rave and electronic dance music scenes. It goes by a lot of monikers, like "e" and "Molly." In addition to being used at free parties, house parties, festivals, and clubs, MDMA is frequently regarded as the drug of choice in the rave community. The drug's sensory effects in a rave setting are frequently greatly enhanced by the lighting and music. MDMA is popular among ravegoers for a variety of reasons, including its psychedelic properties and stimulating effects akin to those of amphetamines. While some users use the drug's inhibition-reducing effects as "party fuel" for all-night dancing, others enjoy the feeling of mass communion that they get from it (Anthony et al., 2017).

Users of MDMA typically take it less than once a week, which is less frequently than other stimulants. Increased dancing enjoyment, illusions of light, sound, and touch, as well as phony emotions of warmth and empathy, are among the effects. Other psychoactive substances like LSD, DMT, psilocybin mushrooms, and 2C-B are occasionally combined with MDMA. Because mentholated products have a cooling effect, users occasionally use them while taking MDMA.

9.2.2 Stimulants

Numerous stimulants are utilized as recreational drugs. Cocaine, methamphetamine, and various amphetamines are used as stimulants. These substances let club patrons dance all night. Cocaine is an effective stimulant of the nervous system. The effects may linger for 15 min, 30 min, or even 1 hour. The amount and mode of administration of cocaine affect how long its effects last. Cocaine can taste bitter and come in the form of fine white powder. It has a numbing effect when injected or inhaled. Cocaine boosts a person's energy and motor activity, sense of competence and sexuality, feelings of well-being and euphoria, and alertness. Although they tend to be more pronounced and shorter-lasting, cocaine's stimulant effects are comparable to those of amphetamine.

Medical Uses

Worldwide, stimulants are widely used as prescription medications and, when not prescribed, illegally or legally as performance-enhancing or recreational drugs. Stimulants are narcotics that, at the end of their effects, cause a noticeable crash or comedown. As of 2013, amphetamine (Adderall), methylphenidate (Ritalin), and lisdexamfetamine (Vyvanse) were the most commonly prescribed stimulants. In 2015, it was estimated that 0.4% of the global population had used cocaine in the previous year. For the category "amphetamines and prescription stimulants" (with "amphetamines" including amphetamine and methamphetamine), the value was 0.7%, and for MDMA, 0.4%.

In medicine, stimulants have been used to treat a wide range of ailments, such as obesity, mood disorders, impulse control issues, sleep disorders, asthma, nasal congestion, and, in the case of cocaine, local anesthetics. The term "anorectics" refers to medications used to treat obesity. These medications typically fall under the general category of stimulants, but they can also include other medications like cannabinoid receptor antagonists. Eugeroics, which include stimulants like modafinil and pitolisant, are used in the treatment of sleep disorders marked by excessive daytime sleepiness, such as narcolepsy. Stimulants are used off-label to treat mood disorders like major depressive disorder and impulse control disorders like ADHD in order to improve mood, focus, and energy levels. Although oral stimulants like salbutamol, theophylline, and epinephrine have been used to treat asthma, inhaled adrenergic drugs are now the preferred option because they have fewer systemic side effects. Pseudoephedrine is used to treat ear congestion brought on by an infection or inflammation of the ears, as well as nasal or sinus congestion brought on by the common cold, sinusitis, hay fever, and other respiratory allergies (Tupper et al., 2015).

Depression

After amphetamines were first introduced to the market in the 1930s, stimulants were among the first classes of medications used to treat depression. However, with the advent of conventional antidepressants in the 1950s, they were mainly abandoned for the treatment of depression. Since then, there has been a renewed interest in depression stimulants in the literature.

Stimulants provide a noticeable, quick-acting, but fleeting mood boost. Accordingly, their efficacy in treating depression is negligible when taken on a regular basis. Furthermore, dosage escalation and dependence have resulted from tolerance to amphetamine's mood-boosting effects. While the efficacy for depression following continuous administration is relatively low, it has the potential to attain statistical significance in comparison to placebo and offer advantages comparable to those of traditional antidepressants. Although the exact causes of stimulant-induced mood enhancements are unknown, they might have something to do with quick tolerance. Both humans and animals have had their tolerance to the effects of stimulants examined and characterized. The symptoms of stimulant withdrawal and major depressive disorder are strikingly similar.

Chemistry

Because stimulants can belong to more than one class and occupy a large number of classes, classifying them is challenging. Ecstasy, for instance, can be categorized as a substituted methylenedioxyphenethylamine, a substituted amphetamine, and subsequently a substituted phenethylamine (Tupper et al., 2015).

Major stimulant classes include phenethylamines, and their daughter class substituted amphetamines.

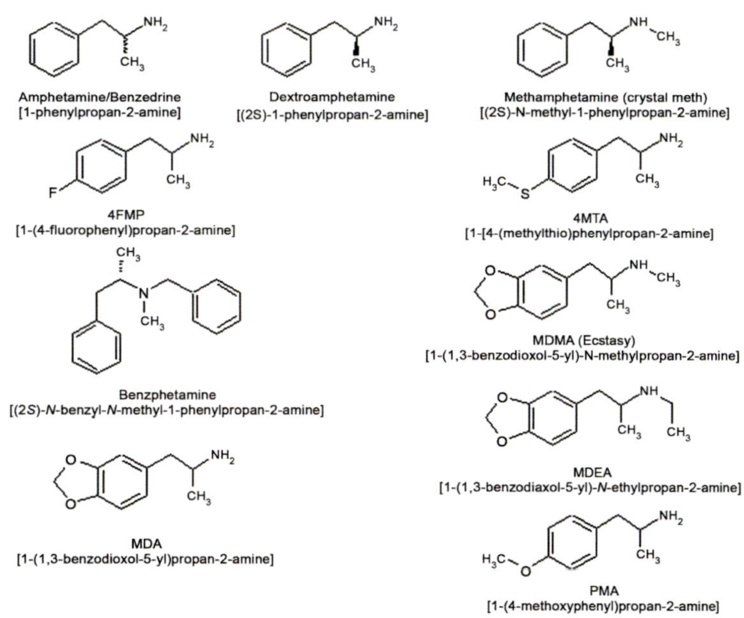

Figure 9.1: A chart comparing the chemical structures of different amphetamine derivatives.

Source: By Shoyrudude555, Public Domain, https://commons.wikimedia.org/w/index.php?curid=2819195

Amphetamines (Class)

A class of compounds known as substituted amphetamines is based on the amphetamine structure and comprises all derivative compounds that are created by substituting one or more hydrogen atoms in the amphetamine core structure. Amphetamine (by itself), methamphetamine, ephedrine, cathinone, phentermine, mephentermine, bupropion, methoxyphenamine, selegiline, amfepramone, pyrovalerone, MDMA (ecstasy), and DOM (STP) are a few examples of substituted amphetamines. A number of medications in this class mainly function by activating the trace amine-associated receptor 1 (TAAR1), which then inhibits dopamine reuptake and releases serotonin, norepinephrine, and dopamine. The release of monoamine neurotransmitter vesicles through VMAT2 is another mechanism of action of some substituted amphetamines. This increases the concentration of these neurotransmitters in the cytosol, or intracellular fluid, of the presynaptic neuron (Black, 2014).

Stimulants similar to amphetamines are frequently used for their medicinal benefits. When patients do not respond well to conventional SSRI medications, doctors may prescribe amphetamine to treat major depression; however, the evidence for this use is either weak or inconsistent. Remarkably, when lisdexamfetamine—a prodrug to amphetamine—is used in conjunction with an SSRI or SNRI for the treatment of major depressive disorder, two recent large-scale phase III trials have not demonstrated any additional benefit over a placebo in terms of efficacy. Several studies have shown how well medications like Adderall, which is a combination of amphetamine and dextroamphetamine salts, work to control the symptoms of ADHD. Substituted amphetamines are easy to get and have quick effects, which makes them very appealing for abuse (Black, 2014).

Cocaine Analogs

There are hundreds of cocaine analogs that have been developed, and they all typically keep a benzyloxy bond to a tropane's third carbon. Different modifications include additions or substitutions in place of the typical carboxylate on the tropane 2 carbon, as well as substitutions on the benzene ring. Other compounds that aren't strictly analogs of cocaine but have structure-activity relationships similar to it have also been developed.

Mechanisms of Action

The majority of stimulants increase catecholamine neurotransmission to achieve their activating effects. Neurotransmitters called catecholamines are involved in regulatory pathways that are linked to motivation, arousal, reward anticipation, task salience, and attention. Classical stimulants cause these catecholamines' circuits to become more active by either stimulating their efflux or blocking their reuptake. Certain stimulants also influence serotonergic transmission; these include stimulants with empathogenic and hallucinogenic effects. By opposing regulatory autoreceptors, certain stimulants, including yohimbine and some amphetamine derivatives, can reduce negative feedback. Ephedrine is one of the adrenergic agonists that works by directly attaching to and activating adrenergic receptors to produce sympathomimetic effects.

A medication may also produce activating effects through additional indirect mechanisms of action. As an adenosine receptor antagonist, caffeine only modifies the brain's transmission of catecholamines in an indirect manner. Pitolisant is an inverse agonist of the histamine 3 (H_3) receptor. Pitolisant increases histaminergic transmission by reducing negative feedback to histaminergic neurons, since histamine 3 (H_3) receptors primarily function as autoreceptors. It is still unclear how exactly some stimulants, like modafinil, work to treat the symptoms of narcolepsy and other sleep disorders.

Notable Stimulants

Amphetamine

The phenethylamine class of powerful CNS stimulants, such as amphetamine, is authorized for the treatment of narcolepsy and attention deficit hyperactivity disorder (ADHD). Amphetamine is also used recreationally as an aphrodisiac and euphoriant, and off-label as a performance and cognitive enhancer. Amphetamine is a prescription drug in many countries, but because of the serious health risks involved in heavy or uncontrolled use, it is often strictly prohibited in the possession and distribution of unapproved forms. Consequently, amphetamine is produced illegally in covert labs in order to be trafficked and sold to users. Methamphetamine production and trafficking are far more common than illicit amphetamine production, according to global drug and drug precursor seizures (Nichols, 2016).

Benzedrine was the first amphetamine to be produced pharmaceutically. It was a brand of inhalers used to treat various ailments. Dextrorotary isomer has stronger stimulant qualities, so formulations that contain all or mostly dextroamphetamine have gradually replaced benzedrine. These days, it is usually prescribed in the form of lisdexamfetamine, dextroamphetamine, and mixed amphetamine salts.

A norepinephrine-dopamine releasing agent (NDRA) is amphetamine. Via the dopamine and norepinephrine transporters (NETs), it enters neurons and, by activating TAAR1 and inhibiting VMAT2, facilitates neurotransmitter efflux. This has emotional and cognitive effects at therapeutic doses, including euphoria, libido changes, elevated arousal, and enhanced cognitive control. Similarly, it causes physical effects like improved muscle strength, resistance to fatigue, and a slower reaction time. On the other hand, amphetamine dosages above the recommended threshold are likely to cause rapid muscle breakdown and cognitive impairment. Psychosis may occur at very high dosages (e.g., delusions, and paranoia), which, even with prolonged use, very seldom happens at therapeutic dosages. Recreational use carries a far higher risk of major side effects, such as dependence, which only rarely occurs with therapeutic amphetamine use. This is because recreational doses are typically much larger than prescribed therapeutic doses.

Ephedrine

Ephedrine is a sympathomimetic amine that shares structural similarities with the well-known drugs methamphetamine and phenylpropanolamine, as well as the crucial neurotransmitter adrenaline. Ephedrine is frequently used to treat hypotension brought on by anesthesia as well as a stimulant, appetite suppressant, aid in concentration, and decongestant.

Chemically speaking, it is an alkaloid present in a variety of plants belonging to the genus Ephedra (family Ephedraceae) that has a phenethylamine skeleton. It primarily functions by enhancing norepinephrine's (noradrenaline's) adrenergic receptor activity. It is most frequently sold as the sulfate or hydrochloride salt. The main active ingredients of the herb *má huáng* (*Ephedra sinica*), which is used in traditional Chinese medicine (TCM), are pseudoephedrine and ephedrine. This might also apply to other herbal remedies that have extracts from different species of Ephedra (Nichols, 2016).

MDMA

MDMA, also known as ecstasy or molly, is

a stimulant, euphoriant, and empathogen belonging to the amphetamine class. After being briefly used as a therapeutic adjunct by some psychotherapists, MDMA gained popularity as a recreational drug. The DEA classified it as a Schedule I controlled substance, which forbade the majority of medical research and applications. MDMA is well renowned for having entactogenic qualities. Hypertension, anorexia (loss of appetite), euphoria, social disinhibition, insomnia (increased wakefulness/inability to sleep), better energy, elevated arousal, and increased perspiration are a few of the stimulant effects of MDMA. When compared to classical stimulants such as amphetamine, MDMA significantly increases serotonergic transmission relative to catecholaminergic transmission. It doesn't seem like MDMA is very addictive or habit-forming.

MDPV

Methylenedioxypyrovalerone (MDPV) is a stimulant-type psychoactive drug that inhibits the uptake of norepinephrine by dopamine (NDRI). A group at Boehringer Ingelheim created it initially in the 1960s. MDPV was a little-known stimulant until 2004 when rumors circulated that it was being sold as a designer drug. Similar to how Spice and K2 are marketed as incense, products labeled as bath salts containing MDPV were previously sold as recreational drugs in American convenience stores and gas stations. There have been cases of psychological and physical injuries linked to MDPV use.

Mephedrone

Mephedrone belongs to the amphetamine and cathinone classes of synthetic stimulants. MCAT and drone are examples of slang terms. It is reportedly made in China and shares chemical similarities with the cathinone compounds present in eastern African khat plants. It is available as tablets or powder that users can inject, snort, or swallow. Its effects are comparable to those of cocaine, amphetamines, and MDMA.

Despite being created for the first time in 1929, mephedrone was not well known until it was rediscovered in 2003. Mephedrone was reportedly being sold online by 2007; law enforcement agencies had learned about the compound by 2008; and by 2010, reports of mephedrone had spread throughout most of Europe, with the UK being the most common location. 2008 saw the outlawing of mephedrone in Israel, and later that year, Sweden also did the same. It was outlawed in several European nations in 2010, and the EU declared it unlawful in December of that same year. It is regarded as an analog of other illegal drugs in Australia, New Zealand, and the US and is subject to legislation akin to the Federal Analog Act. The United States of America temporarily categorized mephedrone as illegal in September 2011, with effect from October 2011.

Mephedrone is a neurotoxic drug with abuse potential. It primarily acts on 5-hydroxytryptamine (5-HT) terminals, causing subjective feelings in abusers that are similar to those of MDMA (Brands et al., 1998).

Methamphetamine

A strong psychostimulant belonging to the phenethylamine and amphetamine classes, methamphetamine (contracted from N-methyl-alpha-methylphenethylamine) is used to treat obesity and attention deficit hyperactivity disorder (ADHD). There are two enantiomers of methamphetamine: levorotary and dextrorotary. Despite being a more potent central nervous system stimulant than levomethamphetamine, dextromethamphetamine is addictive and exhibits similar toxicity symptoms when taken in excessive amounts. Methamphetamine hydrochloride is authorized by the United States

Food and Drug Administration (USFDA) under the brand name Desoxyn, despite the fact that it is rarely prescribed because of the possible risks. Methamphetamine is used recreationally to boost energy, elevate mood, and increase sexual desire. Some users are able to have multiple days of nonstop sex.

Methamphetamine can be sold illegally in two forms: only as dextromethamphetamine, or in a mixture of equal parts right- and left-handed molecules i.e., 50% levomethamphetamine and 50% dextromethamphetamine). Both racemic and dextromethamphetamine are classified as schedule II controlled substances in the US. Furthermore, methamphetamine's inclusion in schedule II of the United Nations Convention on Psychotropic Substances means that its manufacture, distribution, sale, and possession are prohibited or illegal in a large number of other nations. On the other hand, levomethamphetamine is available over-the-counter in the US.

Methamphetamine, when taken in moderation, can improve mood and give tired people more energy, alertness, and focus. Higher dosages have the potential to cause cerebral hemorrhage, rhabdomyolysis, and psychosis. It is well recognized that methamphetamine has a high risk of abuse and addiction. Methamphetamine use for recreational purposes can cause post-withdrawal syndrome, a withdrawal syndrome that can last for months after the usual withdrawal period, or even cause psychosis. Methamphetamine is neurotoxic to humans, harming both dopamine and serotonin neurons in the central nervous system (CNS), in contrast to amphetamine and cocaine. There is evidence that long-term use of methamphetamine in humans causes adverse changes in brain structure and function, including reductions in gray matter volume in several brain regions and adverse changes in markers of metabolic integrity. This is in contrast to long-term use of amphetamine in prescription doses, which may improve certain brain regions in individuals with ADHD. Amphetamine dosages used recreationally, nevertheless, may also be neurotoxic (Martin et al., 2017).

Methylphenidate

Methylphenidate is a stimulant medication that is sometimes used in conjunction with diet restrictions and exercise to treat obesity. It is frequently used to treat narcolepsy and ADHD. At therapeutic doses, it has the following effects: decreased impulsivity, decreased need for sleep, decreased appetite, increased focus, and increased alertness. Though it is rarely used recreationally, methylphenidate has effects that are strikingly similar to those of amphetamines.

Methylphenidate inhibits the norepinephrine-dopamine reuptake by preventing the dopamine transporter (DAT) and the NET from functioning. Methylphenidate primarily causes elevated dopamine levels through inhibited reuptake of dopamine, as it has a higher affinity for the dopamine transporter than for the NET. However, elevated norepinephrine levels also play a role in some of the drug's effects.

Methylphenidate is marketed under several names, such as Ritalin. Additional forms consist of the long-lasting transdermal patch Daytrana and the long-lasting tablet Concerta.

Cocaine

Among SNDRIs is cocaine. The coca shrub, which grows in the mountainous regions of South American nations like Bolivia, Colombia, and Peru, yields leaves that are used to make cocaine. The Aymara people have grown and used coca for centuries in these regions. The most prevalent form of cocaine in Europe, North America, and some regions of Asia is a white, crystalline powder. Although cocaine has stimulant qualities, it is not typically prescribed for therapeutic purposes. However, it is used in clinical settings as a local anesthetic, particularly in ophthalmology.

Since cocaine has a higher potential for abuse than amphetamine and is mostly used recreationally, most jurisdictions strictly prohibit its sale and possession. Although they have not been commercially distributed or used recreationally, other tropane derivative drugs related to cocaine, such as troparil and lometopane, are also known.

Nicotine

The primary chemical component of tobacco is nicotine, which can be found in a variety of forms, including chewing tobacco, cigars, cigarettes, and electronic cigarettes and patches. Nicotine's stimulating and calming properties have led to its widespread use worldwide. Nicotine acts by agonizing nicotinic acetylcholine receptors, which have a number of secondary effects.

For example, it can activate dopaminergic neurons in the midbrain reward system, and one tobacco ingredient, acetaldehyde, can reduce the expression of monoamine oxidase in the brain. Nicotine can lead to addiction and dependence. The most popular source of nicotine, tobacco, ranks sixth most harmful of the 20 drugs evaluated based on a multi-criteria decision analysis. Its overall harm to the user and the self-score is 3% below cocaine and 13% above amphetamines (Darke et al., 2019).

Phenylpropanolamine

As the psychoactive drug belonging to the phenethylamine and amphetamine chemical classes, phenylpropanolamine (PPA; Accutrim; β-hydroxyamphetamine) is also referred to as the stereoisomers norephedrine and norpseudoephedrine. It is used as a stimulant, decongestant, and anorectic. It is frequently found in over-the-counter and prescription cough and cold remedies. Under the brand names Propalin and Proin, it is used in veterinary medicine to treat urinary incontinence in dogs.

Because PPA may raise the risk of stroke in younger women, it is no longer available over-the-counter in the United States. Nonetheless, it is still accessible in some European nations, sometimes over-the-counter and sometimes with a prescription. It was taken off the market in Canada on May 31, 2001. On February 10, 2011, the use of PPA and its formulations by humans was outlawed in India.

Lisdexamfetamine

Lisdexamfetamine, which is found in Vyvanse, etc. is a drug similar to amphetamine that is marketed to treat ADHD. Usually, the effects of it last for 14 hours. The body metabolizes lisdexamfetamine into dextroamphetamine; it is inert on its own. As a result, there is less chance of abuse.

Pseudoephedrine

A sympathomimetic medication belonging to the phenethylamine and amphetamine chemical classes is pseudoephedrine. It can be taken as a stimulant, a nasal/sinus decongestant, or an agent that promotes wakefulness.

Pseudoephedrine hydrochloride and pseudoephedrine sulfate are two salts that are commonly found in over-the-counter preparations. They can be found alone or, more frequently, in combination with guaifenesin, dextromethorphan, antihistamines, paracetamol (acetaminophen), and/or another NSAID (like aspirin or ibuprofen). Additionally, it serves as a precursor chemical in the illicit manufacture of methamphetamine (Darke et al., 2019).

Modafinil

Since modafinil is a eugeroic drug, it encourages alertness and wakefulness. Among other names, Modafinil is marketed under the Provigil brand. Modafinil is used to treat obstructive sleep apnea, shift work sleep disorder, and narcolepsy-related excessive daytime sleepiness. Although it has been used off-label as a supposed cognitive enhancer, there is conflicting evidence regarding its efficacy in this regard. Modafinil has very low risks of addiction and dependence, even though it is a CNS stimulant. While modafinil and stimulant medications share similar biochemical pathways, modafinil is unlikely to have mood-elevating effects. It's unclear whether the effects of caffeine are similar. In contrast to other stimulants, modafinil does not cause a subjective sense of reward or pleasure, which is typically linked to euphoria—a strong sense of wellbeing. Ecstasy may be a sign of drug abuse, which is defined as excessive and obsessive drug use despite negative effects. Modafinil is thought to have a low risk of addiction and dependence because there has been no evidence of abuse potential in clinical trials; however, caution is advised.

Pitolisant

Pitolisant functions as the histamine 3 (H_3) autoreceptor's inverse agonist (antagonist). Thus, pitolisant, a drug that also falls under the category of CNS stimulants, is an antihistamine. Additionally categorized as a eugeroic class medication, pitolisant encourages wakefulness and alertness. Pitolisant is a novel eugeroic medication that functions by inhibiting the H_3 autoreceptor.

Pitolisant has demonstrated efficacy and good toleration in the management of narcolepsy, both in cases with and without cataplexy. In the US, the only non-controlled anti-narcoleptic medication is pitolisant. Research has indicated a low likelihood of abuse.

When the H_3 autoreceptor is blocked, it leads to heightened activity of histamine neurons in the brain. These receptors play a role in regulating histamine levels in the central nervous system and to some extent, in the peripheral nervous system by inhibiting histamine production and release when they bind to naturally occurring histamine. Pitolisant works by preventing the binding of naturally occurring histamine at the H_3 receptor and also produces an opposite response to that of histamine (inverse agonism), ultimately increasing histamine activity in the brain (Hernández-Serrano et al., 2016).

9.2.3 Depressants/Sedatives

Drugs classified as depressants decrease neurotransmission, as well as arousal and stimulation in different brain regions. No one else's mood or mental state is altered by depressants. Since stimulants, also known as "uppers," improve mental or physical performance, they belong to a different pharmacological class than depressants—stimulants, not antidepressants.

Worldwide, depressants are commonly used as both illegal and prescription drugs. One of the most common depressants is alcohol. Ataxia, anxiolysis, pain relief, sedation or somnolence, cognitive or memory impairment, and, in certain cases, euphoria, dissociation, muscle relaxation, lowered blood pressure or heart rate, respiratory depression, and anticonvulsant effects are among the common side effects of depressants. Anesthesia is another effect that depressants have. Cannabidiol, one of the components of cannabis, raises the possibility that it is occasionally a depressant. Like other depressive medications, the latter is recognized for treating muscle spasms, anxiety, and insomnia. Tetrahydrocannabinol, on the other hand, is primarily thought to be a stimulant and primary psychoactive agent that can occasionally cause anxiety, panic, and psychosis, even though it may also slightly slow brain function and lessen response to stimuli. A variety of opioids and benzodiazepines like Xanax are examples of additional depressants. Gabapentinoids, which include baclofen and gabapentin, have anxiolytic, anticonvulsant, and depressant properties. Lamotrigine, phenytoin, and most other anticonvulsants are depressants. Barbiturates and carbamates are related classes of depressants (Hernández-Serrano et al., 2016).

There are several distinct pharmacological pathways by which depressants work, but the most well-known ones involve GABA facilitation and glutamatergic or monoaminergic activity inhibition. Additional examples are substances, the most well-known of which are bromides and channel blockers, that alter the electrical signaling within the body.

Indications

Depressants are used medicinally to relieve the following symptoms:

- Anxiety disorders such as:
  - Generalized anxiety
  - Social anxiety
  - Panic attacks
- Insomnia
- Obsessive-compulsive disorder
- Seizures
- Convulsions
- Depression
- Pain

Types

Barbiturates

Barbiturates work well to relieve the symptoms of the conditions they are intended to treat (seizures, insomnia). They have a significant overdose risk, are physically addictive, and are frequently used for illicit purposes. By the late 1950s, there was a concentrated search for substitute drugs due to worries about the growing social costs of barbiturates, which were starting to outweigh their alleged medical benefits. The majority of people who use barbiturates today do so either to prevent seizures or, in milder forms, to relieve migraine symptoms.

Benzodiazepines

The fundamental chemical structure of a benzodiazepine (sometimes referred to as "benzo" or "BZD") is the union of a benzene ring and a diazepine ring. Leo Sternbach made the initial discovery of this type of medication, chlordiazepoxide (Librium), by accident in 1955. Hoffmann-La Roche then went on to commercialize the benzodiazepine diazepam (Valium) in 1960.

Benzodiazepines have sedative, hypnotic (sleep-inducing), anxiolytic (anti-anxiety), anticonvulsant, and muscle relaxant properties because they increase the action of the neurotransmitter gamma-aminobutyric acid (GABA) at the GABAA receptor. Amnesic-dissociative actions are also observed in the applied pharmacology of high doses of many shorter-acting benzodiazepines. Withdrawal from alcohol, agitation, seizures, anxiety, insomnia, muscle spasms, and premedication for dental or medical procedures are among the conditions for which benzodiazepines are helpful due to these characteristics. There are three types of benzodiazepines: short-, intermediate-, and long-acting. For the treatment of insomnia, short- and intermediate-acting benzodiazepines are preferred; longer-acting benzodiazepines are advised for the treatment of anxiety (Dasgupta, 2017).

While paradoxical effects like aggression or behavioral disinhibition and cognitive impairments are occasionally experienced, benzodiazepines are generally safe and effective in the short term. A minority responds in the opposite way from what is typically anticipated. For instance, taking a benzodiazepine may cause a panic attack to get much worse. Due to negative psychological and physical effects, declining efficacy, physical dependence, and benzodiazepine withdrawal syndrome that occurs after long-term use, long-term use is debatable. Because benzodiazepines have negative side effects when used for extended periods of time, stopping them usually improves both physical and mental health. Senior citizens are more likely to suffer negative short- and long-term consequences.

The safety of benzodiazepines during pregnancy is a topic of debate. They are known to cause withdrawal symptoms in newborns, but it is unclear whether they cause neurobehavioral effects due to prenatal exposure or if they cause cleft palate in a small number of babies. Regardless, they are not major teratogens. Overdosing on benzodiazepines can result in dangerously deep unconsciousness. Even so, benzodiazepines are far less toxic than the barbiturates that came before them, and using them alone rarely results in death. The risk of toxicity and lethal overdose rises when benzodiazepines are taken with other substances that depress the central nervous system, such as alcohol and opiates. Misuse and combination use of benzodiazepines with other addictive substances are common. Additionally, and this is important for clinical practice, all benzodiazepines are included in the Beers List (Dasgupta, 2017).

Cannabis

Cannabis is frequently regarded as belonging in a distinct category or as a mild psychedelic. Tetrahydrocannabinol (THC), a chemical compound present in cannabis, has a variety of depressant effects, including fatigue, sedation, relaxed muscles, and decreased alertness. The exact opposite of what central nervous system depressants do is what happens when cannabinoids activate the CB1 receptor, which inhibits GABA.

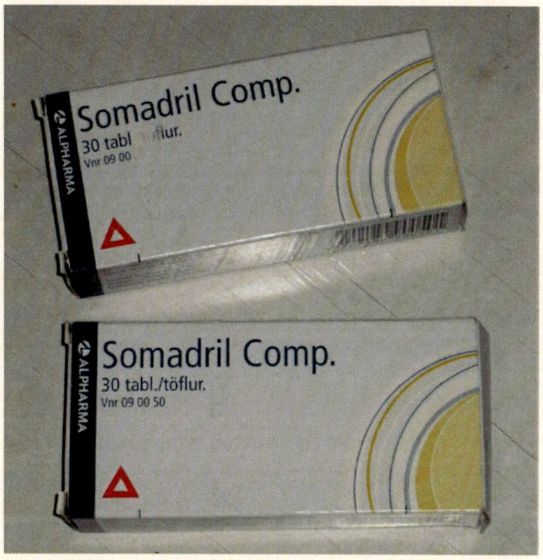

Figure 9.2: Carisoprodol tablets.

Source: By ZngZng - Own work, CC BY-SA 3.0, https://commons.wikimedia.org/w/index.php?curid=14911047

Carbamates

A class of "tranquilizers" or depressants called carbamates are produced from urea. The effects of carbamates include muscle relaxation, analgesia, anticonvulsant, hypnotic, and antihypertensive. They can also be used for withdrawal from alcohol, agitation, and muscle tremors. When used in conjunction with rest, physical therapy, and other measures, their muscle relaxant effects can be beneficial for sprains, strains, and muscle injuries. The synthesis, action mechanism, and effects of carbamates are strikingly similar to those of barbiturates. There are numerous varieties of carbamates; some solely have anticonvulsant properties, while others solely have hypnotic and anxiolytic effects. Drowsiness, dizziness, headache, nausea, diarrhea, flatulence, liver failure, poor coordination, nystagmus, abuse, dizziness, weakness, nervousness, euphoria, overstimulation, and dependence are some of the side effects of carbamates. Hypersensitivity reactions, such as Stevens-Johnson syndrome, embryo-fetal toxicity, stupor, and coma, are uncommon but potentially serious adverse reactions. Because carbamates can be fatal in excess, benzodiazepines have largely replaced them. Long-term use of most carbamates, such as carisoprodol, is not advised because it can lead to physical and psychological dependence.

Launched in 1955, meprobamate metabolizes to carisoprodol. It soon rose to prominence as Hollywood's first psychotropic drug blockbuster, becoming well-known for its supposedly miraculous effects. Since then, it has been sold under more than a hundred trade names, such as Zirpon, Quivet, and Amepromat. Carisoprodol abuse is possible; it is still mostly used for its muscle-relaxing properties. Its mode of action is highly comparable to that of benzodiazepines, alcohol, methaqualone, and barbiturates. Similar to barbiturates, carisoprodol directly activates and allosterically modulates the human α1β2η2 GABAAR ($GABA_A$) in the central nervous system. Chloride floods the neuron as a result of the opening of chloride channels. Communication between neurons and the nervous system is slowed down as a result. When GABA is bound, carisoprodol lengthens the duration of channel opening, in contrast to benzodiazepines, which increase the frequency of the chloride channel opening. The primary inhibitory neurotransmitter in the nervous system responsible for the depressant effects is GABA (Guina and Merrill, 2018).

Overdosing on carbamates can be deadly. Similar to a barbiturate overdose, symptoms usually include impaired thinking, disorientation, a lowered state of consciousness, and a reduction in the effort required to breathe (respiratory depression). If an overdose is combined with another depressant that suppresses breathing, the likelihood of it being fatal increases.

Long-term use of carbamates, especially carisoprodol, can result in both physical and psychological dependence. These days, muscle pain, especially back pain, is the only condition for which carisoprodol is used temporarily. After prolonged use, stopping could have very serious and even deadly consequences. Due to their similar mechanisms of action, alcohol, benzodiazepines, and barbiturates can all cause withdrawal symptoms that are similar to each other. Confusion, disorientation, delirium, auditory and visual hallucinations, insomnia, decreased appetite, anxiety, psychomotor agitation, tachycardia, tremor, and seizures are among the symptoms of discontinuation that can be fatal.

In the 1950s, carbamates were widely used in conjunction with barbiturates. Although worries about the possibility of overdose and dependence have gradually reduced their appeal, newer carbamate derivatives are still being created. Among them is the anticonvulsant felbamate, which was authorized in 1993 and is still widely used today. It is an NR2B subunit of the NMDA receptor blocker and a GABAA-positive allosteric modulator. Sodium channels are blocked by other carbamates. In Europe, phenprobamate is occasionally used for general anesthesia, the treatment of muscular spasticity and cramps, and as an anxiolytic. Robaxin, also known as methocarbamol, is a well-liked medication that is available over-the-counter in some nations (Guina and Merrill, 2018). It is a carbamate that has the ability to relax muscles. Tetrabamate is a controversial medication that combines phenobarbital, febarbamate, and difebarbamate. It is sold in Europe and has been mainly, though not entirely, phased out.

The drug's use was restricted on April 4, 1997, following more than 30 years of use because of reports of acute liver failure and hepatitis. For its muscle-relaxing properties, carisoprodol, sometimes referred to as "Soma," is still widely used today. Additionally, it is widely abused everywhere in the world. In the US, it is classified as a Schedule IV substance. Bruce Lee, the well-known actor and martial artist, passed away from a meprobamate allergy.

Approved

- Carisoprodol/Meprobamate/Tybamate (Soma/Miltown, Solacen) (muscle relaxant, anxiolytic, tranquilizer)
- Difebarbamate (Atrium, Sevrium) (tranquilizer)
- Emylcamate (Striatran) (anxiolytic and muscle relaxant)
- Ethinamate (Valamin, Valmid) (sedative-hypnotic)
- Febarbamate/Phenobamate (Solium, Tymium) (anxiolytic and tranquilizer)
- Felbamate (Felbatol) (anticonvulsant)
- Hexapropymate (Merinax) (hypnotic-sedative)
- Mebutamate (Capla, Dormate) (anxiolytic, sedative, antihypertensive)
- Phenprobamate (Gamaquil, Isotonil) (muscle relaxant, sedative, anxiolytic, anticonvulsant, anesthesia)
- Procymate (Equipax) (sedative, anxiolytic)
- Styramate (Sinaxamol) (muscle relaxant, anticonvulsant)
- Tetrabamate (febarbamate, difebarbamate, phenobarbital) (Atrium, G Tril, Sevrium) (anxiety, alcohol withdrawal, muscle tremors, agitation, depression)

Even after receiving approval, a drug may not always be used as prescribed today.

Not approved

- Carisbamate (anticonvulsant)
- Clocental (hypnotic)
- Cyclarbamate (muscle relaxant and tranquilizer)
- Lorbamate (muscle relaxant and tranquilizer)
- Nisobamate (tranquilizer)
- Pentabamate (tranquilizer)

Gabapentinoids

Voltage-gated calcium channels containing $\alpha_2\delta$ subunits are inhibited by gabapentinoids, a distinct and relatively new class of depressants that bind to the auxiliary $\alpha_2\delta$ subunit (CACNA2D1 and CACNA2D2) site of some VDCCs. $\alpha_2\delta$ is known as the «receptor for gabapentin.». VDCCs are typically closed at resting membrane potential or physiologic potential. Their activation (opening) at depolarized membrane potentials is what gives rise to the term «voltage-gated.». The α_1 and α_2 sites of the α2δ subunit family are bound by gabapentinoids. The archetypal gabapentinoid is gabapentin. Calcium channels of the L, N, P/Q, and R types are all present in the central and peripheral nervous systems, and these channels contain the $\alpha_2\delta$ protein. Presynaptic neurons contain α2δ, which influences calcium channel trafficking and kinetics, starts extracellular signaling cascades, regulates gene expression, and uses thrombospondin 1 to promote excitatory synaptogenesis. Instead of blocking channels directly, gabapentinoids interfere with $\alpha_2\delta$›s regulatory role and its interactions with other proteins. The N and P/Q-type calcium channels that are high voltage-activated mediate the majority of the effects of gabapentinoids. N-type calcium channels are distributed throughout the central and peripheral nervous systems, whereas P/Q-type calcium channels are primarily found in the cerebellum (Purkinje neurons), which may be the cause of the ataxic side effect of gabapentinoids. Gabapentinoids' analgesic effects are primarily due to N-type calcium channels. Ziconotide, a non-gabapentinoid ω-conotoxin peptide, exhibits analgesic properties 1000 times more potent than morphine due to its binding to N-type calcium channels. When binding to the calcium channel complex, gabapentinoids are non-selective, but they are selective for the $\alpha_2\delta$ site. Many excitatory and pro-nociceptive neurochemicals, such as glutamate, substance P, calcitonin gene-related peptide (CGRP), and others, are released less frequently when they act on the $\alpha_2\delta$ site.

The excitatory amino acid transporter 3 and the large neutral amino acid transporter 1 (LAT1, SLC7A5) are primarily responsible for the absorption of gabapentinoids from the intestines. They are among the few medications that make use of these transporters of amino acids. Gabapentinoids share structural similarities with L-leucine and L-isoleucine, two branched-chained amino acids that also bind to the $\alpha_2\delta$ site. The central nervous system uses branched-chain amino acids, such as l-leucine, l-isoleucine, and l-valine, for a variety of purposes. They alter the blood-brain barrier's large neutral amino acid (LNAA) transport and decrease the production of neurotransmitters made from aromatic amino acids, particularly catecholamines from tyrosine and phenylalanine and serotonin from tryptophan. This could have a bearing on gabapentinoids' pharmacology (Graziano, 2017).

Researchers at Parke-Davis created Gabapentin as an analog of the neurotransmitter GABA that could more easily cross the blood-brain barrier. It was initially described in 1975 by Satzinger and Hartenstein and was first approved for epilepsy as an add-on treatment for partial seizures. Gabapentinoids are similar to GABA but do not bind to its receptors or convert into GABA in the body. While Gabapentin activates a potassium channel that enhances its depressive effects, it still mimics GABA activity by inhibiting neurotransmission. Gabapentinoids prevent the delivery of the calcium channels to the cell membrane and disrupt interactions of $\alpha_2\delta$ with NMDA receptors, α-amino-3-hydroxy-5-methyl-4-isoxazolepropionic acid (AMPA) receptors, neurexins, and thrombospondins. Some calcium channel blockers of the dihydropyridine class are used for hypertension weakly blocking $\alpha_2\delta$.

Anxiolytic, anticonvulsant, antiallodynic, antinociceptive, and possibly muscle relaxant qualities are exhibited by gabapentinoids. For epilepsy, pregabalin and gabapentin are mostly used for focal or partial seizures. Generalized seizures cannot be effectively treated with gabapentinoids. Additionally, fibromyalgia, postherpetic neuralgia, neuropathic pain related to diabetic neuropathy, generalized anxiety disorder, and restless legs syndrome are treated with them. Pregabalin and gabapentin are used off-label for a variety of conditions, such as chronic pain, hot flashes, tinnitus, migraines, insomnia, alcohol and opioid withdrawal, smoking cessation, social anxiety disorder, bipolar disorder, and attention deficit hyperactivity disorder. The main purpose of baclofen is to treat spastic movement disorders, particularly those caused by multiple sclerosis, cerebral palsy, and spinal cord injuries. In Russia, Ukraine, Belarus, and Latvia, phenibut is used to treat anxiety and to enhance sleep, including the treatment of insomnia. In addition, it is used to treat a number of other conditions, such as asthenia, depression, alcoholism, alcohol withdrawal syndrome, post-traumatic stress disorder, stuttering, tics, vestibular disorders, Ménière's disease, dizziness, motion sickness prevention, and anxiety reduction prior to or following invasive medical procedures or uncomfortable diagnostic tests. Bodybuilders occasionally use phenibut, along with other GABA B agonists, to raise human growth hormone.

Gabapentinoids are sometimes abused because they have effects that are comparable to those of alcohol, benzodiazepines, and GHB (gamma-hydroxybutyric acid). Regarding severe respiratory issues, the FDA has issued a black box warning for both Neurontin (gabapentin) and Lyrica (pregabalin). It can be fatal to combine gabapentinoids with alcohol, GHB, benzodiazepines, barbiturates, opioids, or any other depressant.

Gabapentinoids frequently cause drowsiness, weakness, dizziness, increased appetite, shortness of breath, urine retention, uncontrollably jerking motions, memory problems, auditory hallucinations, erectile dysfunction, and myoclonic seizures.

Severe sleepiness, severe ataxia, blurred vision, slurred speech, severe uncontrollable jerking motions, and anxiety are typical symptoms of a gabapentinoids overdose. Pregabalin and gabapentin carry a higher risk of suicidal thoughts and actions, similar to that of most anticonvulsants. Similar to all calcium channel blockers, gabapentinoids are known to induce angioedema. The toxic effects of gabapentinoids may increase if they are taken with an ACE inhibitor. Additionally, they might strengthen the effect of some anti-diabetic medications (thiazolidinediones) on fluid retention. If they enlarge the gingiva like other calcium channel blockers, that is unknown. The kidneys primarily excrete gabapentinoids in their original form. When a person has renal failure, gabapentinoids may accumulate in the body. Usually, this manifests as an altered mental state and myoclonus. The safety of gabapentinoids during pregnancy is debatable; some studies suggest possible risks (Fuentes et al., 2020).

Long-term gabapentinoids use does result in physiological or physical dependence. People who stop taking pregabalin and gabapentin suddenly or quickly report experiencing withdrawal symptoms such as headache, nausea, diarrhea, anxiety, depression, pain, hyperhidrosis, seizures, psychomotor agitation, diarrhea, confusion, and gastrointestinal complaints. In addition to acute psychosis, acute withdrawal from baclofen and phenibut can also result in visual and auditory hallucinations. Withdrawal from baclofen may be more severe if it is given intrathecally or over an extended length of time. Extended use of baclofen or phenibut may cause symptoms similar to severe withdrawal from alcohol, GHB, or benzodiazepines. It is best to taper off baclofen or phenibut gradually to reduce withdrawal symptoms. Because of the way that phenibut or baclofen work, stopping abruptly could potentially be fatal. Severe agitation and rebound seizures can result from abrupt withdrawal.

- Gabapentin (Neurontin)
- Gabapentin Enacarbil (Horizant, Regnite)
- Gabapentin Extended-Release (Gralise)
- Pregabalin (Lyrica)
- Phenibut (Anvifen, Fenibut, Noofen)
- Baclofen (Lioresal)
- Mirogabalin (Tarlige) (Japan Only)

Not approved:

- Imagabalin
- Tolibut
- 4-Flurophenibut

- HSK16149
- Trans-4 and cis-4-[18F] fluorogabapentin ($\alpha_2\delta$ PET Imaging)
- 4-Methylpregabalin
- PD-217,014
- Atagabalin
- Arbaclofen
- Saclofen

Endogenous (not Gabapentinoids), endogenous BCAA amino acids that bind to $\alpha_2\delta$):

- Calcium
- Isoleucine
- Leucine
- Valine
- Aspartate

Other α2δ ligands:

- Phenylalanine
- NP-118809
- Gababutin
- Ziconotide (Approved for pain)
- Ethanol
- Dextrothyroxine (Agonist of $\alpha_2\delta$ instead of inhibiting it)
- Ethioninie
- Suloctidil
- Terodiline
- Bepridil

Gamma-Hydroxybutyric acid

A naturally occurring neurotransmitter and depressant medication, gamma-hydroxybutyric acid, or "GHB," is an analog of GABA. Together with ethanol, it is also naturally present in certain alcoholic beverages in trace amounts. Among a few GHB receptor modulators, GHB is the archetypal compound.

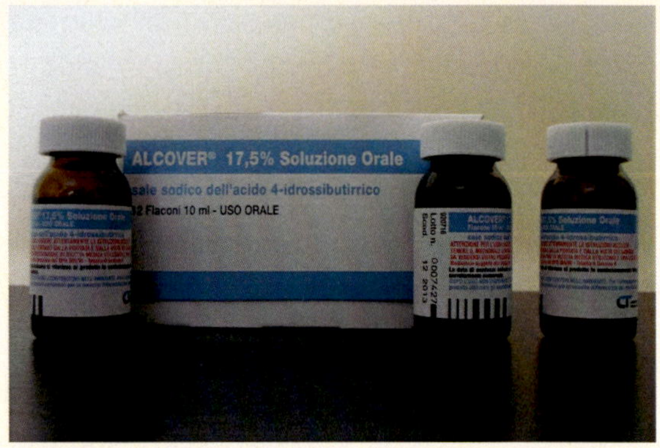

Figure 9.3: GHB that is used to treat alcohol addiction in Italy.

Source: By La Cara Salma - Own work, CC BY-SA 3.0, https://commons.wikimedia.org/w/index.php?curid=19119630

In addition to being used as a general anesthetic, GHB has been used to treat alcoholism, narcolepsy, and cataplexy. These days, sudden muscle weakness, excessive daytime sleepiness, and narcolepsy are frequently treated with sodium oxybate, the sodium salt of GHB. It is offered for sale under the Xyrem brand.

GHB was a depressant that made narcolepsy and muscular weakness worse. However, GHB primarily acts on the GHB receptor at low concentrations. This excitatory receptor releases glutamate and dopamine, which gives GHB stimulant effects—the reverse of depressant effects. However, at high doses, GHB activates the central nervous system's $GABA_B$ receptor, an inhibitory receptor that outweighs the excitatory effects and results in depression of the central nervous system. A few antipsychotics function as GHB receptor agonists (Martin et al., 2017).

Typically, GHB is found as salts of calcium, magnesium, potassium, or sodium. The same conditions as Xyrem are treated with Xywav, a medication that is a combination of all GHB salts. Both Xywav and Xyrem are classified as Schedule III drugs and come with a black box warning due to their high potential for abuse and central nervous system depressant effects, such as bradycardia and hypoventilation. GHB overdose is lethal whether or not other CNS depressants are mixed with it. The most common causes of death from GHB overdoses are coma, seizures, or respiratory depression.

Illegal uses of GHB include aphrodisiac, intoxicant, and performance-enhancing drugs for sports. Because of its potent aphrodisiac and euphoric effects, it is a common club drug in some parts of the world. Bodybuilders use it to raise human growth hormone through GABAB activation, just like they do with phenibut and baclofen. It is also said to have been used as a date-rape drug. As a result, it was classified as a Schedule I substance in the US, Canada, and other nations. In the US, Canada, and other nations, Xyrem—the sodium form of GHB—is classified as a Schedule III drug.

GHB primarily binds to the GHB receptor and only weakly binds to the $GABA_B$ receptor at low doses. An excitatory G protein-coupled receptor is the GHB receptor. GHB is its endogenous ligand because it is a neurotransmitter as well. It also functions as a vitamin B2 transporter. The action of GHB and related compounds, which predominantly act on the GABAB receptor but also display a variety of effects that were found not to be produced by GABAB activity and were therefore suspected of being produced by a novel and at the time unidentified receptor target, was used to predict the existence of a specific GHB receptor. Higher dosages frequently result in seizures. Increased Na^+/K^+ current, as well as increased dopamine and glutamate release, are thought to be the mechanisms mediating this. Absence seizures can also be brought on by GHB; although the exact mechanism is unknown at this time, interactions with the GABAB receptor are thought to be responsible. The possibility that endogenous GHB causes non-convulsive seizures in people is being looked into. The withdrawal from GHB is severe. Physical dependence sets in very rapidly. In addition, it has a strong psychological pull. It is comparable to the stopping of gabapentinoids like baclofen and phenibut because it activates the $GABA_B$ receptor. It has an alcohol withdrawal-like typical depressant withdrawal syndrome. Delirium, tremor, anxiety, tachycardia, insomnia, hypertension, sweating, disorientation, and extreme agitation that may necessitate restraint are among the symptoms. Auditory and visual hallucinations may also occur, and tonic-clonic seizures may result in death.

Patients prefer phenibut and baclofen over benzodiazepines for the treatment of withdrawal because they are more effective than the former.

GHB Receptor Modulators:

GHB receptor agonists:

- Gamma-Hydroxybutyric acid (GHB) (Xyrem)

- Calcium Oxybate, Magnesium Oxybate, Sodium Oxybate (Xyrem), Potassium Oxybate. *Xywav is a mixture of all these salts.*

- 3-hydroxycyclopent-1-enecarboxylic acid (HOCPCA)
- γ-hydroxycrotonic acid, trans-4-Hydroxycrotonic acid (GHC, T-HCA)
- Amisulpride, Levosulpiride, Sulpiride, Sultopride *Antipsychotic GHB receptor ligands*
- 3-Chloropropanoic acid (UMB66)
- 3-phenylpropyloxybutyric acid (UMB72)
- 4-benzyloxybutyric acid (UMB73)
- 4-hydroxy-4-napthylbutanoic acid (UMB86)
- 5-Hydroxypentanoate (UMB58)
- gamma-(4-methoxybenzyl)-gamma-

hydroxybutyric acid (NCS-435)

- 4-(4-chlorophenyl)-4-hydroxy-2-butanoic acid (NCS-356)
- 3-hydroxyphenylacetic acid (3-HPA)
- Catechin, Monastrol *Positive allosteric modulators*

Prodrugs that metabolize into GHB:

- γ-Hydroxyvaleric acid (GHV)

- gamma-Valerolactone, γ-Valerolactone (GVL) *prodrug to GHV*

- 1,4-Butanediol (1,4-BD)
- 1,4-Butanediol acetate (DABD)
- Ethyl acetoxy butanoate (EAB)
- Aceburic acid (GHB acetate)
- gamma-Butyrolactone, γ-Butyrolactone (GBL)
- 2-Furanone, γ-crotonolactone (GCL)
- Gamma-Hydroxybutyraldehyde, γ-Hydroxybutyraldehyde (GHBAL)
- Gamma-Hydroxyvaleric acid, γ-Hydroxyvaleric acid (GHV)

GHB receptor antagonists:

- NCS-382
- Gabazine

Some GHB receptor modulators only bind to the GHB receptor, while others bind to both the GHB and $GABA_B$ receptors.

Nonbenzodiazepines

Nonbenzodiazepines, also known as Z-drugs, are a class of hypnotic depressants primarily used to treat anxiety and insomnia. Benzodiazepines and they share a structural relationship. They are structurally unrelated to benzodiazepines at the molecular level, but they both positively modulate the benzodiazepine site of the GABAA receptor, the primary inhibitory receptor of the central nervous system. To maintain the open chloride channel, nonbenzodiazepines bind to the $GABA_A$ receptor site's benzodiazepine. This floods the neuron with chloride from the intercellular area. The negative charge of chloride makes the neuron rest and stop firing. The central nervous system is consequently calmed and depressed.

Although they have numerous risks and side effects, common nonbenzodiazepines like zolpidem and zopiclone are very effective for treating insomnia. Zopiclone is one of the sleeping pills that has been linked to a higher risk of death (Hernández-Serrano et al., 2016).

Taste disturbance (some report a metallic-like taste); less frequently nausea, vomiting, dizziness, drowsiness, dry mouth, headache; very rarely amnesia, confusion, depression, hallucinations, nightmares; very rarely lightheadedness, incoordination, paradoxical effects, and sleep-walking also reported are among the adverse reactions. Some people who take nonbenzodiazepines have killed people while sleepwalking or been in car crashes. Nonbenzodiazepines are more likely to cause hallucinations and sleepwalking than benzodiazepines. They can induce anterograde amnesia, just like benzodiazepines.

Because nonbenzodiazepines can cause rebound withdrawal symptoms and acute withdrawal reactions that can mimic benzodiazepine withdrawal, it is not advisable to stop taking them suddenly if they have been taken for longer than a few weeks. The course of treatment typically involves tapering the dosage down gradually over a few weeks or months, depending on the patient, the dosage, and how long the drug has been taken. If this method is unsuccessful, a crossover to a long-acting benzodiazepine equivalent dose (such as chlordiazepoxide or, ideally, diazepam) may be attempted, followed by a gradual dosage reduction. Flumazenil may be used as a detoxification tool in extreme cases, especially when severe addiction and/or abuse are evident. Inpatient detoxification may be necessary.

Opioids/Opiates

Opioids are drugs that block opioid receptors in order to lessen pain. In medicine, their main application is in the treatment of pain, including anesthesia. Opioids are highly abused and also produce euphoria. Opiates and opioids are not synonymous. Natural opioids like morphine and codeine are referred to as opioids. All natural, semisynthetic, and synthetic opioids, such as oxycodone and heroin, are referred to as opioids.

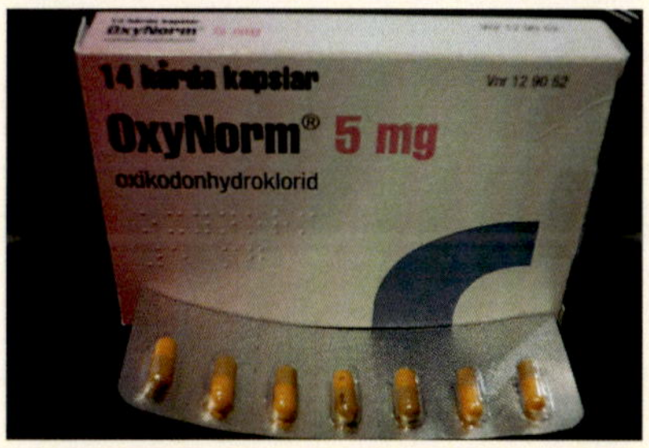

Figure 9.4: Oxycodone is a semi-synthetic prescription opioid.

Source: By Praetorian11 - Own work, CC BY-SA 4.0, https://commons.wikimedia.org/w/index.php?curid=98795982

Opioids do not function as classical depressants, despite what the general public believes. They do cause depression in the central nervous system, but they also cause stimulation in specific regions of the nervous system. Opioids cannot be categorized as "depressants," in keeping with the meaning of the word. Opium derivatives and opioid agonists are categorized differently. These medications are correctly identified as analgesic or narcotic. They do, however, nevertheless exhibit depressing effects.

Opioid receptors fall into three main classes: μ, κ, and δ (mu, kappa, and delta). However, reports of up to seventeen receptor classes have been made, which include the ε, ι, λ, and ζ (Epsilon, Iota, Lambda, and Zeta) receptors. On the other hand, since the opioid inverse-agonist naloxone does not reverse the activation of σ (Sigma) receptors, these receptors are no longer regarded as opioid receptors. One opioid receptor that is involved in pain responses, anxiety, movement, reward, hunger, memory, and many other processes is the nociception opioid peptide receptor (NOP) (ORL1). It has a significant impact on how tolerance to μ-opioid agonists develops.

"Pain" is a signal emanating from the potential injury site. This signal travels up the spinal cord and into the brain, where it is interpreted as "hurt," or nociception, a negative emotion. The brain stem is the structure in the central nervous system that connects the brain to the spine. The first area of the brain to emerge from the neural crest in a mammal is the brain stem. It is also the oldest region of the brain and regulates a wide range of autonomic processes, including breathing, digestion, consciousness, heart rate, and many more. Opioid receptors are specific receptors that block pain. They can bind a large variety of peptides, hormones, and other substances. They are widely distributed throughout the central nervous system, but they are especially concentrated in the brain stem. Activating a receptor can prevent pain from entering the brain and being perceived as such, depending on the receptor. Therefore, opioids only "stop" you from knowing you are in pain—they don't actually "stop" pain. An organism's ability to adapt its pain response to its surroundings is an evolutionary advantage. Research has demonstrated that pain can help an organism escape and survive in circumstances where it would otherwise be rendered immobile by discomfort or injury. Most of the analgesic and stimulatory effects of endogenous and exogenous opioids originate from the midbrain nuclei of the brain stem, which include the reticular formation, rostromedial tegmental nucleus, and periaqueductal gray (Darke et al., 2019).

The opioids' analgesic, euphoric, and harmful effects are caused by the μ-opioid receptor. GPCRs like the μ-opioid receptor. Activation of the μ-opioid receptor results in constipation, constricted pupils, itching, nausea, and pain relief. The μ-opioid, which regulates peristalsis, is found in the digestive system. Constipation results from this, which can be very uncomfortable and problematic. In addition to causing voluntary and involuntary muscle relaxation, activation of this receptor can have unintended consequences, such as difficulty swallowing and urinating. Additionally, the μ-opioid receptor has the ability to lower androgens, which lowers libido and sexual function. Another known side effect of the receptor is "musical anhedonia.".

A vital function of the receptor is in feeding. Opioid receptor-related mechanisms in the ventral pallidum and nucleus accumbens control how palatable food is. The mu-opioid receptors involved in the opioid processes are found on the spiny neurons in the rostromedial shell of the nucleus accumbens. This area is known as the "site of opioid consumption.". Endorphin is one of the numerous endogenous ligands that bind to the μ-opioid receptor.

Within the central nervous system is a G protein-coupled receptor called the Kappa receptor (KOR). Another G-protein coupled receptor is KOR. Compared to most other animals, humans and a few other primates have a higher density of kappa receptors. Nociceptive perception, consciousness, motor control, and mood are all governed by KOR. Addiction to drugs and alcohol has been linked to this receptor system's dysregulation. Dynorphin is the endogenous ligand for KOR. Dysphoria is typically the result of activating KOR; hence, the name dynorphin. Salvinorin A, an alkaloid found in the intoxicating plant *Salvia divinorum*, is a strong and specific κ-opioid (kappa-opioid) receptor agonist. This produces strong delusions. Reversing the effects of the κ-opioid (kappa-opioid) receptor may help treat addiction, alcoholism, depression, anxiety, and stress.

The δ-opioid receptor (DOR) is the third receptor. Of the three primary opioid receptors, the delta receptor has been studied the least. It is a G-protein coupled receptor, and dopamine is its native ligand. The δ-opioid receptor (DOR) may exhibit antidepressant properties when activated. At very high doses, δ-opioid agonists can cause respiratory depression; at lower doses, they have the opposite effect. Seizures may occur from high doses of an δ-opioid agonist, but this is not always the case with delta agonists. The majority of opioids are sedative when they activate the delta receptor, but most opioids stimulate instead.

The regulation of many brain activities, including pain and instinctive emotional behaviors, is mediated by the nociception receptor. NOP is a receptor coupled to G proteins. Numerous biological processes, such as nociception, food intake, memory, heart and kidney functions, spontaneous locomotor activity, gastrointestinal motility, anxiety, and the regulation of neurotransmitter release at peripheral and central sites, are all regulated by the nociception receptor (Tupper et al., 2015).

An overdose of opioids is lethal. When an individual overdoses on opioids or opiates, they may experience respiratory depression, a fatal condition that can result in hypoxia due to shallow, sluggish breathing. The risk of an overdose and respiratory depression rises when opioids are combined with alcohol or other depressants like benzodiazepines. Reduced consciousness, pinpoint pupils and respiratory depression are the results of an opioid overdose. Seizures and spasms of the muscles are additional symptoms. In certain parts of the central nervous system linked to respiratory control, opioids activate μ-opioid receptors. They cause the medulla and pons to become active on μ-opioid receptors. They are found in the area where the brain stem and spine connect. The high density of μ-opioid receptors in this area prevents pain from traveling up from the spine into the brain. The earliest and most basic parts of the brain are located in these regions. They regulate autonomic processes like respiration and digestion. Opioids halt this process, resulting in constipation and respiratory depression. Since the brain stem can no longer sense carbon dioxide in the blood, it is unable to trigger the inhalation reflex, which typically leads to hypoxia. On the other hand, some overdose victims pass away from asphyxia due to choking on their vomit or from cardiovascular failure.

Since naloxone is an μ-opioid receptor antagonist, it interferes with the receptor's ability to function rather than activating it. Naloxone's potent and highly selective nature for the μ-opioid receptor allows it to block the binding of other ligands to the receptor, preventing an overdose. This is particularly useful for potent opioids like fentanyl.

When Naloxone is used, an opioid-dependent person may experience accelerated withdrawal symptoms. Since naloxone prevents all opioids, endogenous or exogenous, from attaching themselves to the μ-opioid receptor. When naloxone is used, this could cause someone to go into withdrawal right away. Withdrawal symptoms such as diarrhea and cold sweats may result from this.

Opioids cause the rostromedial tegmental nucleus (RMTg) to release μ-opioid receptors. A GABAergic nucleus called the retrograde tegmental nucleus serves as a "master brake" for the midbrain dopamine system. Strong anatomical and functional connections exist between the RMTg and the dopaminergic pathways. Opioids disinhibit the GABAergic brake on dopamine networks by reducing the release of GABA. GABA is classified as an inhibitory neurotransmitter because it either prevents or reduces a neuron's ability to fire. Due to GABA's removal, a significant amount of dopamine is released as a result. The rare side effect of opioids that may cause seizures is disinhibition of GABA. Another reason why opioids are not regarded as legitimate "depressants" is the GABAergic disinhibition. The euphoria of opioids is brought on by this stimulation of dopaminergic pathways. The brain receives strong positive reinforcement for doing this, telling it to repeat the action. Addiction and tolerance development are also brought on by the RMTg. This pathway is also stimulated by psychostimulants.

Fentanyl is frequently mixed with other drugs and sold on the streets. The purpose of fentanyl is to make drugs more potent so that the user will pay more for the laced drug. Usually used for post-operative pain, diarrhea, and bronchitis, codeine is a weaker form of natural opiate. When using these drugs excessively is very easy, particularly if you don't have any tolerance. Getting tested for drugs and keeping Naloxone on hand are advised (Anthony et al., 2017).

Natural opiates (*P. somniferum*, Opium)

- Morphine (MS Contin)
- Codeine (Tylenol No. 3)
- Papaverine (Pavabid)
- Noscapine (Narcotine)
- Thebaine
- Oripavine
- Narceine

Semi-synthetic morphinan opioids:

- Oxycodone (OxyContin)
- Heroin (Diamorphine)
- Hydrocodone (Vicodin)
- Oxymorphone (Opana)
- Hydromorphone (Dilaudid)
- Buprenorphine (Suboxone)
- Naloxone (Narcan)

Semi-synthetic opioids are derived from the natural alkaloid thebaine.

Fully synthetic opioids:

- Fentanyl (Duragesic)
- Tramadol (Ultram)
- Methadone (Dolophine)
- Pethidine (Demerol)
- Ketobemidone (Ketogan)
- Pentazocine (Talwin)
- Carfentanil (Wildnil)
- Loperamide (Imodium)
- Dextropropoxyphene (Darvocet)
- Tapentadol (Nucynta)
- Dextropropoxyphene (Darvocet)

Others:

Mitragyna speciosa (Kratom) *Indole alkaloid*

Piperidinediones

One class of depressants that is no longer in use is piperidinediones. Some uses for piperidinediones include the treatment of breast cancer. Barbiturates and the Piperidinedione class share a lot of structural similarities. Glutethimide, Methyprylon, Pyrithyldione, Glutarimide, and Aminoglutethimide are a few examples of piperidinediones. The first three—pyridyldione, methyprylon, and glutathione—depress the central nervous system. Glutethimide, one of the piperidinedione depressants, is a positive modulator of the GABAA anion channel. The medication produces neuro-inhibition of the limbic and cortical systems, which is clinically observed as a sedative-hypnotic effect. It also increases inhibitory GABAergic tone. Additionally, glutathione has a strong inhibitory effect on the liver's CYP 2D6 enzyme. Numerous medications, including beta blockers, antidepressants, opioids, and opiates, are changed into opioids and opiates by this enzyme. It was heavily abused and combined with opioids like codeine because of its effects on the conversion of opioids. For codeine to have both analgesic and psychoactive effects, it must be converted by the liver into morphine. Codeine's effect was increased by mixing it with piperidinedione glutathione, which increased the amount of codeine that the body could convert to morphine. They were referred to as "dors and 4s," "cibas and codeine," and "hits.". Although glutethimide was thought to be less dangerous than barbiturates, the drug caused many deaths. There was a time when demand was high in the US. Glutathione production was shut down in the US in 1993 and in a number of Eastern European nations, including Hungary, in 2006.

Withdrawal from glutathione is severe and similar to that from barbiturates. It induces delirium and hallucinations associated with a depressant withdrawal. There were reports of neonatal withdrawal from glutethimide in the 1970s. Babies born to glutethimide-addicted mothers responded well at first, but about five days later, they experienced a recurrence of symptoms, which included hyperactivity, tremors, hyperreflexia, hypotonus, vasomotor instability, constant crying, and general irritability (Dasgupta, 2017).

Glutethimide withdrawal featured severe agitation, tremors, and seizures, which could be fatal. Overdose causes stupor or coma and respiratory depression.

- Methyprylon (Dimerin, Methyprylone, Noctan, Noludar)
- Pyrithyldione (Presidon, Pyridion, Pyridione, Pyrithyldion, Pyrithyldione)
- Piperidione (Ascron, Dihyprylon, Dihyprylone, Sedulon, Tusseval) (Withdrawan before approval)
- Glutethimide (Doriden)

Quinazolinone

These days, quinazolinones are a rare class of depressants. Quinazolinones possess potent hypnotic, anxiolytic, and sedative properties. Quinazolinone shares a structure with several antibiotics. The primary mode of action of quinazolinone is binding to the GABAA receptor. It does not bind to the ethanol, barbiturate, neurosteroid, and benzodiazepine sites. Rather, it attaches itself to a location on the GABAA receptor that is directly between the GABRB2 (β2) and (α1) GABRA1 proteins. This site may also be bound by the anticonvulsant loreclezole and anesthetic etomidate.

Sometimes quinazolinone overdose results in effects that are the opposite of sedation similar to quinazolinone. Hyperreflexia, vomiting, kidney failure, delirium, hypertonia, coma, myoclonic twitches, somnolence, euphoria, hyperactive muscles, tachycardia, and tonic-clonic seizures are the symptoms of the overdose. 2,764 Americans went to emergency rooms in 1982 as a result of overdosing on quinazolinones, particularly methaqualone. It could be lethal to combine quinazolines with other depressants. The most common cause of death from a quinazolinone overdose is cardiac or respiratory arrest. Overdose is similar to that of barbiturates and carbamates.

When a person who has grown dependent on quinazolinone stops using it, they experience quinazolinone withdrawal. Quinazolinone withdrawal is similar to withdrawal from benzodiazepines, carbamates, ethanol, and barbiturates. The symptoms typically include agitation, tachycardia, insomnia, tremor, hallucinations, delirium, confusion, and seizures. It can also be fatal and include the following symptoms: myoclonic twitches, fever, muscle spasms, and irritability.

Methaqualone hydrochloride, quinazolinone anxiolytics, and hypnotics are referred to as "quaaludes," "ludes," and "disco biscuits." In the Western world in the 1960s and 1970s, methaqualone abuse was rampant. Because it was believed to be safer than barbiturates and carbamates, methaqualone was primarily prescribed for insomnia. Following its introduction in 1965, methaqualone was heavily abused by a large number of people, including celebrities. 1951 saw the first synthesis of methaqualone in India by researchers Indra Kishore Kacker and Syed Husain Zaheer, who were looking for novel antimalarial drugs. "Quaalude" (Methaqualone) is a portmanteau word that combines the terms "quiet interlude.". Methaqualone's psychological addictiveness, widespread abuse, and illicit recreational use led to its discontinuation in the US in 1985. Nowadays, insomnia is treated with benzodiazepines and nonbenzodiazepines. Nowadays, methaqualone is classified as a Schedule I drug. Online sales continue to exist for certain quinazolinone analogs. Seizures are possible with them.

Excessive dosages of Methaqualone may result in sedation, euphoria, disinhibition, increased sexual arousal, sociability, relaxed muscles, and anxiolysis. Methaqualone abuse is a common problem in South Africa these days. Methaqualone is the most well-known celebrity to have used quinazolinone. Bill Cosby acknowledged having casual sex while using methaqualone (Quaaludes) recreationally.

Actress Anissa Jones, 18, passed away at the age of 18 after taking too much cocaine, PCP, methaqualone, and the barbiturate Seconal. Billy Murcia, the rock band New York Dolls' drummer, overdosed on heroin and methaqualone and drowned in a bathtub at the age of 21.

Chloroqualone is a type of quinazolinone that bonded to both sigma-1 and GABAA receptors. It was eventually taken off the market because of the risk of abuse and overdose, even though it had beneficial cough-suppressant properties and less sedative effects than methaqualone.

One quinazolinone that is still in use today is diproqualone. Diproqualone inhibits the COX-1 enzyme, acts as an agonist at the β subtype of the GABAa receptor, is an antagonist at all histamine receptors, and may also act as an agonist at the Sigma-1 and Sigma-2 receptors. These effects contribute to diproqualone's sedative, anxiolytic, antihistamine, and analgesic qualities. Diproqualone is less frequently used to treat neuralgia, anxiety, and insomnia. It is primarily used to treat inflammatory pain related to osteoarthritis and rheumatoid arthritis. Since diproqualone has the same sedative and anxiolytic properties as other medications in its class, it is the only analog of methaqualone that is still widely used in clinical settings. It also has helpful anti-inflammatory and analgesic properties. Diproqualone is not marketed as a pure medication; instead, it is sold as the camphosulfonate salt in combination mixtures with other medications like ethenzamide, raising concerns about the possibility of abuse and overdose.

A depressant in the quinazolinone class is etaqualone. Its effects include sedation, hypnosis, muscle relaxation, and central nervous system depression (Graziano et al., 2017). It was highly addictive and prone to overdosing. Etaqualone hydrochloride salt is the free base that users would snort or smoke.

An analog of methaqualone, methylmethaqualone has sedative and hypnotic properties akin to those of methaqualone. 4-methylation on the phenyl ring is what separates methylmethaqualone from methaqualone.

Only a small amount more than the effective sedative dose causes convulsions. This substance seems to have been marketed as a designer drug analog of methaqualone on the black market in Germany.

A quinazolinone depressant with ten times greater hypnotic and sedative effects than methaqualone is nitromethaqualone.

Quinazolinones:

- Alfoqualone (Arofuto)
- Cloroqualone
- Diproqualone
- Etaqualone (Aolan, Athinazone, Ethinazone)
- Mebroqualone (MBQ)
- Mecloqualone (Nubarene, Casfen)
- Methaqualone (Quaalude, Sopor, Mandrax)
- Methylmethaqualone
- Nitromethaqualone
- SL-164 (Dicloqualone, DCQ)

Methods of Intake

Because it has been suggested that the depressive properties of the central nervous system increase exponentially rather than linearly, combining multiple depressants can be extremely dangerous. Because of this feature, depressants are frequently chosen for intentional overdoses in suicide cases. Overdose deaths among opiate addicts are frequently the result of combining regular doses of heroin with alcohol or benzodiazepines.

9.2.4 Psychedelic Drugs

A psychedelic drug is any of the so-called "mind-expanding" substances that can cause altered states of consciousness and perception, often accompanied by increased awareness of sensory input and decreased control over the experience.

D-lysergic acid diethylamide, also known as LSD-25, is a popular psychedelic substance that was created in 1938 by a Swiss chemist who worked for Sandoz Laboratories. It was discovered that LSD was a very potent drug, hundreds or even thousands of times more potent than drugs like mescaline, psilocin, and psilocybin. LSD hasn't been proven to directly cause death, but it may have sympathomimetic effects like an elevated heart rate. On the other hand, prolonged exposure can cause psychoses, memory problems, or problems with abstract thought. Psychedelic substances have been suggested as therapeutic aids for mental illnesses, alcoholism, and psychotherapy, though their efficacy has not been established. These and other widely used mood-altering drugs seem to function by imitating or replacing the effects of endogenous neurotransmitters, though the precise mechanisms underlying their actions are still poorly understood. LSD shares a chemical structure with serotonin, the dysregulation of which has been linked to a number of mental health issues, including schizophrenia, depression, and OCD. On the other hand, studies have demonstrated that LSD experiences do not entail real hallucinations or psychotic or schizophrenia episodes.

During the 1960s and early 1970s, when drugs like LSD were essential to the "hippie" subculture in Western Europe and the US, psychedelic drugs reached their peak popularity. Although the drugs' appeal waned, they continued to have a following in some areas and cultures, and they saw a resurgence in the 1990s, a decade in which Europe and the United States saw a sizable adolescent population turn to LSD and Ecstasy (Nichols, 2016).

Examples

- Alexander Shulgin first synthesized 2C-B (2,5-dimethoxy-4-bromophenethylamine), a substituted phenethylamine, in 1974. With increasing dosage, 2C-B has greater psychedelic effects and less entactogenic effects. It is a mild entactogen as well. The most well-known member of the 2C family is 2C-B, whose general structure was found by altering the mescaline molecule.
- An indole alkaloid called DMT (N,N-dimethyltryptamine) is present in many different plant species. It has historically been ingested by South American tribes as ayahuasca. In order to prevent monoamine oxidase enzymes in the digestive tract from inactivating DMT when taken orally, a blend of plants containing both DMT and MAOIs—specifically, harmaline—is utilized. In the West, freebase DMT is most frequently vaporized in order to consume DMT. While the effects of Ayahuasca usually last for several hours, inhalation has a much shorter half-life (onset in seconds, duration of effects in minutes). DMT can transport users into a hallucinatory world that is completely detached from reality, especially when vaporized. This realm is often characterized by hyperbolic geometry and is said to be beyond description, both verbally and visually. In this hallucinatory state, users have also claimed to have

encountered and communicated with entities. DMT is the classic example of a substituted tryptamine; it serves as the structural basis for both lysergamides and psilocybin, though to a lesser degree.

- Lysergic acid, which is produced by hydrolyzing ergotamine, is the precursor to LSD (lysergic acid diethylamide). The alkaloid ergotamine is present in the fungus Claviceps purpurea, which mainly affects rye. LSD is the archetypal lysergamide as well as the archetypal psychedelic. Tryptamine and phenethylamine are both present in the structure of LSD, a lysergamide. LSD is more energetic in effect than psilocin, which is not a dopamine agonist and has more sedative effects. This is because LSD agonizes both dopamine and serotonin receptors due to its phenethylamine group.
- Mescaline (3,4,5-trimethoxyphenethylamine) is an alkaloid that phenethylamines found in a variety of cacti species; the most well-known are the San Pedro cactus (*Trichocereus macrogonus* var.) and peyote (*Lophophora williamsii*). syn and pachanoi. pachanoi, or Echinopsis. Mescaline produces effects similar to psilocybin and LSD, but it emphasizes colors and patterns more. Relatively intense spiritual experiences and a low frequency of difficult experiences appear to be the hallmarks of ceremonial San Pedro use.
- The dephosphorylated active metabolite of the substituted tryptamine and indole alkaloid psilocybin, psilocin (4-HO-DMT), is generated by more than 200 different fungal species. Though all psychedelics have varying degrees of potential to induce mystical experiences, psilocybin has garnered the most scholarly attention among the Classical psychedelics. Psilocin's acetylated analog is called O-Acetylpsilocin (4-AcO-DMT). In addition, 4-HO-MIPT and 4-HO-MET are produced when a methyl group at the dimethylated nitrogen is swapped out for an isopropyl or ethyl group, respectively.

Pharmacology

Although the exact mechanism of action of psychedelics is unknown, it is known that they bind to serotonin (5-HT) receptors in different ways and at different levels. They can also be categorized based on how active they are at different 5-HT subtypes, specifically 5-HT1A, 5-HT2A, and 5-HT2C. Almost everyone agrees that psychedelics work by strongly partial agonisting the 5-HT2A receptors to produce their desired effects. It's unclear how this causes the psychedelic experience, but it probably works by making the cortex more excitable, maybe by assisting input from the thalamus, which is the main relay for sensory information input to the cortex. Furthermore, a number of psychedelics have been found by researchers to be strong psychoplastogens, or substances that have the ability to rapidly and persistently promote neural plasticity.

Tryptamines

The central nervous system of mammals contains tryptamine in addition to other trace amines. It is proposed that it functions as a neuromodulator on the classical monoamine neurotransmitters, including epinephrine, dopamine, serotonin, and norepinephrine. In order to release more monoamine neurotransmitter, tryptamine functions as a non-selective agonist of serotonin receptors and a serotonin–norepinephrine–dopamine releasing agent, preferring to release serotonin and dopamine rather than norepinephrine (epinephrine). Tryptamines used in psychedelics include psilocin, DMT, and 5-MeO-DMT, which are found in nature; laboratory-produced tryptamines include 4-HO-MET, 4-HO-MiPT, and 5-MeO-DALT.

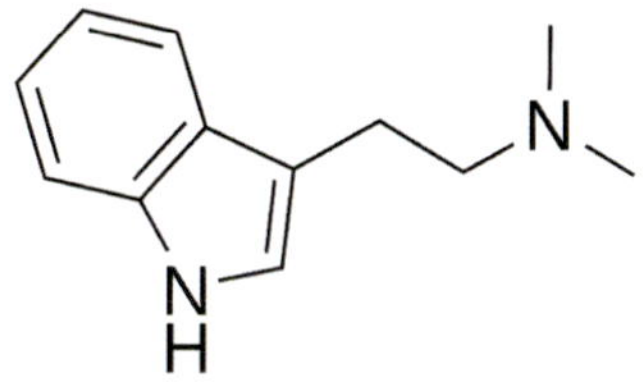

Figure 9.5: N,N-DMT.

Source: By Harbin - Own work, Public Domain, https://commons.wikimedia.org/w/index.php?curid=5336610

Phenethylamines

In the human central nervous system (CNS), phenethylamine functions as a neurotransmitter to a lesser extent than other trace amines. Alternatively, phenethylamine controls monoamine neurotransmission by attaching to trace amine-associated receptor 1 (TAAR1). This receptor is important for controlling neurotransmission in serotonin, dopamine, and norepinephrine neurons in the central nervous system as well as for blocking vesicular monoamine transporter 2 (VMAT2) in monoamine neurons. Monoamine neurotransmitters like dopamine cannot be released into synapses through conventional release mechanisms when VMAT2 is inhibited. Mescaline belongs to the class of substituted phenethylamines and is a naturally occurring psychedelic protoalkaloid (Nichols, 2016).

Lysergamides

Lysergamides, a group of compounds having strong agonist and/or antagonistic effects at different serotonin and dopamine receptors, are the amides of lysergic acid. Tryptamine and phenethylamine structures are both present in the structure of lysergamides. Among the various lysergamides is LSD (Lysergic Acid Diethylamide). In recent times, a diverse array of lysergamides has surfaced, motivated by extant scientific literature. Others have emerged from studies on chemicals. 1P-LSD is a homolog of ALD-52 and a derivative and functional analog of LSD. It alters the LSD molecule by grafting a propionyl group onto the indole nitrogen atom.

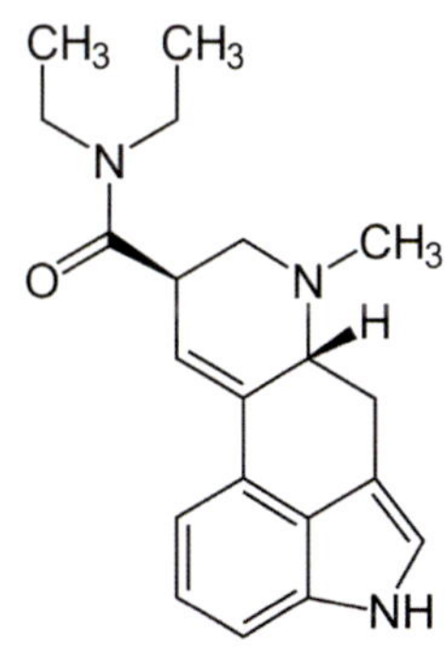

Figure 9.6: Lysergic acid diethylamide (LSD).

Source: By NEUROtiker - Own work, Public Domain, https://commons.wikimedia.org/w/index.php?curid=1760632

Potential Adverse Effects

Contrary to popular belief, psychedelic substances are physiologically safe and do not cause addiction. As of 2016, no fatalities from mescaline, psilocybin, or LSD overdose are known to have occurred.

Though a causal relationship between psilocybin and the onset of psychosis has not been established as of 2011, researchers have called for further investigation into the relationship. Psilocybin-induced states of mind share features with states experienced in psychosis. The majority of reported adverse effects have not been observed in a regulated or medical context, providing evidence against many of the persistently held negative perceptions of psychological risks that are not supported by the available scientific data. In a 2013 population study on the relationship between psychedelic use and mental illness, no evidence was found linking psychedelic use to a higher prevalence of any mental illness.

There is a chance that using psychedelics will cause side effects to resurface, such as flashbacks and hallucinogen-persisting perception disorder. Although there is little research on these non-psychotic effects, the chronic symptoms—also referred to as "endless trip"—are thought to be uncommon. When psychedelics are combined with other serotonergic medications, such as some antidepressants, opioids, CNS stimulants (e.g., MDMA), agonists of 5-HT1 (e.g., triptans), among other things.

Potential Therapeutic Effects

Mescaline, LSD, and psilocybin are psychedelic substances that may be used therapeutically. Some participants in psychedelic scientific trials during the 1950s and 1960s suffered severe, lifelong harm as a result of the trials' lack of informed consent. Subsequently, studies on the efficacy of psychedelic therapy have been carried out in accordance with stringent ethical guidelines, ensuring that participants provide fully informed consent and undergo pre-screening to prevent participation by individuals suffering from psychosis. Despite the fact that the past of these substances has impeded research into their possible medicinal value, scientists can now perform studies and restart research that was put on hold in the 1970s. According to some research, these drugs have been beneficial for treating a variety of mental health conditions, including alcoholism, depression, cluster headaches, PTSD, obsessive-compulsive disorder, and OCD (Hernández-Serrano et al., 2016).

Psychedelics are powerful psychoplastogens that have long been known to enhance neurite growth and neuroplasticity. Psychedelics have been shown to cause neuroplasticity-related cellular and molecular changes, which may be the basis for their therapeutic effects. In animal models of inflammatory diseases such as asthma, diabetes, and cardiovascular disease, psychedelics have also been demonstrated to have strong anti-inflammatory activity and therapeutic effects.

9.2.5 Inhalants

Small bottles of volatile drugs known as "poppers" are inhaled by clubgoers to produce a "rush" or "high.". Poppers got their nickname from the fact that nitrites, like alkyl nitrite, were formerly sold as tiny glass capsules that were cracked open. Due to the "rush" it gives off and the perception that it improves the experience of dancing to loud, bass-heavy disco, the drug first gained popularity in the US during the disco/club scene of the 1970s. The mid-1980s and 1990s rave and EDM scenes saw a resurgence in the drug's popularity. Similar to those who frequent disco clubs, EDM fans, and raver participants took the drug for the "rush" or "high," which they believed improved the experience of dancing to pulsating music and lights.

Nitrous oxide is a dissociative inhalant that can lead to euphoria, dizziness, depersonalization, derealization (the idea that the world is not real), and some sound distortion (flanging). It has a slight aphrodisiac effect and may occasionally induce mild hallucinations. Although access to medical-grade nitrous oxide is restricted to licensed healthcare professionals such as dentists, recreational users frequently acquire the drug by inhaling the nitrous oxide found in whipped cream aerosol cans. Additionally, people who use nitrous oxide purchase tiny canisters called "whippets" that are meant to be used in restaurant whipped cream dispensers. They then "crack" open these canisters to breathe in the gas. Before inhaling the gas, users usually transfer it to a plastic bag or balloon.

Medical Inhalants

A small number of recreational inhalant drugs are pharmaceutical products that are used illicitly.

- Antidote to cyanide poisoning
  - Alkyl nitrites (poppers)
- Inhalational anesthetics used as general anesthetics
  - Nitrous oxide
  - Xenon
- Historical general anesthetics
  - Chloroethane
  - Chloroform
  - Ether

Diethyl ether, which is no longer used medically due to its high flammability and the development of safer alternatives, and nitrous oxide, which is widely used by dentists as an anti-anxiety medication during dental procedures, are two examples of medical anesthetics that are used recreationally. There is a long history of recreational drug use with diethyl ether. The effects of ether intoxication are similar to those of alcohol intoxication but more potent. Also, due to NMDA antagonism, the user may experience all the psychedelic effects present in classical dissociatives, such as ketamine, in the forms of thought loops and the feeling of the mind being disconnected from one's body. Nitrous oxide is a dental anesthetic that is used as a recreational drug, either by users who have access to medical-grade gas canisters (e.g., dental hygienists or dentists) or by using the gas contained in whipped cream aerosol containers. Nitrous oxide inhalation can cause pain relief, depersonalization, derealization, dizziness, euphoria, and some sound distortion.

In Canada, the sale of poppers containing alkyl nitrite was outlawed in 2013. Despite not being classified as narcotics and being lawful to possess or use, they are nonetheless regarded as drugs. Unauthorized sales are now punishable by jail time and fines. Since 2007, only isobutyl nitrite has been banned in Europe; therefore, reformulated poppers containing isopropyl nitrite are sold there. Because of the potential risk to consumers, the sale of goods containing butyl nitrite, pentyl nitrite, or their isomers has been forbidden in France since 1990. This ban was expanded by the government in 2007 to include all alkyl nitrites that weren't allowed to be sold as medications. Following legal action by owners of sex shops, the Council of State invalidated this extension, ruling that the government had not provided sufficient justification for such a broad ban (Darke et al., 2019). The court reasoned that the risks mentioned—which included uncommon accidents frequently resulting from unusual use—were more appropriate justification for required warnings on the packaging.

Poppers are easily obtained and regularly (legally) sold in gay bars and clubs, sex shops, drug paraphernalia head shops, online, and at markets in the United Kingdom. To get around the Medicines Act of 1968, which forbids selling them with advertising for human consumption, they are typically offered as sale as odorizers. Within the U. S. Amyl nitrite was first sold under prescription in 1937 and stayed that way until 1960, when the Food and Drug Administration removed the requirement because of the medication's safety record. In 1969, this requirement was brought back in response to growing evidence of recreational use. The United States banned other alkyl nitrites by the Anti-

Drug Abuse Act of 1988, passed by Congress. There is a legal exemption for business uses. Any use other than the manufacturing of consumer goods containing volatile alkyl nitrites intended for inhalation or other introduction of volatile alkyl nitrites into the human body for euphoric or physical effects is referred to as a commercial purpose. The legislation became operative in 1990. Upon visiting retail locations that sell these products, it is evident that certain manufacturers have subsequently modified their products to comply with the regulations. This involves using the lawful cyclohexyl nitrite as the main ingredient in their products, which are marketed as room odorants, polish removers, and video head cleaners. Methemoglobinemia can be caused by ingesting alkyl nitrites, and inhalation has not been completely ruled out as a cause.

Nitrous Oxide

Since nitrous oxide can produce both visual and auditory hallucinations, it falls under the category of dissociative drugs. Surgery-related anesthetic gases, such as nitrous oxide or enflurane, are thought to work primarily as NMDA receptor antagonists, which are open-channel blockers that attach to the inside of calcium channels on the outside of neurons and provide high levels of NMDA receptor blockade for brief intervals of time.

In contrast to other NMDA antagonists like ketamine, which bind to a regulatory site on the NMDA-sensitive calcium transporter complex and provide somewhat lower levels of NMDA blockade for a longer and much more consistent duration, inhaled anesthetic gases do not cause this side effect.

This makes it easier to achieve a deeper level of anesthesia with anesthetic gases, but it can also make them riskier than other medications used in the same way.

In the US, federal law permits the lawful possession of nitrous oxide, which escapes DEA jurisdiction. However, it is governed by the Food and Drug Administration as per the Food Drug and Cosmetics Act; selling or distributing nitrous oxide for human consumption as a recreational drug is prohibited by its "misbranding" clauses, which may result in prosecution. Laws governing the distribution, sale, and possession of nitrous oxide are in place in many states. These regulations typically prohibit distribution to minors or place restrictions on the quantity of nitrous oxide that can be sold without a permit.

For instance, it is illegal and considered a misdemeanor in the state of California to possess something for recreational purposes. The Medicines Act prohibits the sale or possession of nitrous oxide without a prescription, and the Ministry of Health in New Zealand has issued warnings about this.

It is suggested that only recreational use of the chemical will be legally targeted by this statement, which would seem to forbid all non-medical uses. Nitrous oxide is available in India as Nitrous Oxide IP, which is used for general anesthesia. The gas cylinder regulations in India from 1985 forbid moving gas from one cylinder to another for breathing reasons. Anyone found filling a prescription is required to have a drug manufacturing license in India because the Food and Drug Authority (FDA-India) regulations consider this to be the same as manufacturing a drug.

Although nitrous oxide is thought to be particularly safe, prolonged and heavy use can cause a number of serious health issues, including the breakdown of folic acid and vitamin B12. While they are not toxic in the same way as solvents, some inhalants, such as diethyl ether and amyl nitrite, have medical uses and can still be hazardous when used recreationally (Drake et al., 2019).

Non-medical Inhalants

It is possible to inhale alcohol, specifically ethanol, which is typically drunk. A nebulizer, a device that stirs liquids into aerosols, may be used to transform ethanol from a liquid into a gaseous state (vapor) or aerosol (mist). Some US states have outlawed the sale of nebulizers meant for ethanol inhalation because of safety concerns.

Effects of Inhalants

There is no drug use level that is safe. Any drug use always involves some risk. It is crucial to exercise caution when using any kind of medication.

Inhalants affect everyone differently, based on:

- size, weight and health
- whether the person is used to taking it
- whether other drugs are taken around the same time
- the amount used
- the type of inhalant used
- amount of fresh air breathed while sniffing
- amount of physical activity before and after sniffing

Effects include:

- feelings of excitement and euphoria
- feeling relaxed
- increased risk-taking
- loss of coordination
- dizzy/light-headed
- visual distortions
- confusion
- irritation to eyes/nose/throat
- nausea
- headaches.

Overdose

You run the risk of overdosing if you use an especially potent inhalant or inhale the drug too frequently. Another name for this is "acute intoxication.". If any of the following symptoms apply to you or someone else, call an ambulance right away.

- nausea, vomiting and diarrhoea
- irregular heartbeat
- chest pain
- delirium
- hallucinations
- blackout, seizures, and coma.

Ambulance officers do not need to involve the police.

When recovering from acute intoxication, an individual needs to be kept under close medical observation in a secure environment until they fully recover. If they use inhalants frequently, recovery may take up to four hours.

Sudden Death

Certain substances have been known to cause sudden death upon inhalation. Using inhalants can result in death for the following reasons.

- Sudden sniffing death – when a person who has used inhalants suffers from heart failure or cardiac arrest. Because the heart is sensitive to an increase in adrenaline, inhalant chemicals have the potential to cause cardiac arrest. This is especially dangerous if the person inhales after engaging in strenuous exercise or is under stress.
- Suffocation – this occurs when the

gas inhaled replaces the oxygen in the lungs. It can be caused by using in enclosed areas without access to fresh air, or by engaging in risky behaviors like covering one's head with a plastic bag. Certain substances that are sprayed directly into the mouth have the potential to freeze the airways and throat, suffocating the victim.

Low Aromatic Fuels

In certain isolated and rural Australian communities, low-acid fuels like BP's Opal fuel have replaced unleaded gasoline. While sniffing low-aromatic fuel does not result in a high, it can still have fatal consequences for an individual's health.

9.2.6 Ketamine

Ketamine was one of the most widely used drugs in the New York Club Kid scene and has a long history of use in clubs as a dissociative anesthetic. Ketamine causes a dissociative state known as depersonalization and derealization, which is typified by a feeling of disassociation from one's physical body and the outside world. The effects include hallucinations, altered perceptions of color, durations/time, relative scale, and distances, as well as a slowdown in the visual system's ability to refresh the user's view (Guina and Merrill, 2018).

Medical Uses

Anesthesia

Ketamine's characteristics are reflected in its use in anesthesia. When muscle relaxation is not necessary, it is the preferred medication for quick procedures. Ketamine has a different effect on the respiratory and circulatory systems than other anesthetics. It suppresses breathing far less than the majority of other anesthetics on the market. Ketamine typically stimulates rather than depresses the circulatory system when used at anesthetic dosages. It is occasionally possible to give ketamine anesthesia without taking precautions to protect the airways because protective reflexes for the airways are maintained. The acceptance of ketamine is restricted by psychotomimetic effects; however, the administration of propofol or benzodiazepines can also counteract the reduction of psychotomimetic effects caused by lamotrigine and nimodipine. Ketofol is a concoction of propofol and ketamine.

Ketamine is often administered to patients with severe injuries, and it seems safe in this population. It has been extensively utilized for emergency surgery in combat zones, such as the Vietnam War, under field conditions. The use of ketamine as a sedative in emergency medicine, including during physically taxing procedures, is supported by a 2011 clinical practice guideline. When someone is in traumatic shock and at risk of hypotension, this medication is recommended. Ketamine can raise blood pressure, which makes it useful in treating severe head injuries. It is unlikely to lower blood pressure, which is dangerous for those with such injuries.

In children, ketamine can be used as the only anesthetic for minor procedures or as an induction agent in conjunction with tracheal intubation and neuromuscular blockers. Children with neuromuscular disorders and cyanotic heart disease are particularly well-suited for ketamine anesthesia. Ketamine is useful for anesthesia in patients with severe reactive airway disease, including active bronchospasm, asthma, and chronic obstructive pulmonary disease, because of its bronchodilating effects.

Pain

In emergency rooms and during the postoperative phase for patients with refractory pain, ketamine infusions are used to treat acute pain. Usually referred to as sub-anesthetic doses, the doses are less than those used for anesthesia. Ketamine lowers pain threshold, post-operative nausea and vomiting, and the need for morphine when used alone or in conjunction with it. Patients who are opioid-tolerant and undergoing surgery when severe post-operative pain is anticipated are likely to benefit most from ketamine.

Ketamine is particularly valuable in prehospital situations because of its effectiveness and minimal risk of causing respiratory depression. In emergency department settings, ketamine has been found to have comparable effectiveness to opioids for treating acute pain and managing procedural pain. Additionally, it has the potential to reduce opioid-induced hyperalgesia and postanesthetic shivering (Guina and Merrill, 2018).

Ketamine is used as an intravenous analgesic for chronic pain, especially neuropathic pain. It also has the added advantage of preventing wind-up phenomena, or spinal sensitization, which is a side effect of chronic pain. Ketamine infusions provided short-term pain relief for neuropathic pain, pain following traumatic spinal injury, fibromyalgia, and complex regional pain syndrome (CRPS) in numerous clinical trials. The 2018 consensus guidelines on chronic pain, however, came to the conclusion that, generally, there is either no evidence or weak evidence supporting the use of ketamine for mixed neuropathic pain, fibromyalgia, and cancer pain, and moderate evidence supporting the use of ketamine for CRPS and spinal injury pain. Specifically, there is proof of medium- to long-term pain relief for CRPS alone.

Depression

Ketamine acts quickly as an antidepressant, but its effects wear off quickly. When treatment-resistant depression is administered intravenously, mood can improve within 4 hours, peaking after 24. It has been demonstrated that a single intravenous ketamine dose can produce a response rate of more than 60% as soon as 4.5 hours after the dose (with a sustained effect after 24 hours) and more than 40% after 7 days. Even though there aren't many pilot studies examining the ideal dosage, mounting data indicates that injecting a dose of 0.05 mg/kg over 40 minutes produces the best results. Ketamine's antidepressant effect wears off after seven days, and most users relapse within ten, though a sizable minority report improvements lasting up to thirty days.

The duration of the antidepressant effects following the completion of a course of treatment may be one of the primary issues with ketamine treatment. Ketamine maintenance therapy, which is typically administered twice a week to once every 2 weeks, is one potential option. After the injection, ketamine may reduce suicidal thoughts for up to 3 days.

The European Medicines Agency approved esketamine, a ketamine enantiomer that is commercially marketed under the brand name Spravato, as an antidepressant in 2019. 2019 saw the approval of esketamine as a nasal spray for treatment-resistant depression both domestically and internationally. Esketamine is suggested by the Canadian Network for Mood and Anxiety Treatments (CANMAT) as a third-line treatment for depression.

A Cochrane review of randomized controlled trials in adults with unipolar major depressive disorder discovered that individuals treated with ketamine or esketamine experienced a reduction or remission of symptoms lasting 1 to 7 days when compared to placebo. There was an 18.7% (4.1 to 40.4%) higher likelihood of some benefit reported by those treated with ketamine, with a 9.6% (0.2 to 39.4%) increase in remission within 24 hours. For those receiving esketamine, there was a 2.1% (2.5 to 24.4%)

higher chance of relief at 24 hours and a 10.3% (4.5 to 18.2%) more likely to have fewer or no symptoms. However, these effects did not last beyond one week, and the high dropout rate in some studies makes the duration of the benefit uncertain.

Within 24 hours of starting treatment, but not after three or more days, ketamine may help people with bipolar depression with their depressive symptoms.

One day after treatment, an additional 10 persons with bipolar depression per 1000 may have a brief improvement in their symptoms but not a complete resolution. These projections are based on the scant research that is currently available.

In February 2022, the US Food and Drug Administration warned medical professionals about compounded nasal spray products containing ketamine and meant to treat depression: "At this time, there isn't a ketamine nasal spray product that has been approved by the FDA. Since compounded medications are not FDA-approved, the agency has not assessed their efficacy, safety, or quality before allowing them to be sold."

Near-death Experience

Applying the broadest definition of near-death experience (NDE) to those who were able to recall their dreams while under ketamine anesthesia, the majority of those who did so report having had NDEs.

Features that have been frequently linked to NDEs can be replicated by ketamine. According to a comprehensive study conducted in 2019, written accounts of ketamine experiences were found to be highly similar to written reports of non-destructive experiences when compared to other written reports of drug experiences.

Seizures

Only case studies and no randomized controlled trials support the use of ketamine in the treatment of status epilepticus that has not responded to conventional therapies.

Asthma

When children with severe acute asthma do not respond to conventional treatment, ketamine has been proposed as a potential treatment. Its bronchodilator properties are the cause of this.

Contraindications

Some major contraindications for ketamine are:

- Severe cardiovascular disease such as unstable angina or poorly controlled hypertension
- Increased intracranial or intraocular pressure
- Poorly controlled psychosis
- Severe liver disease such as cirrhosis
- Pregnancy
- Active substance use disorder (for serial ketamine injections)
- Age less than 3 months

Adverse Effects

Adverse psychiatric reactions are experienced by 10–20% of adults and 1–2% of children at anesthetic doses, including dreams, dysphoria, hallucinations, and emergence delirium. Psychotomimetic effects can be reduced with lamotrigine and nimodipine or with a benzodiazepine or propofol before anesthesia. Ketamine anesthesia often causes tonic-clonic movements and rarely hypertonia. Vomiting occurs in 5–15% of patients but can be reduced with propofol. Laryngospasm is rare with ketamine. Ketamine generally increases breathing, though there may be transient respiratory depression in the first few minutes after a high-dose rapid intravenous injection.

Psychiatric side effects are common at lower sub-anesthetic dosages. The majority of people report feeling woozy, weird, or floating, as well as experiencing numbness or visual distortions. Drowsiness, confusion, euphoria, difficulty speaking, and difficulty concentrating are also very common (20–50 %). Six to ten percent of people describe psychotic symptoms like going through a hole, vanishing, feeling as though they are melting, seeing colors, and having hallucinations. The most frequent (>10%) non-psychiatric side effects are dizziness, blurred vision, dry mouth, hypertension, nausea, increased or decreased body temperature, or flushing. By the time the injection is over, all of these negative effects are at their peak, drastically diminish 40 minutes later, and vanish entirely four hours later (Brands et al., 1998).

Urinary and Liver Toxicity

Urinary toxicity is most commonly seen in individuals who use large doses of ketamine on a regular basis, with about 20-30% of frequent users experiencing issues with their bladder. This can lead to a range of problems, from inflammation of the bladder to blockage of the kidneys to kidney failure. Symptoms of ketamine-induced bladder issues typically include frequent urination, painful urination, and a constant urge to urinate, sometimes accompanied by pain and blood in the urine. The damage to the bladder lining resembles both interstitial and eosinophilic cystitis, with a thickened wall and a reduced bladder capacity. Research suggests that ketamine and its byproducts directly harm the lining of the bladder, causing damage to the cells and weakening the protective barrier, leading to the development of these symptoms.

The first step in treating ketamine-induced cystitis is to stop using ketamine. NSAIDs, anticholinergics, and tramadol come next, in case the response is insufficient. Epithelium-protective medications, such as oral pentosan polysulfate or intravesical (intra-bladder) hyaluronic acid instillation, are the second-line treatments. Furthermore. intravesical botulinum toxin is helpful.

Ketamine liver toxicity requires larger doses and repeated administration. It was reported that approximately 10% of chronic high-dose ketamine users experienced liver damage. There are case reports of elevated liver enzymes following chronic pain management with ketamine. Acute kidney injury, hepatobiliary disorder, gastrointestinal disorders, cachexia, and biliary colic have all been linked to chronic ketamine abuse.

Dependence and Tolerance

Some people who regularly use ketamine may develop ketamine dependence, though the incidence of this condition is unknown. Experiments on animals support the possibility of abuse. Furthermore, the quick start of effects after insufflation might make it more likely that people will use it recreationally. The brief duration of the effects encourages overindulging. Even with frequent medical use, ketamine tolerance quickly sets in, necessitating higher dosages. Following their attempts to quit, some daily users reported experiencing withdrawal symptoms, which included anxiety, shaking, sweating, and palpitations. Regular recreational ketamine users showed cognitive deficits along with increased symptoms of dissociation and delusion.

Interactions

Propofol and midazolam both have sedative effects that are amplified by ketamine. Lamotrigine and nimodipine reduce the psychotomimetic effects of a low dose of ketamine, whereas naltrexone amplifies them. Clonidine lessens the rise in blood pressure, heart rate, and salivation that occurs with ketamine anesthesia. It also lessens the likelihood of nightmares. Clinical observations imply that benzodiazepines might lessen ketamine's antidepressant effects. It seems that ketamine and most traditional antidepressants can be taken together without risk.

Pharmacology

Pharmacodynamics

Mechanism of action: Esketamine and arketamine, the two enantiomers that makeup ketamine, are combined in equal proportions. Compared to arketamine, esketamine is a far more effective NMDA receptor pore blocker. Ketamine has anesthetic, analgesic, and psychotomimetic effects due to pore blocking of the NMDA receptor. By preventing central sensitization in dorsal horn neurons, blocking the NMDA receptor causes analgesia; in other words, ketamine's actions disrupt the spinal cord's ability to transmit pain.

Research is currently being done to better understand the mechanism of action of ketamine in treating depression. Esketamine was created as an antidepressant due to the theory that NMDA receptor antagonism is the cause of ketamine's antidepressant effects. Nevertheless, rapastinel, memantine, lanicemine, rislenemdaz, 4-chlorokynurenine, and other NMDA receptor antagonists have not shown any appreciable efficacy in treating depression as of yet. Additionally, studies on animals suggest that the enantiomer arketamine, which has a weaker NMDA receptor antagonistic effect, and the metabolite (2R,6R)-hydroxynorketamine, which has a negligible affinity for the NMDA receptor but a strong alpha-7 nicotinic receptor antagonist effect, may have antidepressant properties. This strengthens the case that ketamine's antidepressant effects may not be exclusively attributable to NMDA receptor antagonism. Another explanation for ketamine's antidepressant effects could be acute inhibition of the lateral habenula, also known as the "anti-reward center," because it is the area of the brain that inhibits the mesolimbic reward pathway.

Ketamine may act directly on the NMDA receptor and indirectly on regulators like mTOR and BDNF as one of its biochemical modes of action. The active metabolite of ketamine, hydroxynorketamine, which does not significantly interact with the NMDA receptor but nevertheless indirectly activates AMPA receptors, may also or alternatively be involved in the rapid-onset antidepressant effects of ketamine. It is unclear whether ketamine alone is sufficient for antidepressant action or whether its metabolites are also important. When NMDA receptors are acutely blocked in the brain, glutamate is released more frequently, activating AMPA receptors. These receptors then modulate various downstream signaling pathways, influencing neurotransmission in the limbic system and mediating antidepressant effects. This process is known as NMDA receptor antagonism. The upregulation of brain-derived neurotrophic factor (BDNF) and the activation of its signaling receptor, tropomyosin receptor kinase B (TrkB), the activation of the mTOR pathway, the deactivation of glycogen synthase kinase 3 (GSK-3), and the inhibition of phosphorylation of the eukaryotic elongation factor 2 (eEF2) kinase are examples of such downstream actions resulting from the activation of AMPA receptors.

Molecular Targets: Ketamine primarily functions as a pore blocker of the ionotropic glutamate receptor known as the NMDA receptor. The dizocilpine site of the NMDA receptor is occupied by the S-(+) and R-(−) stereoisomers of ketamine with varying affinities, the former exhibiting a 3- to 4-fold higher affinity than the latter. Because of this, the S isomer has a stronger anesthetic and analgesic effect than the R isomer.

Through yet another allosteric site on the receptor, ketamine may interact with and inhibit the NMDAR. Apart from a few, ketamine's antagonistic effects on the NMDA receptor are much stronger than its actions at other receptors (Brands et al., 1998).

Ketamine has been proposed to interact with allosteric sites on the monoamine transporters to produce monoamine reuptake inhibition, despite the fact that it is a very weak ligand of the monoamine transporters (K_i > 60 μM). Nevertheless, at concentrations as high as 10,000 nM, neither ketamine nor its metabolites have been shown to inhibit the human monoamine transporters functionally (IC_{50}). Furthermore, there has been no interaction between ketamine and the monoamine oxidase inhibitor (MAOI) tranylcypromine in animal studies or at least three human case reports. This is significant because the combination of an MAOI and a monoamine reuptake inhibitor can cause severe toxicity, including serotonin syndrome or hypertensive crisis. Taken together, these data cast doubt on the role that monoamine reuptake inhibition plays in the physiological effects of ketamine in humans. It has been discovered that ketamine increases dopaminergic neurotransmission in the brain; however, this may occur through indirect or downstream mechanisms, such as NMDA receptor antagonistic effects, rather than dopamine reuptake inhibition.

It is debatable if ketamine is an agonist of D2 receptors. Ketamine was discovered to be a D2 partial agonist with potency comparable to its NMDA receptor antagonism in early research by the Philip Seeman group. Subanesthetic doses of ketamine have been found to dose-dependently increase prolactin levels in humans, but D2 receptor agonists like bromocriptine can quickly and effectively suppress prolactin secretion. Later studies by different researchers, however, found that ketamine had an affinity of >10 μM for the regular human and rat D2 receptors. Human striatal [^{11}C] raclopride binding inhibition by ketamine has been the subject of conflicting imaging studies; while some have reported a significant decrease in this binding, others have not found any effect at all. Nevertheless, rather than ketamine binding to the D2 receptor, variations in [^{11}C] raclopride binding might be caused by variations in dopamine concentrations brought on by ketamine.

Relationships between Levels and Effects: Patients treated with ketamine at plasma concentrations of roughly 100 to 250 ng/mL (0.42–1.1 μM) have reported dissociation and psychotomimetic effects. Ketamine is typically administered intravenously as an antidepressant at low dosages, with maximal plasma concentrations of 70–200 ng/mL (0–29–0–84 μM). It also exhibits analgesic effects at comparable plasma concentrations (70 to 160 ng/mL; 0.29–0.67 μM). Ketamine is injected intravenously quickly to induce anesthesia, and within a minute or two, the plasma concentration of the drug can reach 60–110 μM. The ketamine concentration stabilized at roughly 9.3 μM when the anesthesia was sustained with nitrous oxide and continuous ketamine injection. In a study involving only ketamine anesthesia, subjects started to wake up when the drug's plasma level dropped to roughly 2,600 ng/mL (11 μM), and they started to become aware of time and place when it dropped to 1,000 ng/mL (4 μM). The concentration of ketamine in cerebrospinal fluid, a proxy for the concentration in the brain, varied between 2.8 and 6.5 μM during anesthesia and was about 40% lower than in plasma, according to a single-case study (Fuentes et al., 2020).

Pharmacokinetics

Ketamine's solubility in both water and lipids allows for a wide variety of absorption pathways. The bioavailability of ketamine administered intravenously is 100%, whereas the bioavailability of the drug administered intramuscularly is slightly lower at 93%, and the bioavailability administered epidurally is 77%. Although the subcutaneous bioavailability is unknown, it is thought to be high. The oral route has the lowest bioavailability (16–20%) and the intranasal route (45–50%) among the less invasive methods. At between 25 and 50 %, sublingual and rectal bioavailabilities are deemed intermediate.

Ketamine is quickly absorbed and distributed throughout the brain and other tissues. Ketamine's binding to plasma proteins varies, ranging from 23 to 47%.

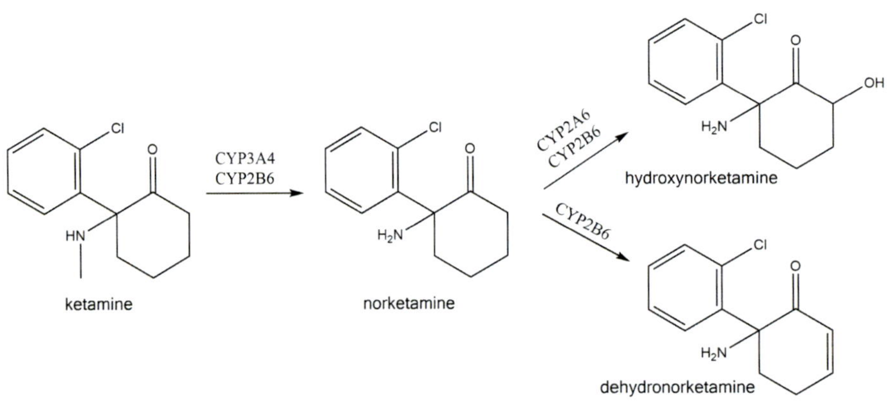

Figure 9.7: Major routes of ketamine metabolism.

Source: By The Sceptical Chymist - Own work, CC BY-SA 4.0, https://commons.wikimedia.org/w/index.php?curid=97478809

Ketamine is extensively metabolized by the body. It is biotransformed into norketamine by CYP3A4 and CYP2B6 isoenzymes. Norketamine is then transformed into hydroxynorketamine and dehydronorketamine by CYP2A6 and CYP2B6. Ketamine's low oral bioavailability is caused by the first-pass effect and potentially by CYP3A4's intestinal metabolism of ketamine. Because of this, after oral administration, norketamine's plasma levels are several times higher than those of ketamine, and norketamine might contribute to the anesthetic and analgesic effects of oral ketamine. This also explains why, in contrast to subcutaneous ketamine levels, oral ketamine levels are not influenced by CYP2B6 activity.

From the feces and urine, 3 % and 91 % of the radioactivity are recovered, respectively, following an intravenous injection of tritium-labelled ketamine. Medication is eliminated primarily as metabolites; only 2 % is excreted unaltered. The most common metabolites found in urine were conjugated hydroxylated derivatives of ketamine (80 %), followed by dehydronorketamine (16 %).

Chemistry

Synthesis

2-Chlorobenzonitrile and cyclopentylmagnesium bromide, a Grignard reagent, react to produce 2-chlorophenyl)(cyclopentyl)methanone. After using bromine to bromate this, the corresponding bromoketone is formed. This is then reacted with methylamine in an aqueous solution to form 1-(2-Chloro-N-methylbenzimidoyl) cyclopentanol, the methylimino derivative, by hydrolyzing the tertiary bromine atom. After heating this last intermediate in decalin or another appropriate high-boiling solvent, an alpha-ketol rearrangement that results in ring-expansion and the creation of racemic ketamine takes place.

Structure

Ketamine is a derivative of arylcyclohexylamine in terms of chemical structure. One chiral compound is ketamine. While the less active enantiomer, arketamine (R-ketamine), has never been marketed as an enantiopure medication for clinical use, the more active enantiomer, esketamine (S-ketamine), is also available for medical use under the brand name Ketanest S. R-ketamine has longer-lasting effects as an antidepressant, but S-ketamine is more potent as an analgesic and anesthetic due to NMDA receptor antagonism.

A given ketamine enantiomer's optical rotation can differ between the compound's salt and free base forms. The free base form of (*S*)ketamine exhibits dextrorotation and is therefore labeled (*S*)(+)ketamine. However, its hydrochloride salt shows levorotation and is thus labeled (*S*)(−)ketamine hydrochloride.

Detection

Ketamine levels in blood or plasma can be measured to support hospitalized patients' poisoning diagnoses, offer proof in cases of suspected drunk driving, or support medicolegal death investigations. Ketamine concentrations in blood or plasma typically range from 0-5.0 mg/L in patients receiving the medication therapeutically (during general anesthesia), 1-2 mg/L in drivers arrested for driving under the influence, and 3-20 mg/L in victims of acute fatal overdosage. When it comes to routine drug use monitoring, urine is frequently the recommended specimen. For the purpose of verifying ketamine consumption, the existence of norketamine, a metabolite with pharmacological activity, is helpful (Fuentes et al., 2020).

9.2.7 Other

Because of their stimulating and psychedelic properties (as well as their chemical affinity for MDMA), synthetic phenethylamines like 2C-I, 2C-B, and DOB have been referred to as club drugs since the 2000s. Derivatives of the psychedelic 2C-X drugs, the NBOMes, and particularly 25I-NBOMe, had become widely available at raves in Europe by late 2012. The drug organization Norconon states that other synthetic drugs used in clubs, or which are sold as "Ecstasy" include harmaline; piperazines (e.g., BZP and TFMPP); PMA/PMMA; mephedrone (generally used outside the US) and MDPV.

Heroin can be found in certain clubs in New York City, though it's far less common than other "club drugs" like MDMA, ketamine, or LSD. Some clubgoers use cannabis products, such as marijuana; some users combine ketamine and Rohypnol powder and smoke the combination.

9.3 Risks of Polydrug Use and Associated Health Complications

Polydrug use, also referred to as polysubstance use, is the term used to characterize the recreational use of multiple substances, either concurrently or sequentially. These mixes may consist of prescription medications, illegal drugs, and/or alcohol. Taking a pill—prescription, recreational, or over-the-counter—and washing it down with a beer or other alcoholic beverage is a common example of polysubstance use.

Other typical ways that polydrug use occurs are as follows.

- Mixing drugs, such as lacing one drug with another
- Using multiple substances to amplify their effects
- Using one substance to counter the effects of another substance
- Using a different substance when the substance you want is no longer available

9.3.1 Understanding Substance Use Disorder

Addictive disorders are another name for substance abuse. Without the substances in question, a person with a substance use disorder is unable to operate normally. Even when abusing this substance has a negative impact on their relationships, finances, legal status, or health, they still use and abuse it.

In order to find new ways to get the desired effect, a person with a substance use disorder may experiment and turn to different substances. They may be so dependent on a particular drug that they have to combine it with something else to achieve the desired "high."

Polysubstance Addiction

The risk of developing an addiction to any substance taken concurrently or simultaneously increases when someone takes multiple substances. Once the brain realizes it needs more than one substance, it will begin to crave them all because addiction alters the brain's general chemistry. Individuals who are addicted to multiple substances may feel different kinds of cravings for each drug. For instance, some people's cravings for nicotine are exclusive to alcohol consumption. Addiction to multiple substances can lead to a higher risk of serious health problems. Every drug has side effects of its own, and combining different substances can negatively impact the body and cause potentially fatal health issues (Fuentes et al., 2020).

9.3.2 Dangers of Polydrug Use

Combining different kinds of drugs can have major negative effects on one's physical and mental health in addition to raising the risk of addiction.

Some of the reasons why a person might decide to mix substances include the following:

- To counter the effects of another substance
- To enhance the "high"
- When their substance of choice is not available
- When someone takes another drug without giving it any thought while already impaired by the effects of the previous one.

Risks of Combining Drugs

All substances have side effects, regardless of whether they are obtained illegally, through over-the-counter purchases, or through medical prescriptions. Combining drugs can be risky and result in serious health problems, both physical and mental.

Some of the side effects associated with polysubstance use and abuse include:

- Depression
- Anxiety
- Hallucinations
- Brain damage
- Organ failure
- Stroke
- Heart attack
- Rapid or slow heart rate

- Breathing issues
- Loss of consciousness
- Respiratory failure
- Uncontrollable muscle spasms
- Memory loss
- Fatal overdose

Since many drug users are unaware that opioids, such as fentanyl, have been added to other illicit drugs, opioid overdoses are becoming a greater concern. Among the most popular drugs that are frequently laced with opiates are cocaine, MDMA, and crystal meth; in many cases, the user is unaware of this.

Combination of Certain Drugs

Although combining substances in any way is regarded as polysubstance abuse, some combinations are more frequently used than others.

Alcohol, depressants, OTC and prescription drugs, stimulants, and alcohol are substances that people frequently mix. Certain combinations have become well-known in popular culture, showing up in songs, films, and other media. because of their ubiquity in the scenes of clubbing and polydrug use. One common mix, for instance, is called a "speedball," and it consists of cocaine and heroin.

Mixing Stimulants

Stimulants can raise blood pressure and heart rate, sometimes to dangerous levels. Examples of these include cocaine, methamphetamines, and ecstasy/MDMA. Combining stimulants may result in:

- Heart attack
- Stroke
- Liver damage
- Brain damage
- Seizures
- Nausea
- Vomiting
- Chest pain
- Increased body temperature
- Psychosis
- Anxiety
- Panic attacks

Mixing Depressants

Depressants slow down the body and brain and shorten breathing. Examples of depressants include alcohol, cannabis, and opiates. Combining depressants can dangerously slow down the central nervous system, which can result in the following effects.

- Brain damage
- Organ damage and failure
- Unconsciousness
- Weak pulse
- Altered mental state
- Confusion
- Increased risk of injury
- Impaired judgment
- Lack of coordination
- Vomiting
- Memory loss
- Irregular breathing

Mixing Stimulants and Depressants

It is untrue for some people to believe that combining stimulants and depressants will neutralize or even cancel each other out. Combining the two may cause the body to experience additional stress, which could result in an overdose and death. Combining stimulants and depressants can put the body under additional strain, which can result in serious health issues like:

- Respiratory issues, including infections
- Heart problems
- Kidney failure
- Dehydration
- Overheating

Mixing Medications

Whether a drug is prescribed or available over-the-counter, there are frequently cautions and guidelines advising against combining particular medications with other substances. Combining different medications can raise your risk of experiencing the following problems.

- Breathing issues
- Drowsiness
- Lack of coordination
- Overdose

Mixing Drugs and Alcohol

Being a depressant, alcohol has many of the same effects as depressant medications. Therefore, combining drugs and alcohol can result in the following problems:

- Drowsiness
- Lightheadedness
- Difficulty concentrating
- Inability to perform basic tasks
- Increased risk of injury
- Liver damage
- Seizures
- Compromised immune system

9.3.3 Polydrug Use in Young People

Compared to other age groups, teens and young adults experiment with drug use more frequently, including mixing substances. According to a study conducted by the Los Angeles-based RAND Research Institute, 29% of senior high school students in California used multiple drugs within the previous year. The following are the primary factors that contribute to teenage polysubstance use, according to the same study.

- Peer pressure
- Pro-drug environment
- Rebelliousness
- Family issues

Additionally, teenage boys are far more likely to engage in polydrug use than teen girls.

The National Institute on Drug Abuse (NIDA) reports that polydrug use is also widespread in the "club scene," which gained notoriety in the 1990s at raves and other events. Clubgoers frequently use polydrugs, which are combinations of psychoactive substances; the most common ones are as follows.

- Alcohol
- MDMA (ecstasy)
- Cocaine
- Ketamine
- Crystal meth
- LSD (acid)
- GHB

9.3.4 Polydrug Use Statistics

According to a June 2020 study, 35 million people in the U.S. meet the criteria for a substance use disorder.

- According to the CDC, in 2019, 50% of all drug overdose deaths involved more than one drug.

- Alcohol is the most common substance involved with polysubstance use.
- Around 11% of the 35 million persons who met the criteria for a substance use disorder also had an alcohol-related polydrug use disorder.
- A 2014 SAMHSA report states that between 2005 and 2011, benzodiazepines and other illegal substances were combined in almost 1 million ER visits.

A Closer Look

Legality of Ephedrine

Canada

Citing a serious risk to health, Health Canada issued a voluntary recall in January 2002 of all ephedrine products containing more than 8 mg per dose, of all ephedrine products combined with other stimulants like caffeine, and of all ephedrine products marketed for bodybuilding or weight-loss purposes. Since it is a Class A precursor, ephedrine is still marketed as a natural health product and is sold as an oral, nasal decongestant in 8 mg pills with a 400 mg maximum per package under the Controlled Drugs and Substances Act.

United States

A regulation limiting the dosage of ephedra (the herb used to make ephedrine) to 8 mg of active ephedrine and no more than 24 mg per day was put forth by the FDA in 1997. Due in part to "concerns regarding the agency's basis for proposing a certain dietary ingredient level and a duration of use limit for these products," this proposed rule was withdrawn in 2000. On April 14, 2005, the U.S. District Court for the District of Utah ruled the FDA did not have proper evidence that low dosages of ephedrine alkaloids are actually unsafe, but on August 17, 2006, the U.S. Court of Appeals for the Tenth Circuit in Denver upheld the FDA's final rule declaring all dietary supplements containing ephedrine alkaloids adulterated, and therefore illegal for marketing in the United States. Moreover, ephedrine is prohibited by the PGA, NFL, MLB, and NCAA. Nonetheless, ephedrine is still allowed in a variety of contexts besides dietary supplements. Currently, purchases are restricted and closely watched; state-by-state variations exist in these policies.

The USA PATRIOT Act was renewed with an amendment passed by the House in 2005 called the Combat Methamphetamine Epidemic Act. ratified by President George W. Bush's act, which was passed on March 6, 2006, changed the US Code (21 USC 830) pertaining to the sale of goods that contained pseudoephedrine, a drug that is closely related to ephedrine. Because both drugs are used as precursors in the illegal manufacture of methamphetamine, the federal statute imposed the following restrictions on retailers selling these goods in order to deter their use:

- A retrievable record, to be retained for two years, of every purchase that includes the name and address of every party.
- Required verification of proof of identity of all purchasers
- Required protection and disclosure methods in the collection of personal information
- Notifications of any regulated product disappearances or suspicious payments to the Attorney General.
- Non-liquid dose form of the regulated product may only be sold in unit-dose blister packs

- Products that are regulated must be sold with restricted access, such as behind a counter or inside a locked cabinet.
- Sales of regulated goods to a single buyer on a daily basis cannot exceed 3.6 grams, regardless of the volume of transactions.
- Sales of regulated products containing no more than 9 g of pseudoephedrine base per month to a single buyer.

Similar rules apply to mail-order purchases under the law, with the exception that the monthly sales cap is 7.5 g.

Ephedrine-containing ma huáng is still legally sold in the US as a pure herb or tea. It cannot be sold as a dietary supplement (pill) or as an additive to other products, such as diet pills, according to the law.

Australia

According to the Poisons Standard, ephedrine and all ephedra species that contain it are classified as Schedule 4 substances. Schedule 4 drugs are classified as Prescription Only Medicines or Prescription Animal Remedy - Substances. According to the Poisons Standard, these drugs must be available from a pharmacist on prescription and used or supplied by individuals authorized by State or Territory law to prescribe.

South Africa

Ephedrine was placed on schedule 6 in South Africa on May 27, 2008, making pure ephedrine tablets prescription-only. OTC schedules 1 and 2 still offer pills with up to 30 mg of ephedrine per tablet when combined with other medications to treat sinus, head colds, and influenza.

Germany

Up until 2001, ephedrine was sold without a prescription in German pharmacies. After that, access was limited because most of the purchases were made for improper purposes. In a similar vein, ephedra is only available via prescription. All products containing ephedrine, including plant parts, have been available only with a prescription since April 2006.

Summary

- Club drugs, also called rave drugs or party drugs, are a loosely defined category of recreational drugs that are associated with discothèques in the 1970s and nightclubs, dance clubs, electronic dance music parties, and raves in the 1980s to today.
- A number of stimulants are used as club drugs. Various amphetamines and methamphetamines are used as stimulants, as is cocaine. These drugs enable clubgoers to dance all night. Cocaine is a powerful nervous system stimulant.
- Depressants are drugs that lower neurotransmission levels or depress or reduce arousal or stimulation in various areas of the brain. Depressants do not change the mood or mental state of others.
- Psychedelic drug, any of the so-called mind-expanding drugs that are able to induce states of altered perception and thought, frequently with heightened awareness of sensory input but with diminished control over what is being experienced.
- "Poppers" are small bottles of volatile drugs that are inhaled by clubgoers for the "rush" or "high" that they can create. Nitrites such as alkyl nitrite originally came as small glass capsules that were popped open, which led to the nickname "poppers."
- Ketamine produces a dissociative state, characterized by a sense of detachment from one's physical body and the external world which is known as depersonalization and derealization.
- In the 2000s, synthetic phenethylamines such as 2C-I, 2C-B and DOB have been referred to as club drugs due to their stimulating and psychedelic nature (and their chemical relationship with MDMA).
- Polydrug use, also known as polysubstance use, describes when a person takes multiple substances (either together or one after the other) for recreational purposes. These combinations can include alcohol, prescription drugs, and/or illicit drugs.
- Mixing different types of drugs can not only increase the chances of the development of an addiction, but it can also cause serious physical and mental health complications.

References

1. Anthony, James; Barondess, David A.; Radovanovic, Mirjana; Lopez-Quintero, Catalina (2017). "Part 1: Psychiatric Comorbidity – Polydrug Use: Research Topics and Issues". In Sher, Kenneth J. (ed.). The Oxford Handbook of Substance Use and Substance Use Disorders: Volume 2. Oxford Library of Psychology. Oxford and New York: Oxford University Press. pp. 27–59. doi:10.1093/oxfordhb/9780199381708.013.006. ISBN 9780199381708. LCCN 2016020729.
2. Black E. Polydrug use: What you need to know about mixing drugs. In: National Drug and Alcohol Research Centre UoNSW, editor. 2014.
3. Brands B, Sproule B, Marshman J. Drugs & Drug Abuse. 3rd ed. Ontario: Addiction Research Foundation; 1998.
4. Darke S, Lappin J, Farrell M. The Clinician's Guide to Illicit Drugs. United Kingdom: Silverback Publishing 2019.

5. Dasgupta A. Alcohol, Drugs, Genes and the Clinical Laboratory An Overview for Healthcare and Safety Professionals: Elsevier Inc; 2017.
6. Fuentes JJ, Fonseca F, Elices M, Farré M, Torrens M. Therapeutic use of LSD in psychiatry: A systematic review of randomized-controlled clinical trials. *Front Psychiatry.* 2020;10. doi:10.3389/fpsyt.2019.00943
7. Graziano S, Orsolini L, Concetta Rotolo M, Tittarelli R, Schifano F, Pichini S. Herbal highs: Review on psychoactive effects and neuropharmacology. *Curr Neuropharmacol.* 2017;15(5):750-761. doi:10.2174/1570159X14666161031144427
8. Guina J, Merrill B. Benzodiazepines: Upping the Care on Downers: The Evidence of Risks, Benefits and Alternatives. Jorunal of Clinical Medicine. 2018;17(7).
9. Hernández-Serrano, Olga; Gras, Maria E.; Font-Mayolas, Sílvia; Sullman, Mark J. M. (2016). "Part VI: Dual and Polydrug Abuse – Chapter 83: Types of Polydrug Usage". In Preedy, Victor R. (ed.). Neuropathology of Drug Addictions and Substance Misuse, Volume 3: General Processes and Mechanisms, Prescription Medications, Caffeine and Areca, Polydrug Misuse, Emerging Addictions and Non-Drug Addictions. Cambridge, Massachusetts: Academic Press, imprint of Elsevier. pp. 839–849. doi:10.1016/B978-0-12-800634-4.00083-4. ISBN 978-0-12-800634-4.
10. Martin, Christopher S.; Chung, Tammy; Langenbucher, James W. (2017). "Part 1: Defining and Characterizing the Nature and Extent of Substance Use Disorders – Historical and Cultural Perspectives on Substance Use and Substance Use Disorders". In Sher, Kenneth J. (ed.). The Oxford Handbook of Substance Use and Substance Use Disorders: Volume 1. Oxford Library of Psychology. Oxford and New York: Oxford University Press. pp. 27–59. doi:10.1093/oxfordhb/9780199381678.013.001. ISBN 9780199381678. LCCN 2016020729.
11. Nichols DE. Psychedelics. *Pharmacol Rev.* 2016;68(2):264-355. doi:10.1124/pr.115.011478
12. Tupper KW, Wood E, Yensen R, Johnson MW. Psychedelic medicine: A re-emerging therapeutic paradigm. *CMAJ.* 2015;187(14):1054-1059. doi:10.1503/cmaj.141124

Chapter 10

EMERGING TRENDS IN SYNTHETIC DRUG DESIGN

Contents

Introduction

The dynamic landscape of pharmaceutical research and development, which is fueled by the growing demand for safer and more effective therapeutics as well as by technological advancements and a better understanding of disease mechanisms. From molecular modeling and computational chemistry to the investigation of new drug targets and delivery systems, these trends cover a wide range of areas in drug design. Keeping up with these developments helps scientists better navigate the tricky problems involved in drug development and discovery, which eventually results in the development of novel drugs with enhanced therapeutic profiles. The use of machine learning algorithms and artificial intelligence (AI) in the drug discovery process is a popular trend in synthetic drug design. With the aid of AI, scientists can now analyze large datasets more quickly, forecast molecular interactions, and more precisely identify possible treatment candidates. Through the application of AI, scientists can expedite the process of identifying potential drug targets, enhance molecular structures, and forecast drug efficacy and safety profiles. This can lead to a more efficient drug development pipeline and lower expenses (Schuster et al., 1998).

Orientation and Directional Terms

Term	Definition	Illustration
Molecular modeling	Molecular modeling is an efficient way of studying protein–protein interactions. It provides detailed information about how protein residues interact with each other at the atomic level.	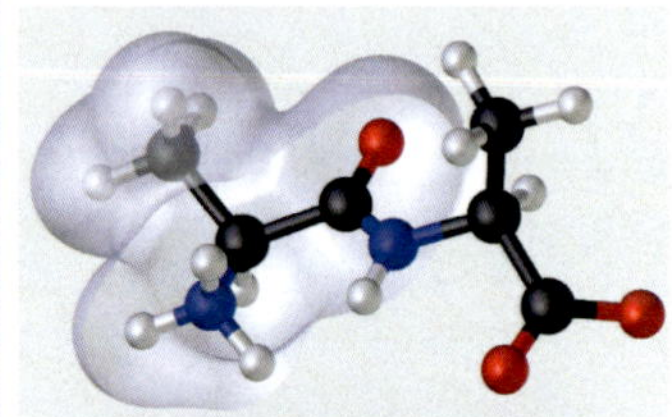
Computational chemistry	Computational chemistry is a type of chemistry that uses computer science to help solve chemical problems.	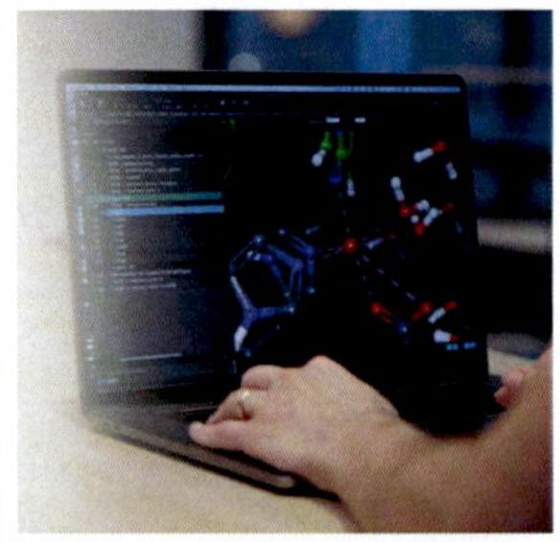
Immune system	The immune system is a complex network of organs, cells and proteins that defends the body against infection, whilst protecting the body's own cells.	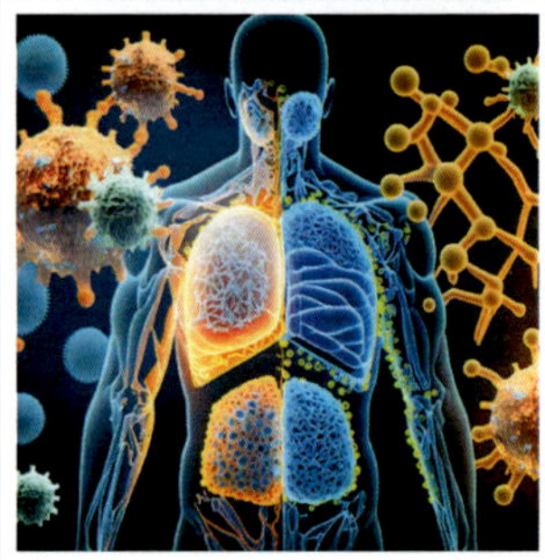
Barbiturates	Barbiturates are a category of sedative-hypnotic medications used for treating seizure disorders, neonatal withdrawal, insomnia, preoperative anxiety, and the induction of coma to address increased intracranial pressure.	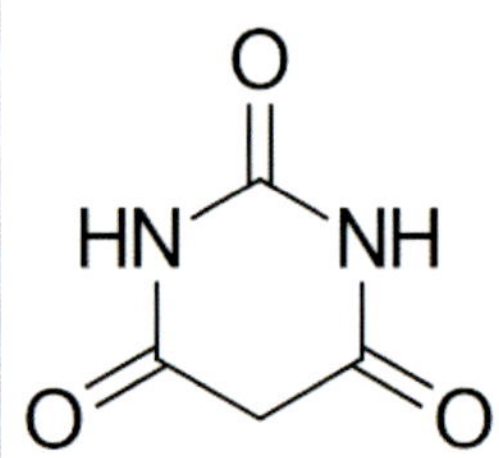
Synthetic drug	Synthetic drugs refer to substances that are artificially modified from naturally-occurring drugs and are capable of exhibiting both therapeutic and psychoactive effects.	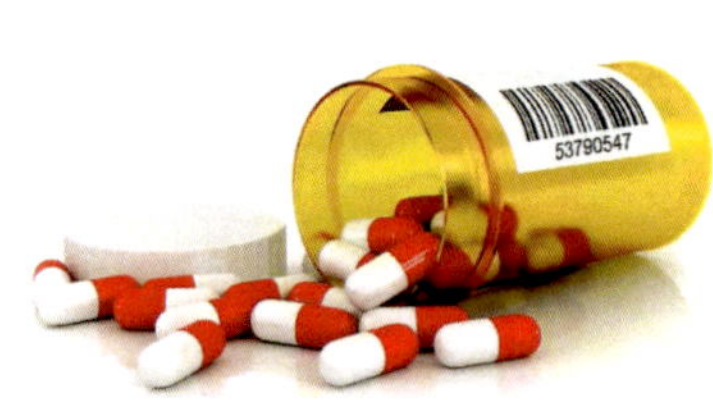

10.1 Advances In The Synthetic Drug Phenomenon

The development of structure-based drug design, which depends on an in-depth understanding of the three-dimensional structures of drug targets, such as proteins or enzymes implicated in disease pathways, is another new trend. Technological developments in structural biology, including cryo-electron microscopy and X-ray crystallography, have made it easier to determine the high-resolution structures of biomolecular complexes. This has allowed for the logical design of targeted therapeutics as well as important insights into the mechanisms underlying disease. Through structure-based drug design, scientists can create compounds that precisely interact with their target, maximizing binding affinity and selectivity while reducing side effects. Additionally, multi-target drug design strategies are becoming more and more important, particularly when treating complex diseases like cancer and neurodegenerative disorders that have heterogeneous pathophysiologies. Multi-target medications attempt to simultaneously modulate several biological targets in order to produce synergistic effects and possibly circumvent drug resistance mechanisms, as opposed to focusing on a single molecular pathway. Developing advanced computational tools and having a thorough understanding of disease networks are necessary for this approach in order to predict the polypharmacological profiles of potential drugs.

Emerging trends in synthetic drug development include the investigation of novel drug delivery systems to improve drug bioavailability, target specificity, and patient compliance, in addition to novel drug design strategies. Drug delivery platforms based on nanotechnology, like liposomes, polymeric nanoparticles, and dendrimers, allow for targeted delivery of the drug to particular tissues or cells and provide precise control over drug release kinetics. Furthermore, developments in gene editing technologies, like CRISPR-Cas9, offer hope for the creation of gene therapies that can rectify genetic mutations that cause disease, potentially providing treatments for inherited and genetic illnesses (ICPO Interpol, 2000; International Narcotics Control Board, 2000).

Chemically manufactured substances intended to imitate or intensify the effects of naturally occurring substances are known as synthetic drugs. These developments have led to more targeted therapies with fewer side effects by greatly increasing the therapeutic options accessible to medical professionals. Precision medicine, which customizes treatments for individual patients based on their genetic composition, lifestyle, and environment, is a significant area of advancement in synthetic drug development. Researchers are able to create highly personalized therapies that are less likely to result in negative side effects and more effective by creating medications that specifically target genetic mutations or biomarkers linked to particular diseases. Treatment advances for diseases like cancer have resulted from this strategy, since targeted medicines can target cancer cells while protecting healthy tissue. The development of synthetic drugs has also led to improvements in drug delivery systems, which have increased the effectiveness and safety of pharmaceuticals. For example, the design of nanoparticles that can deliver medications directly to sick tissues or organs is made possible by nanotechnology, which reduces systemic side effects and enhances therapeutic results. Furthermore, extended-release formulations have been developed as a result of improvements in drug formulation techniques, which enable less frequent dosing and better patient compliance.

Significant advancements have also been made in the field of synthetic drugs in the development of novel drug classes with distinctive mechanisms of action. For example, new treatment options for diseases like cancer, infectious diseases, and autoimmune disorders have been made possible by the development of biologics, which are complex molecules derived from living organisms. Biologic drugs called monoclonal antibodies are becoming more and more significant in targeted therapy because they provide precise means of modifying the immune system and fending off illness. Furthermore, the drug discovery process is now faster and more economical thanks to developments in AI and computational modeling. By mimicking their interactions with biological targets, virtual screening techniques can quickly identify possible drug candidates, reducing the number of compounds that need to be tested in experiments. Large-scale biological data can be analyzed by machine learning algorithms to find hidden patterns and relationships that point researchers in the direction of new therapeutic targets.

10.1.1 Global Overview of Synthetic Drug Markets

Synthetic drug production without authorization, trafficking, and non-medical use are not brand-new issues facing the world. Synthetic drug discovery and proliferation have been facilitated by advancements in the chemical and pharmaceutical industries. Since the beginning of the 20th century, new medications have improved medicine. However, they have also created more opportunities for the illegal supply and use of new mind-altering substances. Examples of these medications include synthetic tranquilizers, stimulants, and anesthetics. The harm caused by the non-medical use of synthetic drugs in the twentieth century was attested to by the adoption of the Convention on Psychotropic Substances of 1971, in which Member States agreed to extend controls over some new synthetic drugs, many of which were of pharmaceutical origin (Thomasius, 2000).

During the past ten years, the number of synthetic drugs on the market has increased. Only a small number of synthetic drugs, mostly ATS, particularly MDMA and methamphetamine, have succeeded in building sizable international markets. Most likely the most supplied and used synthetic drug in the world, methamphetamine is still being produced and used extensively throughout Southeast Asia, North America, South West Asia, Africa, and Europe. Synthetic cannabinoids (SCBs) are a diverse class of constantly evolving compounds that are still available in drug markets worldwide. Other synthetic drugs, such as synthetic opioids like tramadol in North and West Africa and parts of Central Asia and fentanyl in North America, have regionally concentrated markets. A plethora of synthetic drugs (including drugs under international control and non-political substances) have completely changed the heroin-dominated drug market in Eastern Europe and Central Asia. In the near and Middle East, amphetamine in the form of "captagon" is the drug of greatest concern. Meanwhile, the distribution of synthetic drugs, such as ketamine and other NPS stimulants and hallucinogens, has grown in South American drug markets (International Narcotics Control Board, 2000).

10.1.2 Profit-maximizing criminals

Generally speaking, the illegal drug trade functions similarly to other commodities, with profit-driven individuals and organizations controlling the majority of the supply. The fact that drug-related activities are illegal and punishable by law makes a significant distinction, though. In addition to the usual business risks (e.g., inventory and lost investments), but also dangers arising from the illicit nature of the activity (e.g., dangers of violence, arrest, and legal action). They offset these risks by raising markups at every stage of the transaction, which ultimately drives up prices significantly above what they would if the commodities were manufactured lawfully. Operationally and financially, trafficking organizations, like other businesses, aim to minimize operating expenses; as such, they are driven to find ways to lower risk or increase production efficiency. If effective, those cost savings, along with pressure from a competitive market, may eventually result in lower prices for medications sold at retail. Lower retail prices are linked to higher quantities consumed as new entrants into the market increase the total number of consumers and long-term users consume more (Thomasius, 2000).

Certain synthetic drugs provide more ways to lower the risks and operating expenses that criminal actors face when compared to plant-based drugs. Improved synthesis techniques can lower the scale or nature of manufacture, increase yields, or result in the development of new compounds that are more potent than conventional drugs or can evade current controls and detection capabilities. Manufacturing involves the use of chemicals that, for some synthetic drugs, are easily accessible or substitutable. The processing or distribution of synthetic medications as retail formulations can also be advantageous to suppliers, e.g., tablets, which might be enticing to individuals who aren't comfortable injecting drugs. Two other significant benefits that suppliers may receive from the production of synthetic drugs are timeliness and geographic flexibility. Most plant-based drugs require so much space for large-scale production that it is impossible to conceal; as a result, it can only be undertaken in areas where State control is severely restricted or compromised. Contrarily, creating illicit drug mixtures typically doesn't take up much room and can be done practically anywhere. Moreover, the growth of crops requires time, especially coca, which originates from a bush that requires multiple years to reach its maximum productivity.

Natural disasters like blight or drought can wipe out illicit crops, causing significant product losses over the course of a growing season. The time and labor required to produce drugs like cocaine or heroin can result in significant investment losses, which could be reflected in the large amounts of plant-based drugs seized through interdiction. In contrast, it typically takes hours or days to synthesize drugs, so shortages that occur suddenly can be made up for relatively quickly. The benefits of synthetic drugs have not escaped the attention of illicit suppliers. Certain suppliers claimed that when fentanyl and several of its analogs first appeared on heroin markets in some parts of the United States as early as 1979, they were looking into producing less expensive "designer" drugs that could be manufactured with easily obtained ingredients and get around drug laws. However, until recently, the availability of synthetic drugs has been restricted due to the fact that only a small number of highly skilled chemists possess knowledge of chemical synthesis, access to precursor chemicals and related equipment is restricted, and connections to current distribution networks are necessary to bring products to market. In recent decades, many of those obstacles have been significantly removed.

10.1.3 Increasing Availability of Inexpensive Inputs Needed for Synthetic Drug Manufacture

Over the last forty years, the pharmaceutical and chemical industries have expanded rapidly throughout the world, especially in Asia, where the expansion of the industry since the late twentieth century has led to a proliferation of businesses and an increase in the number of people possessing the necessary knowledge of pharmacology and chemical synthesis. According to WHO estimates, with over 2,000 products manufactured and contributing nearly 25% of global output annually, China is the world's largest single producer of active pharmaceutical ingredients by volume. Industry analysis shows that India produces a slightly smaller percentage of active pharmaceutical ingredients. It is difficult for regulators to make sure that suppliers and manufacturers follow handling guidelines and other laws meant to prevent the diversion of psychoactive substances and related precursor chemicals because of the size and speed of these industries. A wide range of inputs required to manufacture drugs are more easily accessible when there is little regulation over large industries or when there are no regulations covering the distribution and advertising of precursors. Because basic chemicals have so many acceptable applications, it can be challenging to regulate their production and distribution. These compounds are sometimes referred to as pre-precursors. Furthermore, some companies produce masked or "designer" precursors in order to evade trade restrictions or control. A large number of those substances are cheap. Prior research by UNODC has revealed that the $9 billion worldwide total in legal sales of other chemicals and controlled precursors required in the production of pharmaceuticals in 2012 represents a very small portion of the total market value (UNODC, 2013). Orders can be placed online and fulfilled by commercial shipment or post. Some non-controlled precursor chemicals are available for incredibly low prices, as advertised by vendors in Asia.

Access to other equipment required for the industrial-scale production of substances facilitates the illicit production of synthetic drugs (e.g., from commercial-grade automated tableting machines to off-the-shelf glassware and custom reaction vessels). Few nations have implemented strong laws governing the sale, transfer, or possession of tableting machines or other equipment of a similar nature, despite the fact that international conventions require governments to take appropriate action to prevent the diversion of supplies and equipment to support the production of illegal drugs. It has been discovered that criminals use this equipment, occasionally locating suppliers online, to make tablets that are illicitly filled with synthetic drugs like ATS, unapproved benzodiazepines, or fentanyl. Both South and East Asia are sources of finished pharmaceutical drugs intended for the black market as well as the precursors required in the manufacture of finished drugs, according to analysis of significant seizures of tramadol and fentanyl.

10.1.4 Improvement of Manufacturing Techniques

The movement of goods and people, the growth of Internet-based communications and encryption technologies, and easier access to chemicals and related equipment have given rise to new channels for drug suppliers and criminal organizations to trade, exchange information, and transact with end users. This has made it easier to trade drugs and chemicals, particularly more recent or "designer" substances that might not raise the attention of law enforcement or customs officials. It has been reported that criminal organizations are utilizing open-access online platforms to locate suppliers of precursor chemicals or other equipment required for the production or processing of synthetic drugs. With the exception of cannabis, most plant-based medications do not work like this. Cultivators of coca and poppies typically trade or sell their harvests directly to criminal organizations. Similarly, online access to patents and medical literature on newly discovered synthetic drugs enables covert chemists to examine and produce novel drugs that were previously investigated as possible medicines but were subsequently withdrawn owing to unfavorable effects or abuse potential. This seems to be the case with a number of synthetic opioids and cannabinoids that were created in the 1970s and 1990s, respectively and later surfaced on black markets for drugs or in physical retail establishments offering NPS. The knowledge needed to manufacture different drugs synthetically using plant-based inputs is also provided by the Internet-based sharing of synthesis and novel drug discovery-related information. Hexahydrocannabinol and other novel, semi-synthetic cannabis-derived compounds are becoming more readily available, and this may be due to the publication and promotion of straightforward synthesis routes that use the CBD present in hemp as a starting material in order to get around national and international regulations (Economic and Social Council, 1997).

Innovative manufacturing techniques can be aided by substitute chemicals that are less hazardous or unmonitored. For instance, a survey of the literature on the ongoing innovation of fentanyl synthesis routes reveals that people engaged in the drug's illicit production are picking up knowledge from patents and published studies. Enhanced synthesis routes for synthetic drugs provide criminals without formal chemistry training with quicker or easier ways to manufacture the drugs. For instance, the examination of fentanyl seizures has revealed that, in Mexico, alternate synthesis routes—which are occasionally more convenient operationally or make use of chemicals that are not under control—have been used. For the first time since 2009, advances in the illicit production of methamphetamine from P-2-P using tartaric acid refinement to increase potency were reported in Europe in 2019. This method has been utilized in Mexico. There may be modifications to the processes used in Southeast Asia to produce methamphetamine illegally, such as the use of P-2-P, which is being seized more frequently, or the combination of tartaric acid and other chemicals to produce ephedrine. Recent large seizures of formic acid, totaling more than 5,800 liters, suggest an evolution in illegal manufacture towards smuggled industrial-grade precursors. Ephedra and diverted cold medication are among the potential precursor inputs used in the manufacture of methamphetamine, which has been reported to come from Afghanistan.

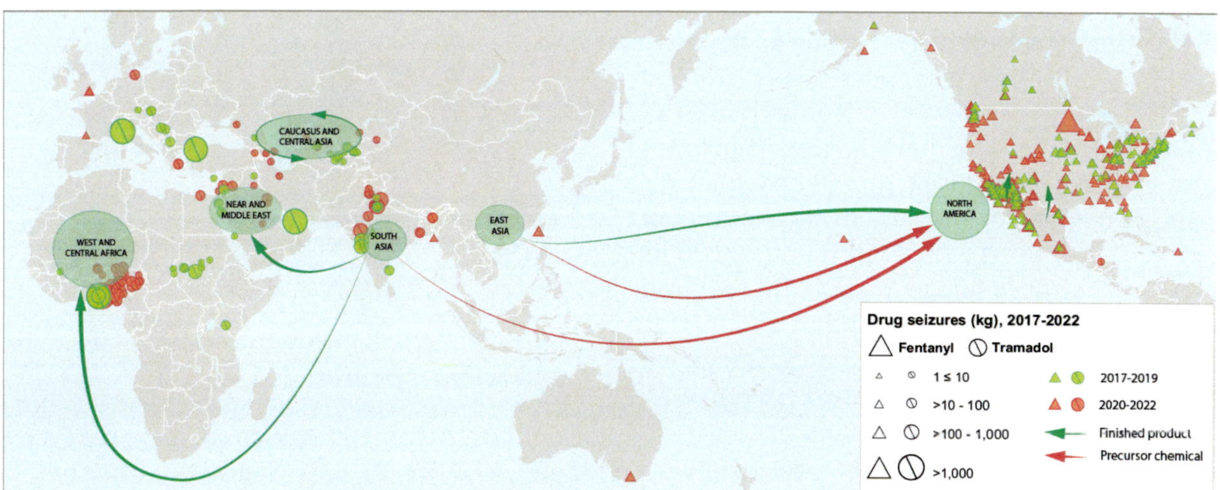

Figure 10.1. Significant individual fentanyl and tramadol seizures over 1 kg in weight, 2017-2022

Source: https://www.unodc.org/res/WDR-2023/WDR23_B3_CH1_Synthetic_drugs.pdf

Although there has been a rise in cocaine and methamphetamine seizures worldwide in recent years, the rise in methamphetamine seizures has been significantly greater, suggesting the scalability and diffusion of the synthetic drug's production. Global methamphetamine seizures nearly tripled and cocaine seizures roughly doubled between 2015 and 2021. Though there may be additional factors influencing trends in seizures, such as improved interdiction strategies, growing markets, etc. Because harvesting and processing take time and are sometimes restricted to specific geographic areas, the production of the majority of plant-based medications cannot easily expand as quickly or widely (Economic and Social Council, 1997).

10.1.5 Pharmacology and Demand-Related Factors

The pharmacology of synthetic drugs may appeal to certain drug users and provide benefits to illicit suppliers. Many synthetic medications have significantly higher potencies than the plant-based counterparts they imitate. This is particularly true for heroin and fentanyl. Maybe 25–50 times as potent as heroin is fentanyl. Because traffickers can more easily conceal smaller quantities of pure fentanyl instead of larger volumes of heroin, this translates into reduced legal risk and, consequently, costs. Compared to roughly 50 metric tons of heroin, it has been estimated that as little as a few tons of pure fentanyl would be required to meet the yearly consumption of opioids sourced illegally in the United States. Smuggling risks can be mitigated by smaller quantities, though occasionally, legal routes are used to transport synthetic drugs with high potencies and purity. For instance, prior to 2019, law enforcement in the United States regularly reported high-purity seizures of fentanyl in the international postal and courier systems, sometimes amounting to as little as 1 g. Because fentanyl is much more potent than heroin, even small amounts of low purity can be smuggled through a variety of channels to meet demand. The benefits of a higher-potency product imply that trafficking groups can disperse the risk of being stopped among numerous lone pedestrians or automobiles. As a result, many synthetic drugs may become more resistant to interdiction, which would lower their retail costs. The fact that the purity-adjusted low-level wholesale price of fentanyl powder produced illegally in the US decreased by more than 50% between 2016 and 2021 is proof of this. Methamphetamine acts more slowly than cocaine in a similar manner. This may result in less frequent redoing, which certain buyers may find appealing. Methamphetamine has additional pharmacological properties that draw some people in. Methamphetamine produces a stronger stimulant effect by increasing dopamine release and inhibiting its reuptake, in contrast to cocaine, which only blocks dopamine reuptake (.

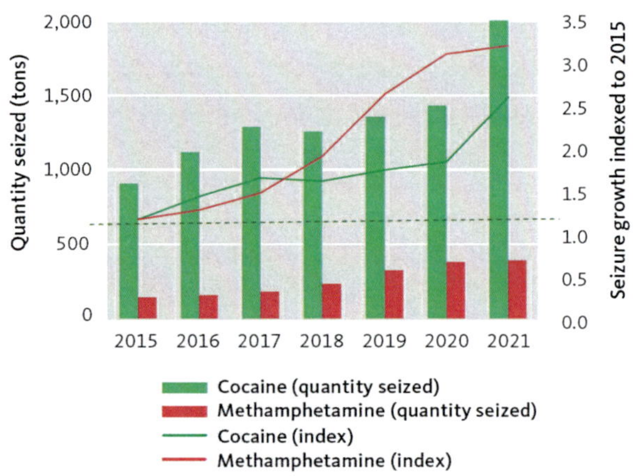

Figure 10.2. Global growth of methamphetamine and cocaine seizures, 2015–2021.

Source: https://www.unodc.org/res/WDR-2023/WDR23_B3_CH1_Synthetic_drugs.pdf

Methamphetamine's increased potency and reduced cost per dose, along with more fruitful sources of production, as documented in North America, Southeast Asia, and Western and Central Europe, indicate that the drug's prevalence is rising. Early warning and drug services monitoring systems indicate that methamphetamine supply is rising in Western and Central Europe, where amphetamine has historically been more prevalent. A combination of supply and demand factors determines the single-drug market dynamics. Purer or less expensive drugs are usually sought after by users, particularly price-sensitive heavy users. If inexpensive drugs appear in tablet form and don't require injection, snorting, or smoking, novice users might be less reluctant to try them. This is especially true if the drugs seem to have been taken out of the pharmaceutical system. It is possible to manufacture and distribute synthetic drugs at a lower cost per dose and formulate them in a way that satisfies current user preferences and behaviors, like taking tablets.

Synthetic drug producers can readily modify mixtures to adapt to changes in supply or demand. According to an analysis of tablet seizures in the US, some drugs—including ones disguised to resemble diverted medications—contain fentanyl produced illegally rather than prescription medication (Al-Sha'er and Taha, 2010). Methamphetamine is frequently found in tablets marketed as MDMA in Afghanistan. Methamphetamine has allegedly been found in tablets marketed as MDMA or as diverted pharmaceutical stimulants, like Adderall, in other US cases. In the Near and Middle East, amphetamine-containing tablets are frequently marketed as "captagon" tablets with pharmaceutical origins. Although diluents and adulterants are frequently added to drugs sold on black markets, suppliers had fewer options in the past. An increasing range of additives can be found in heroin and cocaine sold in Europe and North America, according to a long-term analysis of their impurities. Until recently, the only known additives were caffeine, procaine, and sugars. Occasionally, other tranquilizers—mostly legally prescribed benzodiazepines or other barbiturates—were added. On the other hand, modern drug dealers are combining an increasing number of different drug combinations to offer a range of qualitative and psychoactive effects, frequently hiding the risks from consumers that could have serious health repercussions. A growing percentage of drug seizures in certain opioid markets in North America involve fentanyl mixed with illegal benzodiazepines, xylazine, or veterinary tranquilizers.

Pharmacological aspects of synthetic drugs, such as their duration and mode of action, may also vary more and cater to distinct demand niches. Unlike many plant-based drugs, several synthetic ATS, like MDMA or MDA, can have a range of psychoactive effects. The ease with which new psychoactive effects can be quickly created from synthetic drugs far outpaces the rate at which new naturally occurring drugs are discovered. For instance, users claimed that mephedrone, a synthetic cathinone, was similar to cocaine but better. Mephedrone quickly gained popularity and entry into some European drug markets in the late 2000s and early 2010s. Synthesis enables vendors to investigate novel "research chemicals" intended to replicate the actions of current medications or to offer less expensive substitutes to gullible consumers. These purchasers include those seeking entirely novel drug-induced experiences that differ from those offered by the usual drugs on sale (e.g., psychonauts), people trying to improve their lifestyles in specific dance or party situations (e.g., people having chemsex), or those who desire a drug-induced experience but want to stay under the radar (e.g., people who are being drug-screened) (Al-Sha'er and Taha, 2010). Just a small number of the hundreds of NPS that are presently under surveillance by international and national authorities are plant-based.

10.1.6 Different Supply and Revenue Structures for Naturally Occurring and Synthetic Drugs

Significant variations in the availability of synthetic versus natural drugs are summed up in Table 10.1 and Figure 10.3. Synthetic drug manufacturing, when compared to natural drug origins, provides criminal organizations with structural advantages in the form of shorter supply chains, lower risk, and lower production and risk costs.

Table 10.1. Comparison of drugs of natural and synthetic origin

	Drugs of natural origin	Drugs of synthetic origin
Emergence of new drugs	Rare; would require discovery of new naturally occurring compounds; slow and limited	Chemical development; rapid by comparison and nearly unlimited
Inputs and materials	Crops or other natural inputs that require certain climates or environments; limited State control over growing areas; other related chemicals needed in processing	Precursor chemicals, some of which are controlled, at least in theory. Others can easily be masked or designed to circumvent controls
Scale and scope of production	Large, low-skilled labour supply dedicated to cultivating and harvesting large areas of illicit crops; geographically fixed production centres; extraction and refinement of alkaloids in rudimentary clandestine labs	Only requires a few individuals with knowledge of chemistry or means of carrying out chemical reactions in concealed and small locations; production can be mobile or easily relocated and scaled up or down as needed
Production time	Months. Some illicit crops are harvested only a few times a year, while some have staggered harvests; some plants may take years to reach maturity	Hours or days for reactions and processing
End products	Extracted/isolated and refined alkaloids (cocaine, morphine) or processed plant matter (cannabis, khat, kratom)	A wide array of psychoactive compounds can be produced using a range of precursor inputs
Trafficking	Often involves larger quantities of primary inputs and finished products transported over vast distances or through remote areas, sometimes cross-ing several borders, which enables the authorities to detect and seize such drugs	Can be manufactured close to end markets; small quantities can be posted to end buyers
Forms of administration	Most often injected, snorted or smoked, sometimes ingested	Can be smoked, snorted or injected, but a considerable share is tableted
Pharmacology	Largely understood	Not always known or predictable, even if the chemical structure is known; some new compounds may appeal to different user groups

Source: https://www.unodc.org/res/WDR-2023/WDR23_B3_CH1_Synthetic_drugs.pdf

Manufacturing synthetic drugs is a technological advance that could upend established supply chains and markets. An hourglass-shaped supply chain for conventional plant-based medications can be imagined, with numerous farmers and cultivators at the top. Drugs travel frequently across international borders, from areas of production to areas of consumption, reducing the labor pool for each layer that follows until it reaches exporters and importers. The number of participants rises from there all the way up to the numerous retailers who provide goods to customers. However, the production of synthetic drugs eliminates most of the upper half of the supply chain. Since the marginal return for an additional chemist is significantly higher than that of an additional farmer, the production of synthetic drugs can be scaled up more readily. This has happened with a number of synthetic drugs, including ketamine and methamphetamine, whose production has shifted from small, home-based labs to larger, more sophisticated industrial facilities across Europe, Asia, and North America. From then on, as layers of the supply chain are added, the number of people involved in each level increases.

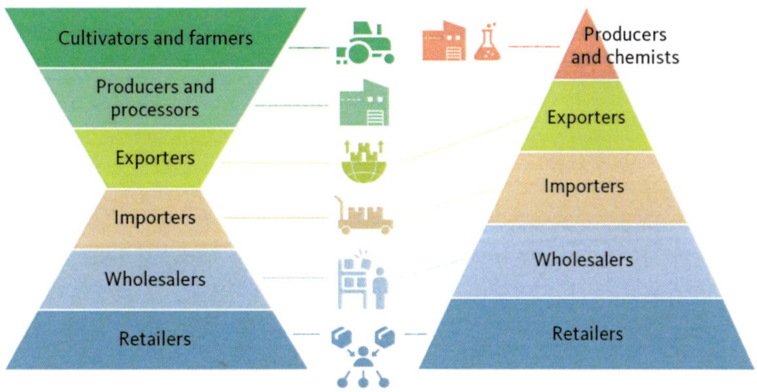

Figure 10.3. Labor supply for drugs of natural and synthetic origin.

Source: https://www.unodc.org/res/WDR-2023/WDR23_B3_CH1_Synthetic_drugs.pdf

Economically speaking, the synthesis of drugs requires more capital than labor-intensive plant-based drug production, though even for synthetic drugs, there may be a minimal capital requirement. To put it simply, chemical synthesis eliminates the need for a vast supply of unskilled labor and tens of thousands of hectares of arable land. The production of illegal plant-based drugs typically depends on impoverished farmers and their families who reside in isolated areas. Because of the nature of this production method, criminal organizations must pay extra expenses. Plant-based drugs are frequently grown in regions with lax governance and the rule of law, and their production frequently depends on non-State actors—many of whom are violent—controlling the extraction and transportation of essential inputs like coca or poppies (Aller et al., 2009). Conversely, synthesis provides suppliers with a number of benefits. Facilities that are simpler to hide from authorities, such as lone homes, warehouses, or labs in isolated locations, ports, or cities, can be the site of clandestine synthesis. Synthetic drug production has persisted on a large scale in both lawless and law-abiding nations; in Europe, for instance, MDMA, amphetamine, and methamphetamine, as well as a small amount of cathinones, are produced primarily to satisfy local or regional demand. European authorities have observed a rise in the production of synthetic drugs on the continent and the subsequent trafficking of these drugs to other areas. The production of synthetic drugs can be easily relocated, sometimes closer to end markets or major commercial hubs with access to imported chemicals or export routes; chemists or cooks can be rotated from one laboratory to another, further reducing the risk of detection, compared with the production of plant-based drugs, which prioritizes control over territory and rural populations.

Shorter supply chains for synthetic drugs can mitigate some risks, particularly if synthesis labs are moved domestically to prevent cross-border movement. Authorities in the US and Canada have found and shut down fentanyl synthesis labs in recent years; these labs are occasionally situated close to end markets. Similar to this, since the early 2010s, end markets in the Middle East have become the focus of illicit "captagon" production instead of East and South-Eastern Europe. A shift in production to meet demand on the continent may have occurred as a result of recent seizures by European authorities of increasing quantities of chemical precursors and the discovery of covert laboratories for a number of synthetic drugs, including ketamine, cathinones, GBL, and gamma-hydroxybutyric acid (GHB). Many of these synthetic drugs originated in Asia before 2020. In some cases, illicit producers have shifted their operations to other developing nations or emerging markets where it is more difficult to detect drugs or check imports for an increasing number of precursors. For instance, there have been recent reports of the illicit production of methamphetamine in African nations, such as South Africa and Nigeria, using precursor materials from Asia with an eye toward regional and international markets. Several large-scale ketamine laboratories that employed teams of foreign cooks and industrial-grade equipment have been dismantled in Cambodia in recent years (Aller et al., 2009). Additionally, compared to earlier reports, countries in Central Asia have noted a notable increase in the discovery of domestic laboratories used for the production of synthetic drugs. Authorities in Kazakhstan reported a 50% increase in laboratory detections between 2020 and 2021. Using progressively more advanced methods and apparatus, 36 laboratories were found to be manufacturing mephedrone and alpha-PVP in 2021.

It is possible to improve drug synthesis to better ensure product pricing and consistency. From one harvest to the next, coca or poppy crops can have different levels of productivity. Economic analyses of illicit drug markets show that because agricultural inputs are volatile and distributors are unlikely to hold large inventories to minimize risk, commodity prices for plant-based drugs are subject to erratic or periodic fluctuations. Because synthetic drugs are guaranteed to have a higher level of purity and because the synthesis process is quick, producers are more likely to be able to react quickly to demand signals and lower the risk of holding inventory, which results in lower price volatility. Actually, data from the US indicates that the price volatility of heroin and cocaine was significantly greater than that of methamphetamine.

In addition, many pharmaceuticals must be diluted and repackaged for retail markets, frequently very close to the point of retail sale. Wholesale distributors typically dilute illegal imports further, which adds to price volatility in retail markets because consumers can't tell the quality of the product until after they've consumed it. The retail distribution of powder that is imported in large quantities enables regional retailers to compete by differentiating their products and building their brands to draw in customers. Drug markets frequently involve dilution, repackaging, and retail-level branding, particularly for powder-based products. While plant-based medications have not typically been available in tablet form, synthetic drugs can. Tableting offers greater product consistency and can be automated from the supplier's perspective. Big-scale commercial tableting machines can create tens or hundreds of thousands of tablets per day with just a few knowledgeable technicians and continuous operation. Even though tablet dosage varies among suppliers, large-scale production might lessen dosage heterogeneity within a single batch. Furthermore, since the product hasn't been traded or trafficked yet, processing for retail purposes can take place at the point of manufacture, where risks are lower than right before the final sale (Economic and Social Council, 1998). Furthermore, the industrial or large-scale tableting of synthetic drugs gives criminal organizations control over branding through the use of stamps, dies, and colors, adding value to the product and potentially boosting export earnings by uniting multiple supply chain tiers.

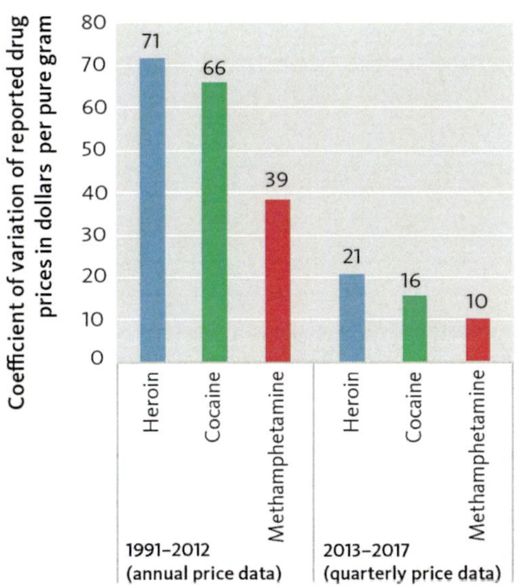

Figure 10.4. Price volatility of heroin, cocaine and methamphetamine in the United States, 1991–2017.

Source: https://www.unodc.org/res/WDR-2023/WDR23_B3_CH1_Synthetic_drugs.pdf

Along the supply chain, revenue retention can change as a result of drug synthesis and tableting. In order to offset the risks involved in the supply chain, the majority of price markups and revenue from the sale of illegal drugs occur at the stages closest to retail.

This is accurate for synthetic drugs, but many (transnational) trafficking organizations tend to concentrate on a single link in the supply chain and do not have complete control over the chain from seed to sale for traditional plant-based drugs. When transporting cocaine or heroin from the mountains of Colombia or Afghanistan to retail street markets in the destination countries, for instance, the product is subject to multiple trades.

10.2 Trends in Clandestine Synthetic Drugs

Drug abuse trends often exhibit cyclical behavior, with specific drugs or patterns of use resurfacing at various times and/or locations. Comprehending these patterns and their fundamental dynamics can thus aid in enhancing policy measures and prompt responses to the recurrence of issues that have already been identified (Economic and Social Council, 1998).

The "synthetic drug phenomenon" has only gained traction in the last ten years, in contrast to the lengthy history of abuse of plant-based drugs like heroin and cocaine, i.e., the worldwide concern has been raised by the widespread recreational use of some psychoactive drugs by a largely young consumer population, who often do so as a part of a particular lifestyle or subcultural group identity. Even though it is now evident that some illicit synthetic drugs are spreading quickly throughout the world, there are still big disparities in the scope of the issue in terms of consumer populations and geography.

10.2.1 From 'Plant-Based' to 'Synthetic' Drugs

The usage of unrefined plant materials for ceremonial, spiritual, or therapeutic purposes that had comparatively low psychoactive potency led to the gradual evolution of the current drug problem. The development of pharmaceutical technology and natural science allowed for the refinement of the (psycho)active compounds (e.g., opium and coca leaf, respectively) of the crude plant products (morphine, cocaine). Although the therapeutic use of those substances was still reliant on the availability of the plant's raw material, the availability of the pure active principle made more dependable and targeted medical applications possible. The production of synthetic therapeutic drugs started to compete with the extraction of active principles from natural raw materials in terms of cost-effectiveness only in the late 19th and early 20th centuries when pharmaceutical research and industry grew to a respectable size and degree of sophistication. Using readily available and inexpensive chemical starting materials, it became possible to produce the pure active principles of several traditionally used plant-based products in laboratories around the world. This allowed for the low-cost distribution of many of those medications to large segments of society (the main developments in the evolution of the modern drug problem are shown in Figure 10.6 below).

The pursuit of pharmaceuticals with improved specificity or potency but comparable or identical therapeutic effects, i.e., with fewer unfavorable side effects, denoted the progression of evolution. Drug design, also referred to as drug modeling, is the process of changing the chemical structure of a known, well-researched parent molecule (Hando and Hall, 1994). It is a fundamental idea in contemporary pharmaceutical research and industrial production. Fentanyl, a class of synthetic opioids used in anesthesia and as analgesics (painkillers), is an example of a contemporary synthetic drug based on the structural properties of morphine. A general enthusiasm for almost all new products characterized the early days of synthetic pharmaceutical drugs. This resulted in a somewhat careless use of these medications, along with easy access to some medications, careless prescribing practices, and/or overprescription. Over time, people started to become more conscious of and concerned about the possible risks connected to the widespread use of some psychoactive medications. Regulations were put in place, medical use was progressively discouraged, and then it began to decline. The primary source of supply for non-medical use then shifted from the legal to the illegal market due to diversion. The creation of covert laboratories resulted from the tightening and enlarging of control measures. Here, illicit manufacturers created counterfeit versions of the desired products using the same chemicals used in the pharmaceutical industry to satisfy illicit demand.

The "design" of new drugs based on a parent substance's chemical structure that yielded the desired effects marked the final stage in the evolution of the contemporary drug problem. Research on pharmaceuticals and this concept are extremely similar. That being said, the objective of covert producers is to produce drugs with pharmacological profiles that the consumer base will find desirable, whereas the pharmaceutical industry seeks to develop safer drugs or to boost specificity for a particular kind of intended therapeutic effect. Creating substances that are exempt from national and/or international control regimes is another motivation for clandestine manufacturers, as it allows them to evade legal action and avoid exposure. Because they are not just illegally produced copies of already-existing substances but rather completely original works created in the clandestine sector, these so-called "designer drugs," which are manufactured in secret, are also sometimes referred to as "synthetic drugs of the second generation."

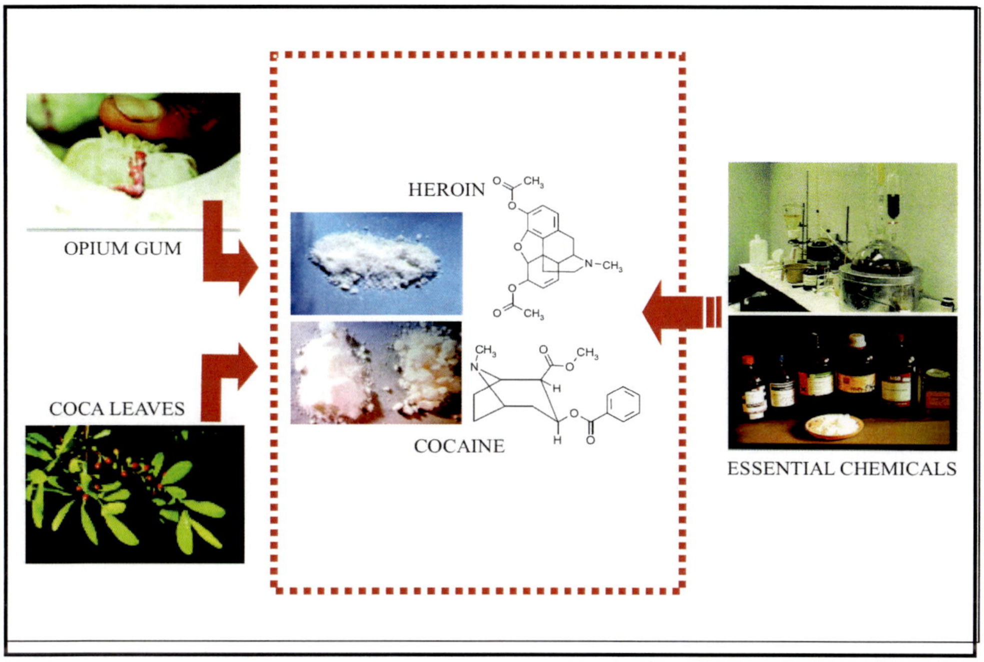

Figure 10.5. Heroin and cocaine can be obtained from natural sources or by chemical synthesis.

Source: https://www.unodc.org/pdf/report_2001-06-26_1/analysis_clandestine.pdf

There are five major classes of designer drugs:

(i) synthetic opioids,

(ii) phencyclidine (PCP) derivatives,

(iii) tryptamines,

(iv) methaqualone derivatives, and

(v) phenylalkylamines (PAAs).

10.2.2 Amphetamine-type Stimulants: A Case Scenario

Social and geographical spread of ATS abuse

Considered the parent drugs of the ATS group, amphetamine and methamphetamine were first used for non-medical purposes in the 1930s, right after they were introduced into medical practice. The Second World War saw soldiers use instruments, and this, along with lax prescribing, contributed to the subsequent public abuse epidemic. The abuse began with certain occupational groups, then spread to athletes, students, and finally, recreational users. Geographically speaking, ATS abuse progressively extended from a small number of nations, such as Sweden, Japan, and the United States, to neighboring nations within the same regions and eventually to additional regions. Abuse of ATS has been seen as a global phenomenon since the mid-1990s, following the beginning of the "ecstasy" epidemic in Europe, albeit with different substances being more common in different regions of the world (Hando and Hall, 1994). The use of ATS for recreational purposes is currently most common in a number of developed nations, especially in Europe. However, it is also rapidly spreading to other regions, especially Southeast Asia, where it was previously more common for instrumental purposes, such as long-distance truck driving.

Sources of supply

Overprescribing and careless prescribing practices contributed to the non-medical use of ATS during the early days when amphetamines were thought to be a cure-all for a variety of illnesses. Following the introduction of regulatory restrictions and the growing concern over the possible risks associated with the widespread use of ATS, large-scale diversion from the licit trade quickly emerged as the main source of supply to meet non-medical demand. What is commonly referred to as the "balloon" effect began in the early 1970s when several traditional ATS were subjected to stricter controls, i.e. supply being moved from one source to another. The term "balloon effect" describes the transfer of resources from the legal to the illegal domain, which in turn gives rise to the covert production of substances such as methamphetamine and amphetamine, and eventually structurally altered designer anti-terrorism drugs (International Narcotics Control Board Report, 2000).

10.3 Clandestine Synthetic Drugs Vis-À-Vis Plant-Based Drugs

It also examines some of the fundamental features that influence the supply and demand for drugs, emphasizing the key distinctions between synthetic and plant-based drugs (as demonstrated by the examples of heroin and cocaine). Access to and availability of the necessary starting materials are critical supply-side factors for a clandestine operator. The production of synthetic drugs usually requires starting materials that are readily available worldwide. The chemicals involved are generally inexpensive, and the desired end product can be produced in a few simple reaction steps. In contrast, the production of classical plant-based drugs, such as heroin and cocaine, is dependent on natural raw materials only produced in certain geographical locations. Risks related to the preservation of cultivation areas are nonexistent, and labor-intensive, drawn-out processes for harvesting, extraction, and isolation are not necessary. The availability of information and the necessary scientific and technical know-how is another crucial component. Synthetic drug manufacturing recipes can be easily obtained online or through specialized underground literature (Hando and Hall, 1994). The spread of covert drug synthesis is actually greatly aided by contemporary information technology, which provides answers to common queries like which chemical precursors to use, where to obtain them, how to avoid detection, and how to set up a basic "kitchen" laboratory. The fact that a typical synthesis involves relatively little technology and a small number of reaction steps makes all of this worse. Yields from synthesis are typically high.

The past ten years have seen a global spread of some synthetic drugs, which can also be linked to financial incentives that influence their production, trafficking, and eventual abuse. From a supply perspective, synthetic drugs are often more profitable in consumer markets than either heroin or cocaine. The production of synthetic drugs is not limited to any particular region; it can happen in close proximity to the final point of consumption. This means that practically all of a synthetic drug's retail price stays in the area where it is used. Additionally, because it permits smaller-scale trafficking, the proximity of locations for covert production and consumption lowers the chance of discovery, for instance, at border crossings. Compared to the production of heroin or cocaine illegally, the fact that synthetic drug laboratories are less noticeable lowers the overall risks for covert operators. On the demand side, a number of factors affect a user's final decision to select a specific drug. The drug's own pharmacological properties, i.e., insofar as they are known to the user, the drug's desired effects balanced against its risks and unfavorable side effects most likely play a big part. Comparably, drugs that are appropriate for delivery methods other than intravenous injection and—more and more—methods other than smoking also appear to be contributing factors. The perception and social portrayal of specific drugs, as well as the accessibility and availability of substitute substances, are additional factors. Cultural, social, and economic factors are also taken into account. As a result, the demand side of the equation is more complicated than the supply side, and customer preferences are subject to change (International Narcotics Control Board Report, 2000).

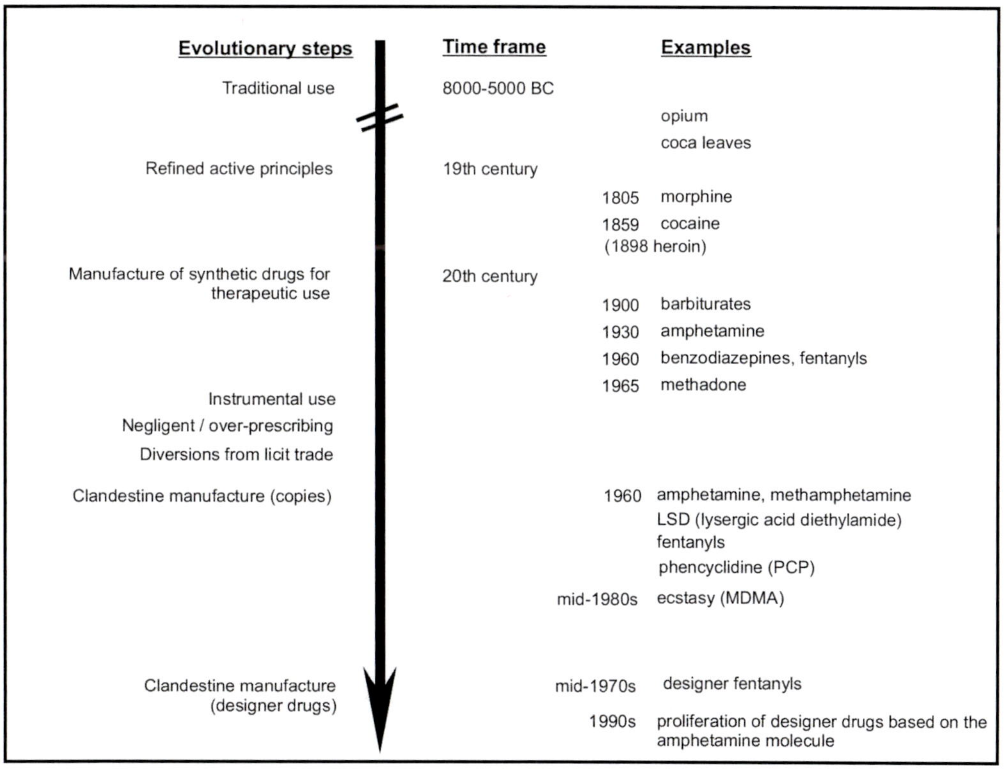

Figure 10.6. Clandestine synthetic drugs: Evolution of a problem.

Source: https://www.unodc.org/pdf/report_2001-06-26_1/analysis_clandestine.pdf

10.3.1 Approaches to Control of Clandestine Synthetic Drugs

The need to maintain the availability of drugs used for legal and medical purposes while preventing their diversion into illicit markets serves as the foundation for the global drug control system. The need to preserve the legal trade in those substances for medical purposes has been taken into consideration in the formulation of procedures to expand control measures to new substances. They comprise estimates for the quantities required for medical and research purposes, as well as a monitoring system of legal transactions involving specific substances that are connected to production, inventories, trade, and use. Any discrepancy or alteration in such a system would be obvious and would eventually lead to caution and corrective action, preventing the leakage of a controlled substance into unapproved channels (Ahlström et al., 2007a; Ahlström et al., 2007b).

Clandestine synthetic drugs challenge the current drug control system in several ways:

- firstly, because they are manufactured clandestinely, there is no legitimate trade, and their distribution cannot be monitored by the traditional drug control system;
- secondly, as a result of the so-called substance-by-substance scheduling approach, the appearance of new substances, which are not included in the schedules of the conventions, cannot be countered immediately with appropriate measures, given that their manufacture, trafficking, and abuse are not 'illicit,' i.e., they do not constitute a criminal offense at that point in time. This offers room for clandestine experimentation or 'research' into individual substances within a class of drugs with similar pharmacological profiles;
- thirdly, as a consequence of the clandestine nature of the substances concerned, usually there is insufficient data available for the required scheduling assessments. The procedure for their inclusion into the control system is thus a lengthy one, and this allows clandestine manufacturers to continue to operate for some time and sell their products without immediately facing legal consequences.

The global community has endeavored to fortify the current drug control framework, which primarily concentrates on finished goods, by utilizing legislative instruments that additionally tackle diversion and the unlawful utilization of precursor materials and additional chemicals needed for covert drug production. The majority of drug control strategies now include precursor control as a fundamental component. It is especially crucial in the case of synthetic drugs because of their versatility in the production process and the abundance of starting materials that can be used in their place. Furthermore, there had been no global system for the control of precursors for synthetic drugs—not even for the most basic materials—prior to the 1988 Convention's implementation. This is not the case for plant-based drugs, where the 1988 Convention only regulates the chemicals needed for the extraction and purification processes, while the 1961 Convention covers immediate starting materials (coca leaf, opium), intermediates (coca paste, morphine), and endproducts (cocaine, heroin). An overview of the various control regimes as they relate to synthetic drugs, plant-based drugs, and the precursors and other chemicals needed for their manufacture is given in Figure 10.7.

Precursors are difficult to regulate to a particularly tight degree due to their many acceptable uses and the often high volumes of licit trade. Furthermore, a great number of businesses worldwide produce and trade a large number of precursors, in contrast to the majority of end products. As a result, there are numerous legal supply sources, which help covert operators (i) quickly adjust to the imposition of stricter regulations in important supplier and transit nations, and (ii) place orders with multiple suppliers worldwide at once. Routes for trafficking and diversion are, therefore, very adaptable. The multiplicity of shipping routes via several middlemen in various nations, which are used to conceal the ultimate destination of the shipment, further complicates the efficient tracking of precursor movements. An additional trend that has emerged in recent years is the growing use of legally obtained, non-controlled substances in the illicit drug trade as replacements for precursors that are already regulated. From the standpoint of drug control, this development raises two issues. Strict regulation of the licit trade of these substances is impractical due to the abundance of viable substitutes, and many of those substitutes have even more acceptable applications than the "traditional" precursor substances. When it comes to synthetic drugs, the situation is more concerning than it is for plant-based ones because even some of the most necessary precursors can be replaced by uncontrolled precursors or synthesized "down the chain" from an uncontrolled pre-precursor (Ahlström et al., 2007a; Ahlström et al., 2007b). While a sufficient supply of opium or coca leaf, respectively, is always necessary for their manufacture, only the chemicals for the isolation, conversion, and purification of heroin and cocaine, respectively, can be substituted with non-controlled alternatives.

10.3.2 The development of a trend - demand pull or supply push

Choices for certain substances (or classes of substances) are the outcome of intricate interactions between social, cultural, economic, and other elements. As a result, they change over time and within and between nations. A new drug trend typically appears when manufacturers investigate the market through covert means and is then embraced by consumers. For a new drug to become popular, it must first satisfy consumer preferences in a particular time and sociocultural context. Consequently, in an expanding market, demand may eventually overtake supply as the primary driver. Globally, the majority of novel trends in synthetic drugs started in Western nations and progressively extended to less developed ones. Changes in societal perceptions of a particular substance are somewhat associated with shifts in drug preferences. This can be partially attributed to the availability of more thorough, precise, and up-to-date information about the risks and adverse effects of using a given substance. Every new generation of drug users appears to rediscover the pleasurable effects of a particular drug in the absence of a sub-cultural memory of the risks associated with its usage. This, along with the later rediscovery and information-sharing regarding detrimental health and psychological effects, is a component of the cyclical pattern that most illicit drug epidemics share.

The new trend in traditional plant-based medications is mostly restricted to altering the mode of administration while also necessitating a change in the drug's presentation (e.g., crack cocaine and cocaine or heroin base and hydrochloride). As a result, customers can only choose from a small selection of products. Contrarily, synthetic drugs make it possible to covertly alter a "successful" drug molecule, usually without altering the desired pharmacological effects for the consumer, which opens up access to a whole class of related substances. Because of their adaptability, synthetic drugs can be a godsend for law enforcement and forensic chemists but also a great fit for situations where trends and fashions change quickly. From a supply and demand perspective, globalization and the internationalization of societies seem to have played a role in fostering an atmosphere that has enabled the illicit trade of synthetic drugs.

On the demand side, there are at least three phenomena that can be observed over the last decade:

- changes in social structures in many societies around the world, which lead, among other things, to an emphasis on individual success and performance;
- a growing global trend towards fashionable lifestyles, short-lived amusement, and a 'consumption culture' that trusts in 'pills' as universal remedies; and
- the spread of modern communication technology.

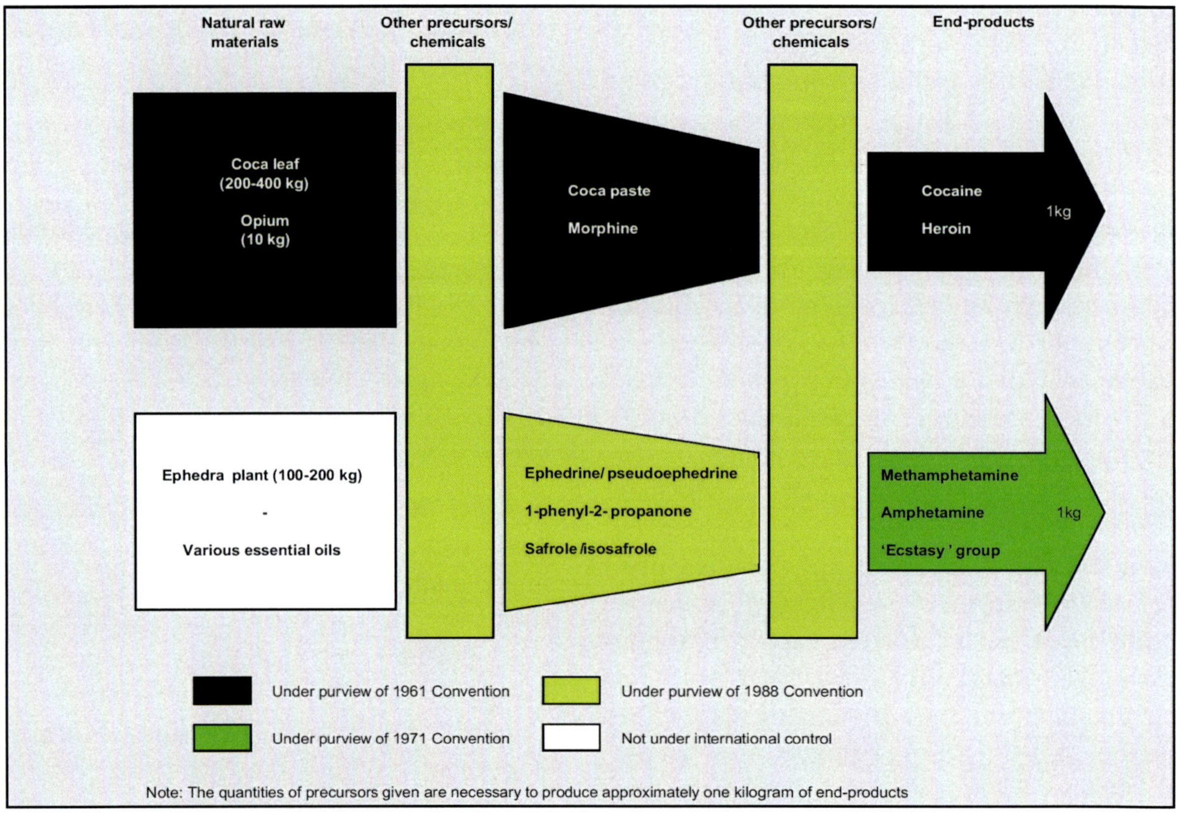

Figure 10.7. Comparison of processing stages and control regimes of selected plant-based narcotic drugs, synthetic drugs, and their precursors / starting materials.

Source: https://www.unodc.org/pdf/report_2001-06-26_1/analysis_clandestine.pdf

The last phenomenon adds to the speed at which synthetic drugs spread and the convergence of consumption patterns across borders, even though the first two phenomena—instrumental/occupational use for the purpose of achieving goals and recreational/social use—may translate into distinct consumption patterns. The media landscape and contemporary communication technologies, particularly the Internet, facilitate the globalization of fashion trends and increase public access to detailed information about a range of drugs, including side effects, availability, and cost comparisons (Alguacil and Pérez-García, 2003).

10.3.3 From the Supply Perspective

From a supply perspective, synthetic drugs allow underground chemists to monitor changes in a consumer market that is influenced by fashion trends and where the drug itself is less important than the customs and myths surrounding its use. A covert chemist, however, would typically prefer not to substitute a less effective medicine for a more effective one that is well-liked by the general public unless absolutely necessary, as in the case of the unavailability of precursor chemicals. A covert chemist will typically create the medications that yield the largest profits and the fewest chances of being discovered among a group of related substances as long as they stay within the parameters of consumer acceptance and preferences. As a result, the emphasis will be on compounds with the highest potencies that can be produced, to the greatest extent feasible, from unreliable starting materials.

Drug type

Due to their low risk and high financial rewards, a number of the substances and substance classes that appeal to recreational drug users also appeal to covert manufacturers. This is especially true for certain artificial stimulants and hallucinogens, as they present chances for pharmacological design and structural alteration. However, there is some risk involved in developing a completely "new" substance class because consumer acceptance is a factor outside the direct control of covert manufacturers. Future trends will, therefore, probably differ from what is already apparent today:

- Increased availability of traditional ATS, such as amphetamine and methamphetamine, to be used for their performance-enhancing effects;
- Re-emergence of other ATS already banned in most countries as a consequence of previous periods of abuse; and/or
- Increase in consumption of new designer ATS or of substances that have so far only appeared sporadically in illicit markets. The so-called phenethylamines (peas), which are close chemical relatives of ATS not controlled in most countries, and which can be expected to produce similar effects, can be included in this category

10.4 Computational Drug Discovery

An efficient method for quickening and streamlining the drug discovery and development process is computational drug discovery. The applicability of computational drug discovery has been expanded and widely applied to almost every stage in the drug discovery and development workflow, including target identification and validation, lead discovery and optimization, and preclinical testing, due to the dramatic increase in the availability of biological macromolecule and small molecule information. Computational drug discovery techniques like sequence-based virtual screening, pharmacophore modeling and mapping, de novo design, molecular docking, and molecular similarity calculation have advanced significantly in the last few decades. The process of discovering and developing new drugs is widely acknowledged to be expensive, risky, and time-consuming. The average drug discovery and development cycle, from concept to market, costs between 0.8 and 1.0 billion USD and takes about 14 years (Alguacil and Pérez-García, 2003).. Combinatorial chemistry and high-throughput screening technologies have advanced quickly, creating a setting that makes it possible to screen and synthesize large libraries of compounds quickly, which has sped up the drug discovery process. Despite the fact that the amount of money spent on developing new drugs has increased dramatically over the past few decades, the output does not positively correspond to the investment due to the high failure rate and low efficiency of drug discovery. As a result, a number of strategies have been created to speed up the drug discovery process while lowering costs and failure rates.Computer-aided drug design (CADD), is one of the best ways to accomplish these objectives.

The acronym CADD is commonly used to refer to sources and computational tools for managing, storing, analyzing, and modeling compounds. It covers a wide range of topics related to drug discovery, such as the creation of digital repositories for researching chemical interactions, tools for methodically evaluating possible lead candidates, and computer programs for designing compounds. Computational tools can be applied to most aspects of the drug discovery and development process in the post-genomic era, thanks to the significant increase in biomacromolecule and small molecule information. This includes target identification and validation, lead discovery, and optimization. The tools can even be applied to preclinical trials, which significantly change the drug discovery and development pipeline. A flowchart illustrating the tasks to which computational approaches have been applied and the computational techniques employed at each stage can be found in Figure 10.8. The cost of developing new drugs could be cut by up to 50% with the use of computational tools.

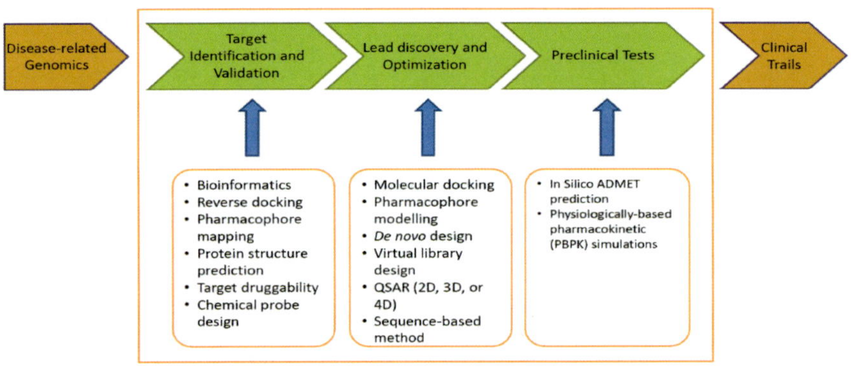

Figure 10.8. Multiple computational drug discovery approaches that have been applied in various stages of the drug discovery and development pipeline, including target identification and validation, lead discovery and optimization, and preclinical tests.

Source: https://media.springernature.com/lw685/springer-static/image/art%3A10.1038%2Faps.2012.109/MediaObjects/41401_2012_Article_BFaps2012109_Fig1_HTML.jpg?as=webp

Three main categories of computational drug discovery approaches are available: sequence-based, ligand-based, and structure-based drug design (SBDD, LBDD). Molecular docking and de novo drug design are two SBDD techniques that depend on the target macromolecule's structure, which is primarily known from crystal structures, NMR data, and homology models. LBDD tools, such as quantitative structure-activity relationship (QSAR), pharmacophore modeling, molecular field analysis, and 2D or 3D similarity assessment, can offer vital insights into the nature of the interactions between drug targets and ligands in the absence of three-dimensional (3D) structures of potential targets. This enables the construction of predictive models that are appropriate for lead discovery and optimization. Sequence-based approaches, which employ bioinformatic techniques to analyze and compare multiple sequences in order to identify potential targets from scratch and conduct lead discovery, have been developed recently to deal with situations where neither the target structure nor the ligand information is available. At the moment, no single technique can meet the practical requirements of drug development and discovery. As a result, combinational and hierarchical strategies that make use of several different computational techniques have been effectively and widely applied (Alguacil and Pérez-García, 2003)..

Numerous technical factors, such as scoring functions, optimization algorithms, conformation generation and sampling, and molecular similarity calculations, have a significant impact on the effectiveness, precision, and speed of these computational techniques. There have been some amazing approaches and systems created for computational drug development and discovery. This section provides an overview of a number of platforms and methodologies related to target identification, virtual library design, scoring functions, conformation sampling, docking-based virtual screening, molecular similarity calculation, and sequence-based drug design. Because these elements are closely related, advancements in one could have a positive impact on all of them (Figure 10.9).

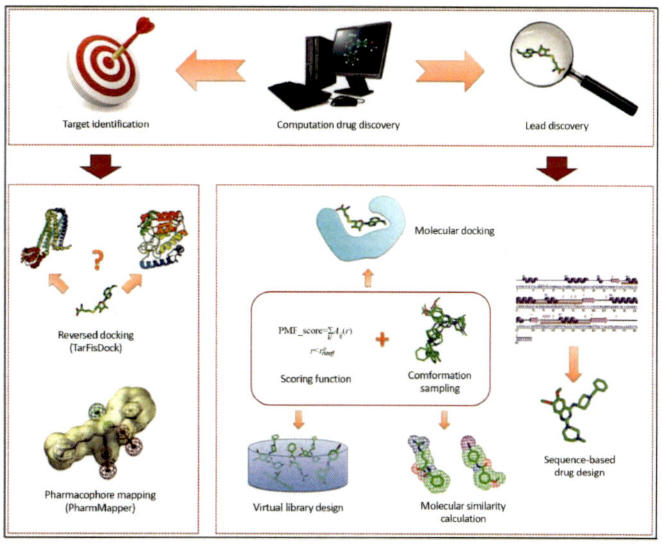

Figure 10.9. Important methodologies and platforms in the computational drug discovery field introduced and discussed in this article, with a focus on target identification and lead discovery fields.

Source: https://media.springernature.com/lw685/springer-static/image/art%3A10.1038%2Faps.2012.109/MediaObjects/41401_2012_Article_BFaps2012109_Fig2_HTML.jpg?as=webp

10.4.1 Target Identification

Finding potential drug targets among a large number of candidate macromolecules is a crucial and difficult first step in the drug discovery process. Currently, the most popular methods for identifying targets are time-consuming and laborious proteomic and genomic techniques. Consequently, computational platforms and tools, such as reverse docking and pharmacophore mapping, have been developed to supplement the experimental methods. TarFisDock is a web server that finds potential drug targets by searching for every binding protein for a specific small molecule using a reverse docking technique. The popular docking program DOCK (version 4.0) served as the foundation for the creation of TarFisDock. This platform uses MySQL as the database system and a front-end web interface written in PHP and HTML. Reverse docking uses DOCK as a back-end tool. TarFisDock has a clear benefit in that it can be a useful tool for locating possible targets for a drug that is currently on the market, a newly isolated natural product, or a compound with known biological activity but an unclear pharmacological mechanism. Furthermore, this platform can identify putative targets that may be accountable for a drug's toxicity and adverse effects, potentially enabling the prediction of a drug candidate's off-target effects. Indeed, research indicates that the high attrition rate in drug development has been primarily caused by off-target effects. In addition, TarFisDock might offer useful data for building drug target networks, which would enable a more methodical investigation of the drug-target interaction. By determining the putative binding proteins of vitamin E and 4H-tamoxifen, the methodology's dependability has been evaluated. According to the findings, TarFisDock was able to forecast 50% of the corresponding targets that were reported (Shulgin and Shulgin, 1991). This approach does, however, still have some drawbacks: (1) the number of protein entries is insufficient to fully capture the protein information of genomes associated with diseases; (2) the flexibility of the proteins is overlooked during the docking process; and (3) the scoring function, designed to assess small molecules, might not be precise enough to assess reverse docking.

For TarFisDock, a web-accessible potential drug target database (PDTD) was created. At present, the Protein Data Bank provides over 1100 protein entries in this database that feature 3D structures. General information about these proteins was taken from a number of online databases, including TTD, DrugBank, and Thomson Pharma, as well as from published works. More than 830 possible drug targets are covered in this database, each of which has structures available in both PDB and MOL2 formats. Additionally, data on linked biological processes, diseases, and signaling pathways have been gathered. Each target was categorized based on its function and associated diseases. A keyword search feature for PDB IDs, target names, and disease names is available in PDTD. It could be utilized for virtual screening, in silico drug target identification, and the identification of side effects for currently approved medications as a comprehensive and distinct database of drug targets (Shulgin and Shulgin, 1991).

Determining the optimal mode of interaction between the small molecule probes and the prospective target candidates is a crucial aspect of target identification. Pharmacophore mapping and modeling are additional techniques that can be utilized in addition to reverse docking to determine the ideal interaction mode. The spatial arrangement of characteristics required for a molecule to interact with a particular target receptor is known as a pharmacophore model. PharmMapper is the first web application that predicts possible drug targets against any given small molecule using a "reverse" pharmacophore mapping technique. But in order for the PharmMapper server to function, there must be a substantial quantity of pharmacophore models on the internet that explain how recognized ligands bind to specific binding sites. As a result, PharmTargetDB, a sizable internal database of pharmacophore models annotated with target information, was created. From the DrugBank, BindingDB, PDBBind, and PDTD databases, the target protein structures in complex with small molecules were carefully extracted. Based on the complex structures, over 7000 pharmacophore models (covering data for over 1500 drug targets) were generated. To find the pharmacophore that best fit the task, a sequential combination of genetic algorithm (GA) optimization and triangle hashing (TriHash) was used. PharmMapper is a computationally efficient and high throughput screener that leverages the robust and highly efficient triangle hash mapping method. The interface is easy to use, and the algorithm is highly automated. Experienced users can freely customize the candidate targets subset and optional parameters that control speed and accuracy (Shulgin and Shulgin, 1991). The pharmacophore database exclusively contains drug targets with PDB structures that have a co-crystallized ligand, which is the program's main drawback. On the other hand, PharmTargetDB is updated on a regular basis as more structures are deposited in PDB.

10.4.2 Docking-Based Virtual Screening

Molecular docking-based virtual screening has emerged as one of the most popular SBDD techniques. The conformational searching method has a significant influence on the three main criteria for any docking method: docking accuracy, scoring accuracy, and computational efficiency. Since molecular docking is a common optimization problem, finding the global optimum solution is challenging. The binding energy, shape complementarity, or chemical complementarity are examples of the single objectives that the majority of conformational optimization techniques in docking programs are only able to address. When it comes to solving real-world problems, which typically have several goals, this kind of approach is ineffective. Therefore, there is an urgent need for an optimization algorithm that combines multiple objectives and produces more reasonable and robust binding modes between macromolecules and ligands.

GAsDock, a recently developed docking methodology, optimizes the binding poses between small molecules and macromolecule receptors using an entropy-based multi-population GA. Contracted space was utilized as the convergence criterion and information entropy was utilized in the GA for optimization, guaranteeing that GAsDock can converge quickly and consistently. According to a validation test, GAsDock is more accurate than other docking programs like GOLD, FlexX, DOCK, Surflex, and Glide. The test involved docking known inhibitors into the binding pockets of thymidine kinase (TK) and HIV-1 reverse RT. An enhanced adaptive genetic algorithm that supports a flexible docking method has been developed in order to improve the process' accuracy and speed. This algorithm included several sophisticated techniques, including quasi-exact penalty, entropy-based searching with self-adaptation, and multi-population genetic strategy. This method is much faster than the previous one because a new iteration scheme was also used in conjunction with these techniques to accelerate the optimization and convergence processes. Furthermore, two sets of MOSFOM (Multi-Objective Scoring Function Optimization Methodology) multi-objective optimization (MO) methods were developed that take into account the energy score and the contact score at the same time. Rather than accurately predicting the binding free energy, MOSFOM focuses primarily on a new strategy to obtain the most reasonable binding conformation and increase the hit rates (Agnese et al., 2007).

10.4.3 Conformation Sampling

Understanding the bioactive conformations of small molecules, which dictate their physical and biological properties, is one of the most important aspects of drug design and development. A lot of the techniques used in drug discovery involve conformational sampling to create conformations of small molecules in the binding pocket and a scoring phase to rank these conformations. Examples of these techniques include molecular docking, pharmacophore construction and matching, 3D database searching, 3D-QSAR, and molecular similarity analysis. An efficient conformation ensemble should ensure that the conformers span the conformational space in a reasonable amount of time and with reasonable energy. The process of generating conformers through the application of complex criteria like pharmacophore and binding pocket mapping has resulted in a multi-objective optimization process for conformation generation (Agnese et al., 2007).

Based on the multi-objective evolution algorithm (MOEA), a highly efficient conformational generation method named Cyndi has been developed. Cyndi can search the conformational space in almost constant time and sample the Pareto frontier at which the energy and diversity features are favored by using multiple objectives to control both geometric diversity and energy accessibility. The torsional energy terms and the VDW are two unique goals for separating the generated conformers in energy space using the Tripos force field. The conformers are encoded into GA individuals with information on the dihedral torsions of the rotatable bonds. Rather than focusing on a single criterion, Cyndi makes sure that the generated conformation ensemble simultaneously satisfies several criteria, including low energy and geometric diversity. The MMFF94 force field was recently added to Cyndi in order to improve the rationale behind the conformational energy assessment. A comparison of Cyndi and MacroModel integrated in Maestro V7.5 (Schrodinger Inc.) has been carried out, with an emphasis on the conformational costs in relation to the employed algorithm method and the sampling depth of the conformational space. When it came to finding bioactive conformations quickly, Cyndi outperformed MacroModel in terms of conformation sampling efficiency, but MacroModel was found to be equally effective at retrieving the bioactive conformations.

10.4.4 Scoring Function

One crucial element of virtual screening is the scoring function. The knowledge-based scoring method is a prominent scoring technique that involves the extraction of structural information from experimentally determined protein-ligand complexes. The Bolztmann law is then utilized to convert the atom pair preferences into distance-dependent pairwise potentials. Expected to be more applicable is the potential of mean force (PMF) scoring function, which can translate structural information into free energy without requiring knowledge of the binding affinities. This approach implicitly balances a number of competing binding contributions, including interaction enthalpy, conformational entropy, and solvation effects. The following introduces a few noteworthy approaches that are concentrated on these fields. To evaluate the binding of ATP-competitive kinase inhibitors, a kinase data set of 872 complexes from the PDB database was used to create a kinase family-specific PMF scoring function called kinase-PMF. The functional form and atom type of PMF04 are inherited by this scoring function. In contrast to eight other widely used scoring techniques, kinase-PMF demonstrated the highest success rate in distinguishing crystal conformations as well as positive compounds from decoys. As a result, this technique might help scientists identify and refine hit compounds for kinase inhibitor development (Agarwaland Fishwick, 2010).

A newly defined atom-typing scheme using 23 redefined ligand atom types, 17 protein atom types, and 28 newly introduced atom types for nucleic acids has been used to create the improved PMF scoring function known as KScore. It is based on multiple diverse training sets. The pairwise potentials for various atom types used in KScore have greatly improved when compared to the current PMF potentials, such as PMF99 and PMF04. This is especially true when it comes to reflecting experimental phenomena, such as the interaction distances and strengths of hydrogen bonding, electrostatic interactions, VDW interactions, cation-π interactions, and aromatic stacking. KScore can be used for large-scale virtual screening and is an effective tool for identifying strong binders from a group of compounds. Additionally, tweaking the atom-typing scheme and using a variety of training sets ought to enable further advancements. GAsDock, the molecular docking program mentioned earlier, now includes KScore. IPMF, a knowledge-based scoring function, was created using a new iteration technique and the PMF concept and formalism. Additional experimental binding affinity data is integrated into the knowledge base by this scoring function as supplementary data to the widely used structural information. In order to produce a "enriched" knowledge-based model, the 3D structural information and the binding affinity information are extracted using an iteration method. By assigning scores to a variety of 219 protein-ligand complexes and contrasting the outcomes with seven widely-used scoring functions, the effectiveness of IPMF was assessed (Agarwaland Fishwick, 2010). Thus, in the activity prediction test, the IPMF score does the best. Furthermore, IPMF showed only slight improvements over the other assessed knowledge-based scoring functions when it came to re-ranking binding poses. These findings imply that scoring functions can be improved in their capacity to predict binding affinities as well as be developed using the additional binding affinity information. Applying the IPMF approach to other knowledge-based scoring functions may yield a well-defined scheme for incorporating binding information into standard statistical potentials.

10.4.5 Molecular Similarity Methods

Molecular similarity is a key idea in LBDD since it forms the basis of structural clustering analysis and the structure-activity relationship (SAR). Considered one of the most potent instruments in medicinal chemistry, similarity-based virtual screening and candidate ranking have been effectively used in numerous instances. Programs that search for similarities can be broadly divided into two categories: 2D and 3D similarity, depending on whether or not 3D conformation information is taken into account. Complementary compound profiles can be swiftly and effectively created using 2D similarity methods. To some extent, though, it might return distinct results for the same queries because different 2D similarity definitions focus on different informational dimensions. Additionally, this approach often finds close structural analogs rather than new scaffold hits. However, several aspects of the 3D conformation, such as pharmacophores, molecular shapes, and molecular fields, are usually taken into account by 3D similarity methods. Scaffold hopping to identify novel compounds is a convenient application of 3D methods.

The pharmacophore matching approach, which served as the basis for the aforementioned PharmMapper Server, has led to the development of a quick 3D molecular similarity calculation method called SHAFTS (SHApe-FeaTure Similarity). In order to combine the benefits of volumetric similarity and pharmacophore matching, this method uses hybrid similarity metrics of molecular shape and colored (or labeled) chemistry groups annotated by pharmacophore features for 3D calculation and ranking. The fast molecular alignment poses are counted using the triplet hashing technique. Alignment modes are ranked and scored using the hybrid similarity, which is composed of pharmacophore feature fit values and overlaps between shape densities. SHAFTS outperformed other ligand-based techniques in terms of overall and early stage enrichments of known actives and chemotypes. ChemMapper Server now incorporates SHAFTS (unpublished result).

A collection of orthogonal spherical functions known as the spherical harmonic (SH) can be used to accurately depict the form of a closed curve surface, like a molecular surface. Virtual screening, protein-ligand recognition, binding pocket modeling, molecular fragment similarity, and other applications have all benefited from the effective application of SH expansion theory. A novel molecular shape similarity comparison technique based on SH expansion is called SHeMS. This method yields a clear contribution from both overall and detailed features to the final score by weighting the SH expansion coefficients to calculate similarity. Furthermore, the user has the ability to configure the reference set for optimization, enabling customized and system-specific comparisons. Retrospective VS experimentation using principal component analysis (PCA) and the Directory of Useful Decoys (DUD) database shows that SHeMS outperforms both the original SH (OSH) and ultra-fast shape recognition (USR) methods by a significant margin (Acharya et al., 2011).

10.4.6 Virtual Library Construction

The goal of de novo drug design is to chemically occupy target macromolecules' binding sites. The process presents several critical challenges, one of which is to identify fragment sets with the highest potential to form novel drug leads for a particular target. One solution to this problem has been proposed: the creation of virtual libraries, such as primary screening libraries, targeted libraries, and focused libraries. Establishing appropriate criteria for product evaluation presents another difficulty. Drug-likeness and structural diversity have been incorporated into library design to address this issue, allowing for smaller libraries with higher screening efficiency.

Targeted libraries are made to look for drug leads against specific targets, whereas focused libraries focus on a single target and are constructed using a lead compound or pharmacophore. To create, optimize, and evaluate focused libraries, a new, effective method was developed that incorporates technology from drug-like analysis and docking-based virtual screening while embracing the benefits of both targeted and focused libraries. Using the new method, a software package called LD1.0 was developed successfully. Building blocks are chosen to construct a number of virtual libraries from pre-given fragment databases. Next, using library-based GA, the virtual libraries are optimized and assessed according to predetermined standards like molecular diversity, docking energy, and drug-likeness. In order to form the next generation of focused libraries, GA keeps the libraries that have higher scores and creates new ones. GA optimization comes to an end when the termination condition is met (Acharya et al., 2011).

10.4.7 Sequence-Based Drug Design

Most proteins' three-dimensional structures are unknown, and many of them lack known ligands altogether. Research on drug discovery and development cannot be done in this scenario using either structure-based or ligand-based methodologies. Thus, there is an urgent need for a way to predict ligand-protein interactions (LPIs) without access to 3D or ligand information. Recently, the support vector machine (SVM) technique was used to build a sequence-based drug design model for lipophilic inhibition (LPI) that was based only on the primary sequence of proteins and the structural characteristics of small molecules. 15 000 LPIs between 626 proteins and more than 10,000 active compounds gathered from the Binding Database were used to train this model. Using only the target's sequence, nine novel active compounds against four pharmacologically significant targets were discovered in the model's validation test. This is the first instance of a sequence-based drug design campaign that has been successful.

10.4.8 Position of Computer-Aided Drug Design in the Drug Discovery Pipeline

Compared to traditional HTS and combinatorial chemistry, CADD employs a far more focused search, which can increase the hit rate of new drug compounds. It seeks to forecast potential derivatives that could enhance activity in addition to elucidating the molecular underpinnings of therapeutic activity. Three main goals are typically achieved with the use of CADD in a drug discovery campaign: (1) reduce large compound libraries into smaller sets of anticipated active compounds that can be tested experimentally; (2) direct lead compound optimization, whether the goal is to improve affinity or drug metabolism and pharmacokinetics (DMPK) properties, such as absorption, distribution, metabolism, excretion, and potential for toxicity (ADMET); and (3) design novel compounds, either by growing starting molecules one functional group at a time or by assembling fragments into novel chemotypes. Figure 10.10 shows where CADD is in the pipeline for drug discovery.

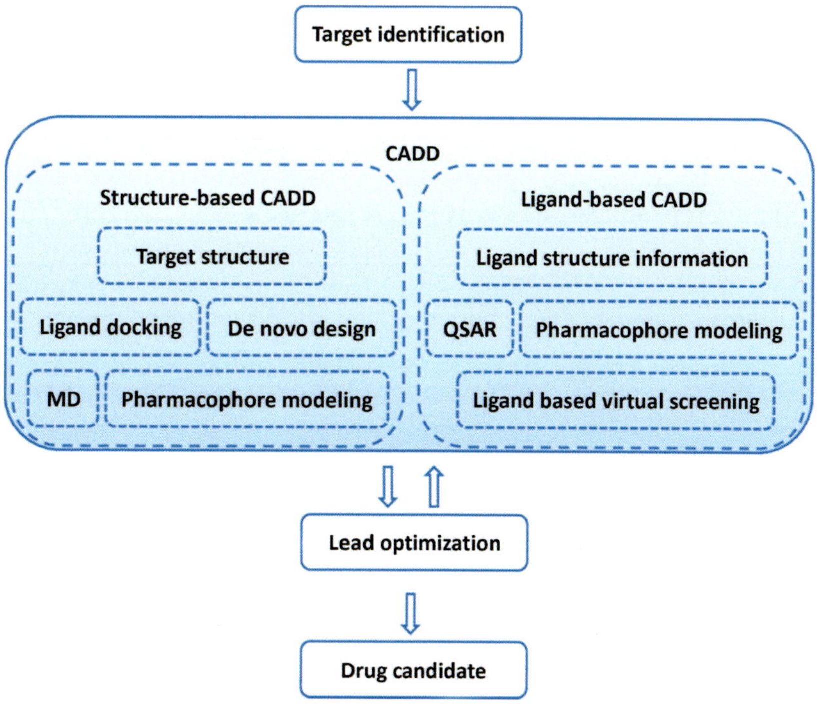

Figure 10.10. CADD in drug discovery/design pipeline. A therapeutic target is identified against which a drug has to be developed. Depending on the availability of structure information, a structure-based approach or a ligand-based approach is used. A successful CADD campaign will allow identification of multiple lead compounds. Lead identification is often followed by several cycles of lead optimization and subsequent lead identification using CADD. Lead compounds are tested in vivo to identify drug candidates.

Source: https://www.ncbi.nlm.nih.gov/pmc/articles/PMC3880464/bin/pr.112.007336f2.jpg

Structure-based and ligand-based CADD can be broadly divided into two groups. While ligand-based CADD uses the knowledge of known active and inactive molecules to generate predictive, QSAR models or conduct chemical similarity searches, structure-based CADD depends on the target protein structure knowledge to calculate interaction energies for all compounds tested. When the target protein's high-resolution structural data are available, structure-based CADD is typically recommended, i.e., in favor of easily crystallized soluble proteins. When structural information is lacking or nonexistent, ligand-based CADD is typically recommended, especially for targets that are membrane proteins. Creating compounds that bind firmly to the target is the main objective of structure-based CADD, i.e., with a significant decrease in free energy, enhanced DMPK/ADMET characteristics, and targeted specificity, i.e., possess fewer off-target consequences. If these techniques are applied successfully, the compound produced will have undergone in vitro and in vivo validation, and its binding location will have been verified—ideally using a cocrystal structure.

Virtual compound library screening, or virtual high-throughput screening (vHTS), is one of the most popular applications of CADD. This enables experimenters to concentrate their efforts on examining substances that might exhibit any interesting activity. This allows a researcher to screen significantly fewer compounds while still finding an equal number of hits because compounds that are highly confidently predicted to be inactive may be skipped. Saving time and money by avoiding a large population of inactive compounds allows for a significant reduction in the size of the experimental HTS without sacrificing a significant number of hits.

vHTS can take many different forms, such as virtual docking of compounds into targets of interest (also known as structure-based docking) or chemical similarity searches by fingerprints or topology. It can also select compounds based on their predicted biological activity using pharmacophore mapping or QSAR models. These techniques enable the virtual compound library's "hits" to be ranked for acquisition. When it comes to docking, the ranking can represent the lowest energy scoring pose for each ligand bound to the target of interest, or it can reflect a property of interest like percent similarity to a query compound or predicted biologic activity. Frequently, initial hits are rescored and ranked with computationally complex methods that take too much time to implement for full-scale vHTS. It is significant to remember that the goal of vHTS is to find leads with chemotypes that have not yet been linked to a target, not to find a drug compound that is ready for clinical testing. This bears similarities to a conventional HTS in which a compound is deemed successful if its activity is near 10 μM. A molecule is initially transformed into a "lead" with greater affinity, some comprehension of its structure-activity-relation, and preliminary testing for DMPK/ADMET properties through iterative rounds of chemical synthesis and in vitro testing. Compounds attain acceptable DMPK/ADMET properties and clinically appropriate potency only after undergoing additional rounds of iterative lead-to-drug optimization and in vivo testing.

The cost benefits of incorporating computational tools during the lead optimization stage of drug development are significant. Developing new drugs can be incredibly expensive, ranging from $400 million to $2 billion, with the synthesis and testing of lead analogs being a major cost driver. Utilizing computational tools for hit-to-lead optimization allows for a more extensive exploration of chemical space while reducing the number of compounds that need to be synthesized and tested in the lab. Computational optimization can involve a variety of techniques, such as analyzing docking poses and energy profiles, screening for compounds with similar structures or improved biological activity, and predicting favorable DMPK/ADMET properties. The relatively low cost of computer-aided drug design compared to traditional methods makes it an attractive option for focusing, streamlining, and diversifying chemical exploration.

De novo drug design is an additional tool in CADD methods that focuses on designing new compounds instead of screening libraries of previously synthesized ones. To sample the chemical space, a structure generator is required. Because there are more than 1060 molecules in the search space, heuristics are used to narrow down the focus of these algorithms to molecules that are expected to be highly active, easily synthesized, free of unwanted characteristics, frequently derived from an initial scaffold with proven activity, etc.

Furthermore, when working with large search spaces, efficient sampling techniques like simulated annealing, metropolis search, and evolutionary algorithms are employed. In general, the construction algorithms are classified as growing or linking techniques. Small fragments or functional groups like rings, acetyl groups, esters, etc., are docked in linking algorithms.

fragments from nearby sites are then linked to specific binding sites. By contrast, growing algorithms start with a single fragment in the binding site, to which additional fragments can be added, subtracted, or altered to increase activity. Similar to vHTS, the goal of de novo drug design is to create a lead compound that can be further refined rather than a single compound with nanomolar activity and suitable DMPK/ADMET characteristics.

10.4.9 Ligand Databases for Computer-Aided Drug Design

Virtual HTS screens massive chemical databases, and ranks compound for synthesis using high-performance computing. Structure-based screening of up to 100,000 molecules per day using parallel processing clusters is possible thanks to current hardware and algorithms. However, in order to conduct a virtual screen, a virtual library needs to be made accessible for screening. Virtual libraries come in different shapes and sizes; general libraries are suitable for screening against any target, focused libraries are made for a group of related targets, and targeted libraries are made for a single target. Numerous computational and combinatorial tools are available for building general libraries. Early systems generated all possible structures for a fixed number of atoms by using the molecular formula as the only constraint on structure generation. Further limitations are imposed because it is not and will not be possible to perform a thorough computational enumeration of all chemical space. Chemical entities that are difficult to synthesize or that are anticipated or known to cause adverse DMPK/ADMET properties are typically excluded. Fink and others. suggested using connected graphs filled with C, N, O, and F atoms and pruned according to molecular structure constraints and the removal of unstable structures as a generation method for building virtual libraries. 26.4 million chemical structures that have been used for vHTS are included in the final database that this method generates, known as the GDB (Generated a DataBase). A more recent version of this database, known as GDB-13, has 970 million compounds and contains the atoms C, N, O, S, and Cl (F is not included in this variation to speed up computation).

Preparation of Ligand Libraries for Computer-Aided Drug Design

Enriching ligands for drug-likeness or

specific desirable physiochemical properties appropriate for the target of interest is a common method used to construct ligand libraries. Eliminating non-drug-like, unstable, or unfavorable compounds can save time, even with fast docking algorithms, which still need a significant amount of resources to dock millions of compounds. Lipinski's rule of five, states that an orally active drug should generally have no more than one violation of the following criteria—a maximum of five hydrogen bond donors, a maximum of 10 oxygen and nitrogen atoms, the molecular mass of less than 500 Da, and a maximum of five octanol-water partition coefficient—is commonly used to evaluate drug-likeness (Acharya et al., 2011). It is reasonable to anticipate poor adsorption if two or more of the requirements are broken. Similarly, oral absorption and brain penetration are also determined by the polar molecular surface. Prior to starting a vHTS campaign, it is customary to filter molecules based on expected DMPK/ADMET properties. Ligand-based approaches to predict DMPK/ADMET properties model biologic processes such as oral bioavailability, intestinal absorption/permeability, half-life time, distribution in human blood plasma, etc., using statistical and learning methods, molecular descriptors, and experimental data.

A specific target or family of targets is frequently the focus of compound library enrichment. Compounds that meet particular geometric or physicochemical constraints are added to a library through the use of physiochemical filters that are derived from observed ligand-target complexes. These libraries are created through ligand similarity searches with established active ligands. The Cambridge Structure Data Base has a number of target-specific libraries, including sets that are kinase-, GPCR-, and ion channel-biased. Furthermore, to prepare a small molecule library, steps like assigning the correct stereo isometric and protonation state and performing conformational sampling are necessary. Since molecules are malleable in a solvent environment, conformational flexibility representation is a crucial component of molecular recognition. Protein and ligand conformations are frequently precomputed via simulation or knowledge-based techniques.

Representation of Small Molecules as "SMILES"

Methods that are universally applicable to the virtual representation of small molecules are necessary for the development and effective use of ligand databases. For the purpose of clearly and consistently representing molecules computationally, SMILES (Simplified Molecular Input Line System) was created. It was created as an upgrade from the Wiswesser Line Notation, which had a complex set of rules but was favored because it represented molecular structure as a linear string of symbols that computer systems could read and store with ease. Typically, SMILES assumes that hydrogens make up the remaining portion of an atom's lowest normal valence and do not explicitly encode hydrogen atoms (hydrogen-suppressed graph). Enclosed in square brackets are the atomic symbols of all non-hydrogen atoms. It is possible for atoms to be listed without square brackets, indicating that hydrogens are present. Specifically, formal charges are denoted with + or −, and are followed by an optional digit enclosed in brackets. Atomic symbols in lowercase are used to designate aromatic atoms. The symbols"-,""=,""," and":," respectively, stand for single bonds, double bonds, triple bonds, and aromatic bonds. The way to specify branched systems is to put them inside parentheses. In order to depict a cyclic structure, a ring is broken at a single or aromatic bond, and the atoms on either side of the break are assigned numbers. For instance, the SMILES string C1CCCCC1 represents cyclohexane. Periods divide disconnected compounds, and ionic bonds are disconnected structures with complementary formal charges c.

An extended version of Huckel's rule (all atoms in the ring must be sp^2 hybridized, and the number of available π electrons must satisfy 4N + 2) can be used by SMILES algorithms to detect the majority of aromatic compounds. Thus, it is not always necessary to define aromaticity in advance. Tautomeric structures, however, need to be stated clearly as distinct SMILES strings. Both mobile hydrogens and tautomeric bonds lack SMILES definitions. As a molecular file format, SMILES was created with good human readability in mind. For the same structure, there are typically numerous distinct but equally valid SMILES descriptions. Compounds are most frequently stored and retrieved using it on various computer platforms Abrams CF, Vanden-Eijnden.

SMARTS (SMILES ARbitrary Target Specification) is an extension of SMILES that allows for variability within the represented molecular structures. This provides substructure search functionality to SMILES. In addition to the SMILES naming conventions, SMARTS includes logical operators, such as "AND" (&), "OR" (,), and "NOT" (!), and special atomic and bond symbols that provide a level of flexibility to chemical names. For example, in SMARTS notation, [C,N] represents an atom that can be either an aliphatic carbon or an aliphatic nitrogen, and the symbol "~" will match any bond type.

Small Molecule Representations for Modern Search Engines: InChIKey

The International Chemical Identifier, or InChI, is a structure representation algorithm that was made available as open source in 2005 with the goal of integrating searches conducted with various chemical databases via contemporary internet search engines. It is currently capable of supporting chemical elements up to 112. It is maintained by the InChI Trust. The goal of InChI and its hash-key variant, InChIKey, is to offer a machine-readable, nonproprietary code that is unique for all chemical structures and can be indexed without modification by major search engines like Google. This protocol allows researchers to look for chemicals in a systematic and uncomplicated way. Chemical searches across several databases using standard search engines were unreliable prior to the creation of INChI. Since different databases have adopted different unique SMILES, SMILES-based searches are likewise inadequate because different systems have their own proprietary identification method for indexing chemicals (KyushuOkinawa Summit Meeting, 2000).

Several layers that represent various classes of structural information make up InChI. Only general information, such as the chemical formula and connections, are included in the first two layers. Further optional layers represent more specialized conformational data, like stereochemistry, tautomerism, and isotopic information.

Depending on the required level of specification, bonds between atoms can be divided into up to three sublayers. The bonds to nonbridging hydrogen atoms, immobile hydrogen atoms, and mobile hydrogen atoms are represented by these layers in that order. To produce a distinct and reliable chemical representation, the InChI algorithm employs six normalization rules that apply characteristics like variable protonation and the recognition of tautomeric patterns and resonances.

A shortened SHA-256 cryptographic hash function is used in InChIKey, a hash-key variant of InChI, to produce two blocks. As a result, there is little possibility of two distinct molecules having the same hash key, and the keys can 27 characters long with strong collision resistance. When InChIKeys were used to search multiple databases using standard search engines, there was very little false positive data. Chemists can draw molecules and use an automatically generated InChIKey to search the web with web applets that are accessible to the general public.

10.4.10 Target Data Bases for Computer-Aided Drug Discovery/Design

For structure-based CADD to work, it is necessary to understand the target protein's structure. The Cambridge Crystallographic Data Center and the Protein Data Bank (PDB), which was founded in 1971 at Brookhaven National Laboratory, are two of the most widely used databases for protein structure information. There are currently over 81,000 protein structures stored in PDB, most of which were found by X-ray crystallography, with a smaller number found by NMR spectroscopy. It is frequently possible to build a comparative model based on the experimental structure of a related protein in cases where an experimentally determined structure of a protein is unavailable. The relationship most often has its roots in evolution, which is where the term homology model originated. For homology modeling, one of the most popular web-based tools is the Swiss-Model server. All structure-based design techniques were initially applied to static protein structures. On the other hand, proteins are collections of various conformational states rather than static structures. The protein spends more time in conformations with lower free energies as it fluctuates through this ensemble based on the relative free energies of each of these states. Ligands are hypothesized to stabilize conformational populations in the ensemble by interacting with certain conformations but not others. Because the selected conformation might not be indicative of the conformation that is able to bind the ligand, docking compounds into a static protein structure can be misleading. Utilizing extra computational resources to simulate and assess a protein's conformational space, such as molecular dynamics and molecular mechanics, has recently advanced to the state of the art. A set of snapshots that represent the range of fluctuations the ligand might experience in vivo can be used in place of a single structure thanks to conformational sampling. This method has been shown to be very helpful in the CADD identification of new HIV integrase inhibitors. There is no need for snapshot ensembles when using certain methods, like ROSETTALIGAND, which can incorporate protein flexibility during the actual docking process (KyushuOkinawa Summit Meeting, 2000).

Beyond the non-covalent interactions between ligand and protein, a series of events takes place when a ligand binds a receptor. Binding free energies are influenced by ligand and binding pocket desolvation, changes in the conformational ensembles of the ligand and protein, and rearranging of water molecules within the binding site. For important mechanistic processes and binding, water molecules must be taken into account as an essential component of binding sites. These water molecules cause an overall change in free energy upon binding by either dislodging the ligand into more advantageous direct interactions with the protein or by facilitating specific noncovalent interactions between the ligand and protein. The accuracy of computational methods can be increased by including more accurate representations of physiochemical interactions thanks to advancements in computational resources.

10.4.11 Benchmarking Techniques of Computer-Aided Drug Design

In order to evaluate the accuracy and performance of CADD algorithms, reliable benchmarks are necessary. When comparing new CADD methods with existing ones, the selection of quality measures, size and composition of active and inactive chemicals, and number and type of target proteins in the benchmark design all matter. Scientific benchmarks typically entail screening a compound library that contains a subset of known actives along with known inactive compounds, counting how many known actives were found using the CADD technique, and assessing the results. Using receiver operating characteristic curves, performance is typically reported by comparing expected and experimentally observed activities. Plotted on the y-axis is the number of true positive predictions, while the x-axis shows the number of false positive predictions. Plotting a random predictor would produce a line with a slope of 1, while curves with high starting slopes above this line show rising performance scores for the tested method. Thus, the analysis of receiver operating characteristic curves involves finding the area under the curve, enrichment (a benchmark that normalizes positive predictive value by the background ratio of positives in the dataset), and positive predictive value (the ratio of true positives in a subset chosen in a vHTS screen).

Decoy molecules are now frequently used in structure-based CADD to test a method's capacity to separate actives from inactives at a high resolution. It comprises a set of carefully selected decoys and experimental data for about 3000 ligands covering up to 40 distinct targets. The purpose of these decoys was to mimic positive ligands in appearance but not in topology. However, these decoys are only hypothesized to be "inactive" against the targets; there is no experimental validation for this claim (Acharya et al., 2011).

A Closer Look

Structure-Based Drug Design

Structure-based drug design (SBDD) is a powerful approach in pharmaceutical research that relies on the detailed knowledge of the three-dimensional structures of biological targets to guide the rational design of therapeutic agents. At the core of SBDD are techniques such as X-ray crystallography, nuclear magnetic resonance (NMR) spectroscopy, and homology modeling, which provide insights into the spatial arrangement of atoms within proteins and other biomolecules. X-ray crystallography is a widely used method for determining the atomic structure of proteins by analyzing the diffraction patterns produced upon passing X-rays through a crystallized sample.

This technique allows researchers to visualize the precise arrangement of amino acid residues and ligands within the protein's binding site, providing crucial information for designing small molecule inhibitors or modulators that can interact with the target protein with high affinity and specificity. Similarly, NMR spectroscopy enables the determination of protein structures in solution by measuring the interactions between atomic nuclei and magnetic fields. NMR provides valuable information about protein dynamics and flexibility, which is particularly useful for designing drugs that can accommodate conformational changes in the target protein upon ligand binding.

Additionally, homology modeling, also known as comparative modeling, is a computational technique used to predict the 3D structure of a protein based on its amino acid sequence and the known structure of related proteins. Homology modeling is especially valuable when experimental structures of the target protein are unavailable, allowing researchers to generate accurate structural models for virtual screening and structure-based drug design.

By integrating these techniques, researchers can elucidate the structural and functional characteristics of drug targets, identify druggable binding sites, and optimize lead compounds through rational design and structure-activity relationship studies. SBDD has led to the discovery of numerous successful drugs across various therapeutic areas, highlighting its importance in modern drug discovery and development. However, challenges such as protein flexibility, solubility, and selectivity still exist, underscoring the ongoing need for innovation and refinement in SBDD methodologies to address complex biological targets and improve the success rate of drug candidates.

Summary

- Structure-based drug design allows researchers to design molecules that interact specifically with the target of interest, optimizing binding affinity and selectivity while minimizing off-target effects.
- Synthetic drugs are chemically produced compounds designed to mimic or enhance the effects of naturally occurring substances. These advancements have significantly expanded the range of therapeutic options available to healthcare professionals, leading to more precise treatments with fewer side effects.
- The field of synthetic drugs has also seen significant progress in the creation of novel drug classes with unique mechanisms of action.
- Developments in the pharmaceutical and chemical industries have contributed to the continued discovery and proliferation of synthetic drugs.
- Compared with plant-based drugs, some synthetic drugs offer greater means of reducing the risks and operational costs faced by criminal actors.
- The global pharmaceutical and chemical sectors have developed very rapidly in the last four decades, in particular in Asia, where industry growth since the end of the twentieth century has resulted in the proliferation of firms and an increase in the number of individuals with the requisite knowledge of chemical synthesis and pharmacology.
- Alternative chemicals that are not monitored or are less dangerous can facilitate new means of manufacture. For example, a review of the literature on the continuous development of synthesis routes for fentanyl has shown that those involved in the illegal manufacture of the drug are learning from published research and patents.
- The pharmacology of synthetic drugs can offer advantages to criminal suppliers and might be attractive to some people who use drugs. Several synthetic drugs are substantially more potent than the plant-based products they mimic.
- Synthetic drug manufacture represents a technological advancement, possibly disrupting markets and traditional supply chains. The supply structure for traditional plant-based drugs can be thought of as having an hour-glass shape, with many cultivators and farmers at the top.

References

1. "Anti-Drug Conference, Tokyo, 2000», Japan, January 2000; 33rd ASEAN Ministerial Meeting, Bangkok, Thailand, July 2000; G8 KyushuOkinawa Summit Meeting, Japan, July 2000; International Congress "In pursuit of a drug-free ASEAN 2015, Sharing the vision, leading the change», Bangkok, Thailand, October 2000.
2. Abrams CF, Vanden-Eijnden E. (2010) Large-scale conformational sampling of proteins using temperature-accelerated molecular dynamics. Proc Natl Acad Sci USA 107:4961–4966
3. Acharya C, Coop A, Polli JE, Mackerell AD., Jr (2011) Recent advances in ligand-based drug design: relevance and utility of the conformationally sampled pharmacophore approach. Curr Comput Aided Drug Des 7:10–22

4. Agarwal AK, Fishwick CW. (2010) Structure-based design of anti-infectives. Ann N Y Acad Sci 1213:20–45

5. Agnese V, Bazan V, Fiorentino FP, Fanale D, Badalamenti G, Colucci G, Adamo V, Santini D, Russo A. (2007) The role of Aurora-A inhibitors in cancer therapy. Ann Oncol 18 (Suppl 6):vi47–vi52

6. Ahlström MM, Ridderström M, Zamora I, Luthman K. (2007. b) CYP2C9 structure-metabolism relationships: optimizing the metabolic stability of COX-2 inhibitors. J Med Chem 50:4444–4452

7. Ahlström MM, Ridderström M, Zamora I. (2007. a) CYP2C9 structure-metabolism relationships: substrates, inhibitors, and metabolites. J Med Chem 50:5382–5391

8. Alguacil LF, Pérez-García C. (2003) Histamine H3 receptor: a potential drug target for the treatment of central nervous system disorders. Curr Drug Targets CNS Neurol Disord 2:303–313

9. Aller SG, Yu J, Ward A, Weng Y, Chittaboina S, Zhuo R, Harrell PM, Trinh YT, Zhang Q, Urbatsch IL, et al. (2009) Structure of P-glycoprotein reveals a molecular basis for poly-specific drug binding. Science 323:1718–1722

10. Al-Sha'er MA, Taha MO. (2010) Elaborate ligand-based modeling reveals new nanomolar heat shock protein 90α inhibitors. J Chem Inf Model 50:1706–1723

11. Economic and Social Council (ECOSOC) (1998), Youth and Drugs: A Global Overview, United Nations (E/CN.7/1998/8).

12. Economic and Social Council (ECOSOC) resolution 1995/20; Comprehensive reviews of the ATS phenomenon in recent years include (i) the study by UNDCP on 'Amphetamine-type Stimulants: A Global Review' (UNDCP/TS.3, 1996); (ii) a WHO Meeting and report on 'Amphetamines, MDMA and other Psychostimulants', November 1996; and (iii) a book edited by H.Klee on 'Amphetamine Misuse: International Perspectives on Current Trends', Harwood Academic Publishers, 1997.

13. Hando, J. and Hall, W. (1997), Patterns of Amphetamine Use in Australia, in: Amphetamine Misuse: International Perspectives on Current Trends (H. Klee, ed.), Harwood Academic Publishers, The Netherlands.

14. ICPO Interpol, 1999 Trends and Patterns of Illicit Drug Traffic, prepared for 43rd Session of the Commission on Narcotic Drugs, Vienna, 6-15 March 2000.

15. International Narcotics Control Board (INCB), Report 2000, United Nations, New York, 2001, para321.

16. Political declaration and action plan on international cooperation on the eradication of illicit crops and on alternative development, adopted at the Special Session of the General Assembly Devoted to Countering the World Drug Problem Together, 8-10 June 1998 (Resolution S-20/1).

17. Schuster. P., et al., Is the use of ecstasy and hallucinogens increasing?, European Addiction Research, 4, pp. 75-82, 1998.

18. Shulgin, A. and Shulgin, A. (1991), PIHKAL, A Chemical Love Story, Transform Press, Berkeley; Shulgin, A. and Shulgin, A., (1997), TIHKAL, The Continuation, Transform Press, Berkeley.

19. Thomasius, R. (2000), Ecstasy: eine Studie zu gesundheitlichen und psychosozialen Folgen des Missbrauchs, Wissenschaftliche Verlagsgesellschaft mbH Stuttgart, 2000.

INDEX

D

E

FSC
www.fsc.org
MIX
Papier | Fördert gute Waldnutzung
FSC® C083411

Kolibri 360 GmbH
Ferdinand-Jühlke-Straße 7
99095 Erfurt, Deutschland
produktsicherheit@kolibri360.de